48 95
5.0

Literacy and Deafness

The Development of Reading, Writing, and Literate Thought

Peter V. Paul

The Ohio State University

Allyn and Bacon

Boston • London • Toronto • Sydney • Tokyo • Singapore

Executive Editor: Stephen D. Dragin
Editorial Assistant: Elizabeth McGuire
Editorial-Production Administrator: Joe Sweeney
Editorial-Production Service: Walsh & Associates, Inc.
Composition Buyer: Linda Cox
Manufacturing Buyer: David Suspanic
Cover Administrator: Suzanne Harbison

Copyright © 1998 by Allyn & Bacon
A Viacom Company
160 Gould Street
Needham Heights, MA 02194

Internet: www.abacon.com
America Online: keyword: College Online

Library of Congress Cataloging-in-Publication Data

Paul, Peter V.
    Literacy and deafness : the development of reading, writing, and
literate thought / Peter V. Paul
        p.   cm.
    Includes bibliographical references and index.
    ISBN 0-205-17576-7
    1. Deaf—Education. 2. Hearing impaired—Education. 3. English.
language—Composition and exercises—Study and teaching.
4. Reading. 5. Literacy. I. Title.
HV2469.E5P38   1998
371.91′2—dc20   97-21431
                                                          CIP

Printed in the United States of America

10   9   8   7   6   5   4   3   2   1   00   99   98   97

Contents

Preface

This text is intended to be a comprehensive treatment of the acquisition of English literacy skills in children and adolescents with severe to profound hearing impairment. Although the focus is on this cohort of individuals, there is some discussion of children with less severe hearing impairment, also known as children who are hard of hearing. One of the most important features is the inclusion of a chapter on literary critical theory and its relevancy to deafness. This line of thinking has led to the importance of developing literate thought for individuals who are deaf and has provided some impetus for the establishment of ASL/English bilingual and second-language learning educational programs.

It is axiomatic to assert that the development of reading and writing skills is important for success in school and in mainstream society. It might be heretic to suggest that literacy skills are not *necessary* for the development of literate thought, that is, the ability to think critically and reflectively. Based on a synthesis of metatheories, theories, and research, the text provides some insights into the relationship between literacy and literate thought. Perhaps the major goal of education should be the development of literate thought, which can be manifested via the use of the conversational form of a language (i.e., speech or signs), written language, and even computers. The critical requirement for literate thought is the acquisition and development of a bona fide language and concomitant cognitive skills at as early an age as possible.

Chapter 1 provides an overview of the major aspects of literacy and deafness that are elaborated upon in the rest of the text. The reader is introduced to major perspectives on literacy, the role of teaching, and on deafness. It is argued that holding a certain view on deafness influences the development of theories, the type of research methods, and the content of instructional practices.

Chapter 2 addresses the research on hearing students, and Chapter 3 focuses on students who are deaf. There is an attempt to discuss research in the major areas of reading such as word identification and comprehension, especially from a reading-comprehension perspective. The development of higher-level reading skills is shown to be dependent on the reciprocity between word identification and comprehension. That is, word identification facilitates comprehension and comprehension facilitates word identification during fluent reading. In essence, the reciprocity at this level is dependent on an individual's acquisition and knowledge of the alphabetic code (e.g., consonants and vowels), the system on which written language is based.

Chapter 4 focuses on the development of writing in both hearing and deaf students. The two bipolar views of writing are discussed. The traditional, or product, view deals with the development of mechanics such as grammar, punctuation, and spelling. The emerging view of writing is the process approach that emphasizes higher-level skills such as organization, intent, and audience. Perhaps the deeper revelation is the notion that reading and writing share underlying processes. This is often construed as the reading-writing connection and makes the case that there is a reciprocal, developmental relationship between these two entities.

Chapter 5 presents an overview of the major tenets of the literary critical perspective, which has been influenced by critical theories. This perspective has provided some support for the ASL/English bilingual movement, but most particularly for the use of American Sign Language as the first language and major medium for communicative exchange between and among individuals who are deaf and individuals who are hearing. Literary critical theorists are interested in issues such as empowerment, enlightenment, instrumental rationality, and oppression.

The main intent of Chapter 6 is to provide a comprehensive overview of the theory and research on second-language development of English literacy. There is also a discussion of the failure of several ASL/English bilingual programs to consider the extant theory and research conducted on literacy and hearing students. In addition, some of these proponents have misinterpreted the salient principles of first-language and second-language literacy theories. Another important issue covered in this chapter is the notion of similarity/difference relative to the development of second-language literacy. That is, it is critical to know if the development of English first-language literacy is similar to or different from the literacy development in English as a second language. This has important implications for the use of instructional practices and curricular materials.

The text devotes two chapters to the teaching of literacy in English as a first or second language—Chapters 7 and 8. In addition to providing instructional examples and guidelines, the chapters also cover issues such as the teachability/learnability dichotomy and the notion of a best method or effective methods. It is emphasized that most of the instructional strategies shared in these chapters are heavily influenced by the cognitive interactive theory of literacy—the authors' bias.

The main focus of Chapter 9 is on reform in assessment. Here, it is argued that educators need to consider alternative measures of *achievement* rather than continuing the heavy reliance on paper-and-pencil, objective, standardized tests. In addition to discussing traditional concepts such as reliability, validity, and practicality, the chapter illustrates that many current literacy assessments have not kept pace with the emerging views of reading and writing. Some alternative measures that are discussed and recommended are those involving curriculum-based measures, ecologically based assessments, and mediated learning situations (e.g., based on Vygotsky's zone of proximal development). One of the common denominators of these alternative tests is that they are considered to be performance-based and diagnostic-oriented, thus more suitable for meeting the student's needs within a classroom setting.

Chapter 10 reemphasizes at least three major issues relative to the development of literate thought: (1) the interrelations of metatheory, theory, research, and practice; (2) the reciprocal relations between word identification and comprehension and between the conversational and written forms of a phonetic language such as English; and (3) the contributions of a well- and early-developed language to the subsequent development of literate thought. It is concluded that literate thought should be the ultimate goal for all students who are deaf—indeed *all* students.

I would also like to thank the following reviewers for their time and input: Martha Gaustad, Bowling Green State University, and Harry G. Lang, National Institute for the Deaf, Rochester Institute for Technology.

Introduction to Literacy and Deafness

Reading must be seen as part of a child's general language development and not as a discrete skill isolated from listening, speaking, and writing. (Anderson, Hiebert, Scott, & Wilkinson, 1985, p. 20)

Critical literacy, the literate use of language to problem solve and communicate, should be the primary aim of the elementary years of schooling. (Calfee, 1994, p. 19)

. . . my demonstrations depended on our ability to read and write, and this makes our communication even more impressive by bridging gaps of time, space, and acquaintanceship. But writing is clearly an optional accessory; the real engine of verbal communication is the spoken language we acquired as children. (Pinker, 1994, p. 16)

The above passages capture the manner in which literacy and deafness are discussed in this text. The reader should obtain a deep understanding of and appreciation for the interrelations between cognition, the conversational form of a language, and literacy, that is, the ability to read and write. With literate thought in the subtitle of this text, it is clear that a key goal of education is to enable students who are deaf (indeed, all students) to think critically and reflectively. This is evident in the preceding passage by Calfee (1994). However, acquiring a high level of literate thought (or critical literacy) is dependent on the acquisition of the spoken or conversational form of a language at the earliest possible age. Many students who are deaf have problems with reading and writing because of their difficulty in acquiring "the real engine of verbal communication" (Pinker, 1994, p. 16), that is, the conversational form (spoken and/or signed) of the language in which they are trying to read or express via writing.

The purpose of this introductory chapter is threefold. One aim is to provide the reader with a brief introduction and background to the major areas of literacy and deafness discussed in the rest of this text. It is argued that the selection and presentation of these areas are dependent upon the overall metatheoretical (or metaanalytic) perspectives of the writer. After this background information, the second aim is to provide a brief discussion of literacy. Specifically, the reader should become familiar with current perspectives, for example, reading-comprehension, literary criticism, and the influences of phenomenological and social-constructionist theories. The chapter also presents introductory information on second-language development and second-language literacy. The third, and final, aim is to describe deafness from two bipolar perspectives, clinical and cultural. On one level, an understanding of this dichotomy is critical for understanding the major impetus for establishing American Sign Language/English bilingual education programs. However, the major intent of this section is to show how adherence to a particular philosophical perspective on deafness affects the acceptance and use of specific literacy theories, research thrusts, and instructional practices.

Metatheorizing in Literacy and Deafness

The various forms of metaanalyses, particularly metatheorizing, are critical for understanding the condition of literacy and deafness. In fact, it is argued that understanding is not possible without a metatheoretical perspective. For example, it has been stated elsewhere (Paul & Jackson, 1993) that it might not be possible for proponents of *oralism* and proponents of *total communication* to communicate effectively to each other because each side represents a different philosophical (perhaps, metatheoretical) perspective. At present, it is not clear whether oralism or total communication represents a specific type of metatheorizing. The intent of the ensuing paragraphs is to (1) discuss briefly the notion of metaanalysis and (2) show the utility of such analyses.

Types of Metaanalyses

Metaanalysis refers to the systematic analysis or synthesis of the available theories, research, and other types of data, for example, syntheses, methodologies, policies, assessments, curricula, and instructional practices. This analysis might employ the use of the scientific method (e.g., quantitative or qualitative analyses) or the critical method (e.g., literary critical theory; discussed later in this chapter and in Chapter 5). One common type of metaanalysis is meta-data-analysis (e.g., Glass, McGaw, & Smith, 1981). The focus of this type is on analyzing (actually, reanalyzing) statistical results across a range of research studies. The main goal is to synthesize these results. Similar procedures can be done with the array of methods for collecting data (e.g., survey, observational, experimental) or with data from qualitative studies (e.g., interpretative, descriptive, ethnographic data; see discussion in Lincoln & Guba, 1985). Translative research, that is, deriving practices based on a specific theory or several theories, is also a common form of metaanalysis. Traditionally, these analyses have adhered to scientific or systematic inquiry guidelines that are similar for conducting integrative theoretical and research reviews. The possible steps of this type of review include: (1) formulation of a problem or hypothesis, (2) selection and collection of data, (3) analysis and interpretation, and (4) presentation of the results (e.g., see discussion in Cooper, 1982).

Consider the following example based on a published, refereed journal article (Paul & O'Rourke, 1988). The intent of this article was to examine the relationship of word knowledge, particularly knowledge of multimeaning words, to reading comprehension. The following remarks are relative to the guidelines delineated above.

Example Based on Paul & O'Rourke (1988)

1. The investigators were interested in several problems in this area: (a) the prevalence of polysemic (multimeaning) words in reading materials, (b) the comprehension of the meanings of these words by deaf and learning-disabled readers, and (c) the relationship between vocabulary instruction and reading comprehension.

2. To answer *a,* the researchers studied the information in several sources (i.e., compilations of frequency and meanings) that have been cited frequently in the literature (e.g., Carroll, Davies, & Richman, 1971; Dale & O'Rourke, 1981; Durkin, 1981; Johnson, Moe, & Baumann, 1983; Kucera & Francis, 1967; Searls & Klesius, 1984). To address *b* and *c,* the researchers conducted a review of the literature from 1969 to 1987, covering journal articles, ERIC documents, and theses. The emphasis was on empirical articles, although research syntheses were also included. For *b,* all of the available literature was included whereas for *c,* a sample was selected for review and synthesis. [In retrospect, the selection of the sample for *c* was not random; however, it could be argued that the names of the researchers and scholars were well known in this area. Because of this, it is doubtful that the results were not representative and accurate.]

3. Despite some differences in the data for *a,* the researchers were still able to synthesize the common findings regarding prevalence of multimeaning words in both the spoken and written language of young children. Although all of the empirical studies in *b* and *c* involve quantitative analyses (i.e., group comparisons), the samples, designs, and procedures were not similar, thus, it was difficult to conduct a meta-data-analysis. However, there was sufficient information in the studies for the researchers to make general, synthesized statements regarding both the comprehension of multimeaning words and the relationship of vocabulary instruction to reading comprehension. A good discussion of this issue relative to hearing students, based on a metaanalysis, was provided by Stahl and Fairbanks (1986).

4. The results of the Paul and O'Rourke (1988) research synthesis were presented in *Remedial and Special Education;* these results are discussed later in the text.

Note: The numbers 1, 2, 3, and 4 correspond to the four steps of the scientific method mentioned previously.

Utility of Metaanalyses

Several arguments can be put forward to support the utility of the various types of metaanalyses (e.g., Ritzer, 1991, 1992), especially in the area of literacy and deafness (e.g., Paul, 1994a; Paul & Quigley, 1994a). One of the biggest arguments is that there is a growing body of theoretical and research data in the area of literacy, making it difficult for theorists, researchers, and practitioners to keep abreast of the new developments and, more importantly, to synthesize the information to obtain a reasonable understanding. For example, our understanding of literacy has been influenced by the numerous models that have been developed in cognitive psychology, linguistics, philosophy, and literary criticism. Most of the reading-comprehension theories have been based on the cognitive metatheory, with information-processing models serving as its most prominent metaphor. Naturalistic theories have been influenced by the cognitive models of Piaget and Vygotsky. Literary critical theories derive their knowledge base from *social* theories, especially within a qualitative, interpretative framework. From one perspective, synthesizing the prevailing, available thinking on literacy is critical if it is agreed that there is or should be interrelations among metatheory, theory, research, assessment, curriculum, and instruction or practice. In addition, with the advent of a variety of theories and models, metaanalysis can help us make sense of this proliferation of information.

Perhaps a major reason for conducting these types of analyses is to reduce what can be described as a *crisis* (Ritzer, 1991, 1992) or *distrust of theorizing and research*. These *feelings* lead to the sense that there is a widening gap between theory and practice and that there are too many theoretical models, many of which do not correspond to reality. To minimize problems such as establishing policy on limited data, relying substantially on testimonials, and misinterpreting the major tenets of theories and research, it is critical for scholars to engage in metaanalyses, particularly metatheorizing. Examples of these problems in the field of deafness include the use of a *whole-language approach* as the only and best way to teach or develop literacy skills (e.g., see discussions in Dolman, 1992; Paul, 1993a, 1993b; Samuels & Kamil, 1984) and the establishment of ASL/English bilingual programs, many of which do not seem to be based on second-language theory and research (e.g., see Paul, 1993b, 1994b; Paul & Quigley, 1994b). However, as noted in Chapters 5 and 6, these ASL/English bilingual models are based on some aspects of literary critical theories.

Relative to deafness, another important reason for conducting various forms of meta-analyses is due to the limited data on specific areas of concern, for example, literacy and ASL/English bilingualism. Despite the importance of developing literacy skills, few empirical research investigations have been reported in the literature (e.g., see King & Quigley, 1985; Paul & Quigley, 1994a; Quigley & Paul, 1989). Given the absence of well-formed *deafness* theories of literacy, it is possible, and indeed necessary, to use the theoretical and research results from the literature on hearing children in conjunction with the little existing research on deaf children to obtain a better understanding of the problem of literacy and deafness.

From the foregoing discussion, the reader can infer that there are general similarities in the development of language and literacy for both children who are deaf and children who are hearing. This implication has been supported by several lines of research (e.g., see research reviews in Hanson, 1989; Paul, 1993a, 1993b; however, cf. Lane, Hoffmeister, & Bahan, 1996). In addition, it is also assumed that such a comparison should be made from an ethical or cultural point of view. For example, can and should educators compare the literacy levels of both groups? Can and should the standards for students who are deaf be the same as those established for students who are hearing? Can and should the *definition* of literacy be the same for both groups? These issues are briefly addressed later in the section on perspectives on deafness in this chapter and are discussed in depth in Chapter 5 dealing with literary critical theories.

Perspectives on Literacy

It is no surprise that there are several perspectives, indeed multiple, interdisciplinary perspectives, on the answer to the question, What is literacy? (Another view on this question is presented in Chapter 5). Literacy can be described to include reading, writing, computer, and mathematics, although there is a tendency to emphasize reading and writing, or text-based literacy skills (Douglas, 1989; Garton & Pratt, 1989; Paul, 1993a). Some scholars opined that literacy should include both spoken and written language (e.g., Garton & Pratt, 1989; see also, the *psycholinguistic guessing game* discussion in Goodman, 1976, 1985). This view is also echoed in some literary, or literary critical, models (e.g., see discussions in Calfee, 1994; Ellsworth, 1994; Ray, 1984). Although they are aware of and receptive to the notions of computer and mathematics literacy, most educators view literacy as the ability to read and write at either a functional level or a highly literate level (e.g., see discussion in Paul, 1993a).

There are two broad groups of remarks to be made about literacy perspectives. First, the problem of defining literacy is not new. In fact, much can be learned about the present debate on, for example, reading perspectives by reexamining early theories of reading, particularly during the eighteenth and nineteenth centuries (e.g., Bartine, 1989, 1992). As remarked by Bartine:

> . . . in that period as now, the interest in reading was highly interdisciplinary. Contributors to theory building then, as now, were deeply concerned with rhetoric, literary criticism, linguistics, psychology, and pedagogy. Then, as now, there was debate concerning the relative usefulness of aesthetic and pragmatic analyses of texts and of reading as process; a "unit of meaning" in ongoing discourse was variously defined; and theorists struggled with the relation of thought to language and of spoken language to written language. (1989, p. 2)

The second group of remarks concerns the importance and influence of possessing a perspective. If a perspective is philosophical or has the status of a metatheory, discussed previously, it will exert a tremendous influence on theory, research, practice, and assessment. For example, the notion of including both spoken and written language in the literacy framework has several implications. One, based on sociocultural analyses, it can be argued that the two systems are interrelated (e.g., Garton & Pratt, 1989). Two, there are similar processes underlying the development of both modes (e.g., Garton & Pratt, 1989; Goodman, 1976, 1985). Thus, learning to read and write depends on the prior development of spoken language. In addition, it is asserted that good literate persons make use of context cues better than poor literate persons (i.e., readers). This perspective provides the conceptual framework for one whole-language approach to reading, or what is commonly known as the psycholinguistic-guessing game (Goodman, 1976, 1985). It is also related to naturalistic views of literacy (e.g., Antonacci & Hedley, 1994).

In this text, literacy is defined narrowly as the ability to read and write. However, it is also opined that literacy is one aspect, albeit a very important one, of the ability to engage in literate thought, or what is commonly referred to as being literate (e.g., Calfee, 1994; Garton & Pratt, 1989; Olson, 1989). Literate thought is the ability to engage in reflective and critical thinking and can be expressed in or manifested by various modes, for example, reading, writing, computer, mathematics, and the conversational form of a language (i.e., spoken and/or signed).

It is difficult to categorize theories and models of literacy. Any categorization scheme is dependent on the metatheoretical perspectives of the individual who has developed categories (e.g., see discussions in Paul, 1994a; Ritzer, 1991, 1992). Nevertheless, it is possible to capture the current understanding of literacy by proposing two broad labels: reading comprehension and literary (or literary critical). Although there might be a consensus that there are two groups of *theories*, it is also possible that these labels are *metatheories* (Lemley, 1993; Paul, 1994a; Paul & Quigley, 1994a). The use of these two labels captures the essence of much of the debate on the broad *dichotomies* or *either–or* situations that exist in the literature for both first- and second-language literacy. Examples include empiricism versus rationalism (McCormick, 1988; for language development, see Steinberg, 1982), reductionism versus constructivism (Douglass, 1989), social versus cognitive literacy views (Bernhardt, 1991; McLaughlin, 1987), and the debate on how literacy should be researched (e.g., Bernhardt, 1991; Bereiter & Scardamalia, 1983, 1987; Bloome, 1989; McLaughlin, 1987) with a focus on two broad groups of so-called dichotomous views. On one side of the continuum are concepts such as reductionism, positivism, experimentalism, and mainstream science. On the other side are notions such as constructivism, interpretativism, hermeneuticism, and action science (e.g., see discussions in Alexander & Colomy, 1992; Argyris, Putnam, & Smith, 1985; Lincoln & Guba, 1985; Priest, 1991). In essence, to obtain an understanding of present instructional practices as well as theoretical and research thrusts, a brief explanation of some of these terms relative to the two broad groups of literacy perspectives is undertaken. This discussion also covers writing and second-language literacy.

Reading-Comprehension Framework

Within a reading-comprehension framework, theorists and researchers are interested in understanding literacy processes and in developing or improving the literacy proficiency of children, adolescents, and adults. Most of the theories are based on the cognitive metatheory, expressed with an information-processing metaphor (Baars, 1986; McCarthey & Raphael, 1992; Samuels & Kamil, 1984). Information processing focuses on the representation, transformation, and retrieval of "knowledge." As described by Baars:

> . . . psychologists observe behavior in order to make inferences about underlying factors that can explain behavior. . . . cognitive psychologists often talk about the representations that organisms can have of themselves and of their world, and about the transformations that these representations undergo. "Transforming representations" is sometimes called information processing. (1986, p.42)

It is possible to categorize reading-comprehension theories into three broad groups: bottom-up (text-based), top-down (reader-based), and interactive (parallel-processing) (e.g., Grabe, 1988, 1991; King & Quigley, 1985; Samuels & Kamil, 1984). A brief description of each group, including some metatheoretical underpinnings, is provided in the ensuing paragraphs. A more detailed description with instructional examples is presented in Chapter 2. The reader should keep in mind that these are general, prototypal descriptions of the models, rather than a description of a specific model.

Bottom-Up Models

In bottom-up models, the emphasis is on the identification of words and their parts—phonemes (roughly vowels and consonants; example: /c/ /a/ /t/ has three phonemes) and morphemes (roughly smallest meaning parts; example: cats has two morphemes: /cat/ and /-s/). This process is considered bottom-up because it begins at the bottom with letters and ends at the top with comprehension by the reader. It should also be emphasized that these models assert that meaning is in the text and the reader must *decode* words in order to access it.

Three terms that characterize bottom-up models are linear, hierarchical (Lipson & Wixson, 1991; Samuels & Kamil, 1984), and empiricism (McCormick, 1988). The models are linear and hierarchical because there are several levels of analyses through which readers must proceed in a hierarchical fashion. That is, readers begin with the processing of the smallest units of analysis (e.g., letters) and work their way up to the next largest level. The sum (i.e., synthesis) of all analyses reveals the meaning of the passage.

Empiricism refers to a philosophical position that "experience is the source of all knowledge" (Chaplin, 1975, p. 172). This means that there is a separation of knowledge and the knower. Thus, knowledge or information is objective and can be accessed via sense experience. Bottom-up theories are related to empiricism relative to "the question of control in reading" (McCormick, 1988, p. 56). That is, the text contains information and directs or controls the reading process. The text, which represents knowledge or information, is outside the reader, who represents the knower and must process the text in order to obtain an understanding of it.

Debates aside, empiricism is often considered the trademark of the scientific method because of the focus on discovering objective facts through the use of observation and experimentation. This notion seems to proceed in tandem with that of reductionism, to be discussed later. More important, as will be shown in subsequent chapters, both empiricism and reductionism have implications for instructional practices as well as for theory and research.

Top-Down Models

In top-down models, the emphasis is on the information or knowledge that is in the reader's head (Lipson & Wixson, 1991; Samuels & Kamil, 1984). This process is considered top-down because the processing begins at the top in the reader's head, with predictions and inferences, and proceeds downward to the text to confirm these predictions or inferences or generate new ones. Many top-down models view reading/writing as a language-learning process in which readers sample the text in order to build a model of what it means. As with learning a first language, no explicit instruction of reading or reading subskills (e.g., word identification skills) is necessary or, from another perspective, such instruction should be minimized. Indeed, this type of instruction might be detrimental to the acquisition process. Much of the *instruction* that seems to occur focuses on *meaning making* and *use of context* (e.g., see discussion in Lipson & Wixson, 1991, p. 10).

Similar to bottom-up models, top-down models are also considered to be linear and hierarchical (Samuels & Kamil, 1984). In this case, readers focus on the largest unit of processing and move toward the smallest unit. Relative to the issue of *control*, these models can be labeled as examples of the philosophical position of rationalism (McCormick, 1988). Rationalism exemplifies the position that "reason is extoled as a means of arriving at the truth" (Chaplin, 1975, p. 440). In addition, there is an emphasis on *a priori* or *innate* knowledge. Thus, in this view, the reader brings meaning and knowledge to the text. This reader-based knowledge and meaning directs or controls the process of reading.

Several top-down models seem to be influenced by theoretical and research constructs such as interpretativism and constructivism, which are discussed later in this chapter. In fact, these influences seem to create another view of literacy known as the naturalistic approach (e.g., Antonacci & Hedley, 1994; McCarthey & Raphael, 1992) with a focus on reading/writing connections. This issue is discussed in depth in Chapter 4.

Interactive Models

The third group of models is labeled interactive, or parallel processing (e.g., Grabe, 1988; Lipson & Wixson, 1991; Mason & Au, 1986; Samuels & Kamil, 1984). In this view, it is asserted that reading is an interactive process between the reader and the text. In other words, good readers integrate information from the text with their own knowledge to construct meaning. This is an active process requiring the coordination of both bottom-up and top-down skills. Good readers engage in high-level comprehension strategies such as applying prior knowledge, making inferences, and thinking about what they know and do not know in relation to the text (e.g., cognitive and metacognitive skills).

Two terms that characterize the interactive models are parallel-processing (Rumelhart, 1977, 1980; Rumelhart, McClelland, & the PDP Research Group, 1986) and phenomenological (McCormick, 1988). Parallel-processing refers to processing that might proceed in both directions, that is, bottom-up and top-down. One implication of this interaction is that bottom-up skills facilitate top-down processing and top-down skills facilitate bottom-up processing. As is discussed in Chapter 2, this seems to dispute the either-or syndrome involving word identification (i.e., bottom-up processing) and comprehension (i.e., top-down processing). However, most interactive models assert that word identification skills should be mastered at as early an age (or grade) as possible, preferably by the end of second or third grade.

Relative to philosophical perspectives, interactive models represent the interaction of both empiricism (e.g., bottom-up or text-based) and rationalism (top-down or reader-based). In this sense, it is said to have something in common with phenomenology, which is often used to described other models such as social-constructionist and literary-critical theories (McCarthey & Raphael, 1992; McCormick, 1988; Ray, 1984). It is difficult to describe phenomenology, which was a reaction against British empiricism as formulated by Locke, Berkeley, and Hume. Phenomenology is termed *radical empiricism* and has a slogan of *back to things themselves* (e.g., see McCormick, 1988). This notion employs the use of terms such as *intentionality* and *consciousness* and focuses on the study of events that occur immediately in experience without interpretation (Chaplin, 1975). However, phenomenologists are concerned with the understanding of meaning, which is important for our purposes.

Where does meaning occur? McCormick provides one perspective of this situation with a passage from another source:

> Phenomenology . . . is neither a science of objects [empiricism] nor a science of the subject [rationalism]; it is a science of experience. It does not concentrate exclusively on either the objects of experience or on the subject of experience, but on the point of contact where being [the objects] and consciousness [the subject] meet. (Edie, in McCormick, 1988, p. 59)

Thus, what phenomenology has in common with interactive theories is it ". . . implies that both the text and the reader must be fully acknowledged; but further, such acknowledgment will be adequate only if the text and the reader are considered as bound up together in an interactive relationship" (McCormick, 1988, p. 64). A better understanding of phenomenology should provide more light on the nature of interactive models of reading and, possibly, the implications for instruction in reading and writing.

It has been argued that interactive theories of reading seem to be "too closely tied to Cartesian or Newtonian philosophical dualism, the paradigm that treats human beings and nature as separate entities" (Rosenblatt, 1989, p. 154). Within this view, the construction of meaning is seen as an interaction between the reader and the text; however, meaning ultimately is constructed from pre-existing elements in the mind. In essence, the reader's interpretation should match the author's intention, which can be related by the author or by experts on the author's style. In this sense, interactive theorists are motivated by a reductionist point of view (see later discussion of reductionism).

A summary of the major points of the three groups of reading-comprehension models presented in this section is provided in Table 1-1.

TABLE 1-1   Summary of salient points associated with the three groups of reading-comprehension models

Bottom-Up Models

- Characteristics based on linearity, hierarchy, and empiricism
- Sum of all analyses from smallest to largest units reveals meaning
- Text contains meaning and controls the reading process

Top-Down Models

- Characteristics based on linearity, hierarchy, and rationalism
- Emphasis is on the information in reader's head; reader controls the reading process
- Influences include notions such as interpretativism and constructivism

Interactive Models

- Characteristics based on parallel processing and phenomenology
- Process entails both bottom-up and top-down aspects; the reading process is controlled by the interactions of the reader and the text
- Representation of interaction between empiricism and rationalism

Literary Critical Framework

The focus of Chapter 5 is on the literary critical framework with implications for understanding literacy and deafness. For individuals schooled in the traditional framework of teaching reading and writing skills, it might be confusing to encounter terms such as phenomenology (mentioned briefly previously), structuralism, reader-response, and deconstruction. It might be even more difficult to understand what this framework has to offer for the teaching of literacy.

Prior to offering implications, it is necessary to discuss briefly here the nature of this concept and the manner in which it has been applied to deafness and literacy. A few examples of the influence of literary critical theory on understanding literacy and deafness are offered. The approach to discussing these topics here is meant to be taken as an introduction to the more detailed discussion of literary critical theory in Chapter 5.

Critical Theory

There is no unified critical theory; rather, there are critical theories (e.g., Gibson, 1986). The existence of several theories reflects the varying disagreements among proponents. Critical theorists argue that social and human knowledge are not value free or objective. Knowledge is socially constructed and, typically, reflects the values of the group in power. There are no *universal* interests or values; thus, there is always conflict and tension because of the varying interests of numerous groups. The best way to phrase this issue is to inquire, "Whose interests are being served?" (Gibson, 1986, p. 5).

Critical theorists argue that certain groups need to recognize that they are being oppressed because of the standards or values that they are forced to adhere to. For example, let us assume that literacy is an unrealistic goal for some subgroups in the population because of their extreme difficulty in accessing this form. This lack of access might also lead to an impoverished development of cognition and/or subject these individuals to what can be called *second-class citizenship*. Even more interesting is the fact that many members of these subgroups might be able to obtain a high level of literate thought (thinking creatively and reflectively); however, they cannot demonstrate this level in the text-based literate mode (i.e., reading and writing). In this sense, if text-based literacy is the major requirement for graduation credentials (e.g., high school and colleges) and also for access into such professions as medicine, law, or academe, it can be argued that this requirement represents an oppressive situation.

Critical Theory and Literacy

Relative to literacy, the influence of critical theory is most often associated with the interpretation and understanding of literature (e.g., Bartine, 1992; Gibson, 1986, Ray, 1984). Critical theorists proffer provocative assertions regarding the timeless, universal truths expressed in great literature, for example, the works of Shakespeare, Goethe, and Dickenson. According to critical theorists, there is no such thing as great literature (Gibson, 1986). In essence, these works, and others, are constructed at particular times in particular contexts to express particular values. Typically, these works promote values and interests of a dominant group or dominant groups during a specific period.

In this text, the concern is with critical theory as it applies to an understanding of reading and writing. This concern is with the meaning and function (or context) of literacy.

There is an intense preoccupation with meaning, implying that there is no such thing as absolute, static meaning associated with a particular text. In fact, it is asserted that there is no connection between word and meaning. These points should highlight some of the basic assumptions of social-constructivist theories of literacy. As is discussed in Chapter 5, these assumptions do not support literacy instruction of the *author's* meanings as determined by *experts*.

The second area of concern refers to the context of the application of skills associated with reading and writing (e.g., Lemley, 1993; McCormick, 1988; Olson, 1989; Ray, 1984; Wagner, 1986). There are several dimensions to the notion of *context*, for example, literature, history, socioculture, and sociopolitics. As discussed previously, any construction of meaning by the individual is dependent upon these dimensions; there is no meaning separate from context. More important, the construction of meaning is not dependent upon the written text itself.

Within this perspective, the skills of reading and writing are subsumed under the broad notion of literacy (or being literate). In some societies, being literate might include the ability to read or write as *one* expression of literate thought (e.g., Olson, 1989; Wagner, 1986). Literate thought refers to the ability to engage in critical and reflective thought, which, according to the quote at the beginning of this chapter (Calfee, 1994), should be a major goal of education. In addition, the broad notion of literacy also includes the views and beliefs of affected societies toward the functions of reading and writing. This broad perspective makes it difficult to construct a theoretical framework because of the varying views that exist across societies. Obviously, critical theorists assert that there is no *universal* theoretical framework.

Literary Critical Theory and Deafness
The reader should be most interested in the application and influence of literary critical theory on understanding deafness and literacy, including the *teaching* of reading and writing skills. Only a few remarks are made here; an in-depth discussion occurs in Chapter 5.

One application of literary critical theory has been the use of the reader-response perspective to explain how readers who are deaf, particularly children, participate in the story world of print (e.g., Lemley, 1993; see also, the discussion of research in Chapter 4 on writing). Lemley has argued that previous research, especially studies influenced by reading-comprehension theories, have focused on the *deficiencies* of deaf readers. Her study was an initial investigation of how readers who are deaf interacted with print, particularly within the framework of reader-response theory.

This focus on the perspective of individuals who are deaf has also been supported by other scholars (e.g., Padden & Ramsey, 1993). For example, Padden and Ramsey argued that literacy is different (actually, broader) than reading and writing skills. Reading and writing skills focus on the individual whereas literacy is essentially a social phenomenon. Relative to deafness, they argued that it is important to consider the relationship between literacy and Deaf culture. A deeper understanding of this relationship might result in the improvement of reading and writing skills.

Paul (e.g., Paul, 1993a; Paul, 1994a; Paul & Quigley, 1994a) has attempted to address the question of literacy pertinent to some of the fundamental aspects of critical theory as discussed by Gibson (1986) previously. The discussion in this text (Chapter 5) is motivated by two broad questions (Paul & Quigley, 1994a, p. 299):

TABLE 1-2   Summary of salient points of the literary critical perspectives

Literary Critical Perspectives

- Knowledge is socially constructed; it reflects the values of groups in power.
- Literary critical perspectives are characterized by the question, Whose interests are being served?
- There is no such thing as absolute, static meaning associated with a particular text.
- Literate thought refers to the ability to engage in critical and reflective thought.
- Reader response theory focuses on the reactions of the individual to the text during a reading or storytelling session.
- Concerns include oppression and accessibility.

1. Is it possible to develop literate thought without possessing high-level skills in text-based literacy, that is, the ability to read and write printed materials?
2. Is literate thought sufficient for participation in a scientific, technological society such as the United States?

Within this perspective, the importance of text-based literacy is acknowledged. However, it might be a value-laden answer, especially if a high-level of thought is possible without an accompanying level of proficiency in text-based literacy. For example, the emphasis on text-based literacy for individuals who are deaf might be oppressive because (a) text-based literacy is difficult for the overwhelming majority and (b) it prevents many from either reaching or demonstrating literate thought.

A summary of the major points of the literary critical perspectives and their relations to deafness is presented in Table 1-2.

Perspectives on Writing

It is quite difficult to answer the questions, What is writing? and How do children learn to write? (Czerniewska, 1992; Hillocks, 1986; Mosenthal, Tamor, & Walmsley, 1983; Rubin & Hansen, 1986). In this text, there will be a focus on two broad aspects of writing: product and process. More specifically, the topic of writing, as manifested in reading/writing connections, is discussed from three perspectives: cognitive information processing (i.e., reading comprehension), naturalism, and social constructionism; the latter two have been influenced by literary critical theories (e.g., see discussion in McCarthey & Raphael, 1992; see also Chapter 4).

The Products of Writing
Traditionally, theorists and researchers, studying students who are deaf and students who are hearing, have focused on the products of writing (e.g., see discussions in Czerniewska, 1992; Laine & Schultz, 1985; Paul & Quigley, 1994a). The products of writing refer to the contents of written language samples examined for vocabulary, grammar (syntax, use of pronouns, etc.), and mechanics such as punctuation, capitalization, and legibility. Much of the research on children with hearing impairment has been described relative to the products of writing (e.g., see discussion in Paul & Quigley, 1990, 1994a). That is, the written language samples

of children with hearing impairment contained quantitatively fewer grammatical elements (e.g., nouns, verbs, complex sentences) than those of their hearing counterparts. Another popular tenet of this view is that writing should be *taught* after reading has been adequately established. This view spawned several beliefs, for example, good readers have the potential to become good writers; however, good writers were invariably good readers.

Although the products of writing are considered low-level skills, similar to bottom-up skills of reading, two general statements can be averred. First, if writers are struggling with lower-lever skills, they might find it difficult to apply the top-down, or composing, aspects of writing such as organization and style. Second, within a psycholinguistic framework, influenced by the work of Chomsky (e.g., 1957, 1965, 1975, 1988), it can be asserted that many children with severe to profound hearing impairment are operating with a rule system that is not acceptable, standard English. At best, this line of research on the products of writing made it clear that these children have not internalized the grammatical rules of English.

Writing as a Process

Nevertheless, too much emphasis on the products of writing has resulted in the use of instructional methods and materials that might have been responsible for some of the stilted written productions of children with severe to profound impairment. Although knowledge of the products is important, a more complete understanding of writing can be gleaned from the perspective of writing as a process. In one sense, viewing writing as a process means emphasizing higher-level skills such as organization, intent, audience, and style. In a deeper sense, the process view is interpreted to mean that writing is a social process. Writing is an aspect of language whose meaning, role, and value vary across contexts and communities. Writing is not an attempt to reflect reality; writing is the construction of reality (Bereiter & Scardamalia, 1983, 1987; Czerniewska, 1992; Rosenblatt, 1989).

The process view of writing has led theorists and researchers to define and explore the relationships between reading and writing. Writing facilitates the development of reading, and reading facilitates the development of writing. Research seems to show that there are many parallels between reading and writing (e.g., Tierney & Pearson, 1983).

This view proffers three subprocesses or stages of writing: planning, composing, and revising (i.e., within a cognitive interactive view). Roughly, planning refers to generating and organizing ideas, establishing a purpose, and identifying the audience. Composing is the actual production of a first draft. Revising refers to the reviewing and editing processes. It should be mentioned that these stages are not always mutually exclusive. For example, one can revise the organization of ideas during the planning or composing stage. In addition, this view acknowledges that writing can be used to help students become better readers. That is, reading does not need to be adequately developed before one engages in writing. In fact, the reciprocity between writing and reading has been documented in a classic study by Durkin (1966), who remarked that children's early involvement with writing (starting with illegible marks on the page) was related to their later reading achievement level.

Within a literary critical, particularly naturalistic and social-constructionist, perspective, the process of writing is articulated quite differently (e.g., Rosenblatt, 1989). As an example, the notion of transactional theory is discussed briefly (Rosenblatt, 1989). This theory has been influenced by the view of constructivism. According to this viewpoint, the implications for the *teaching* of reading and writing and for researching the literacy process are pervasively different from those proffered by cognitive theories (i.e., within the reading-comprehension framework).

As argued by Rosenblatt (1989), there are both similarities and differences between reading and writing. In her view, the *composing* metaphor (i.e., Tierney & Pearson, 1983) neglects critical differences between the two processes. Rosenblatt has also argued that her transactional paradigm is a reaction against the duality expressed in *interactive* theories, indeed in any theory based on the traditional scientific approach in which there is a separation of the observer and the entity being observed.

A better understanding of reading and writing can be gleaned from the transactional nature of language and the notion of selective attention. Based on Vygotsky's views (see discussion in Vygotsky, 1962), language is a social process, which is internalized as a result of the individual in transaction with a particular environment (i.e., the development of *internal speech*). This view has also been articulated in a social-constructivist theory of language development (see discussion in Bohannon & Warren-Leubecker, 1985).

Selective attention, also referred to as the cocktail-party syndrome, refers to the allotment of attention to a particular, selected area. Within a transactional framework, this is not a mechanical process in which an individual chooses to focus on an entity "from among an array of fixed entities; rather, . . . (it is) a dynamic centering on areas or aspects of the contents of consciousness" (Rosenblatt, 1989, p. 157).

Considering the transactional view of language and selective attention, Rosenblatt (1989) describes reading as:

> . . . an event, a transaction involving a particular reader and a particular time in a particular context. Certain organismic states, certain ranges of feeling, certain verbal or symbolic linkages, are stirred up in the linguistic reservoir. From these activated areas, selective attention—conditioned by multiple personal and social factors that enter into the situation—picks out elements that synthesize or blend into what constitutes "meaning." Meaning does not reside ready-made in the text or in the reader; it happens during the transaction between reader and text. (1989, p. 157)

Finally, in discussing the writing transactional process, Rosenblatt (1989) avers that:

> An important difference between readers and writers should not be minimized, however. . . . the reader has the physical pattern of signs to which to relate the symbolizations. The writer facing a blank page may start with only an organismic state, vague feelings and ideas, which require further triadic definition before a symbolic configuration—a physical text—can take shape.
>
> But writing, which is often spoken of as a solitary activity, is not a matter simply of dipping into a memory pool. Writing, we know, is always an event in time, occurring at a particular moment in the writer's biography, in particular circumstances, and under particular external and internal pressures. In short, the writer is always transacting with a personal, social, and cultural environment. . . . Thus the writing process must be seen as always embodying both personal and social environmental factors. (1989, p. 163)

Further discussions and descriptions of writing are presented in Chapter 4 of this text.

Second-Language Literacy

Based on the difficulties that students who are deaf have in acquiring English as a first language, a number of educators and researchers have advocated for the development of American Sign Language/English bilingual programs or English-as-a-second-language (ESL) programs (e.g., Luetke-Stahlman, 1983; Paul, 1991; Paul & Quigley, 1994b; Reagan, 1985; Strong, 1988a, 1988b). It is assumed that English might be easier to acquire as a second language or in conjunction with American Sign Language (ASL) in a bilingual education program. There is much debate on what type of program should be established, how much time and exposure should be allotted to the two languages (i.e., ASL and English), and who should be candidates for such programs. Some unanswered questions include (Paul & Quigley, 1994b, p. 220):

1. Should ASL and English be developed (or taught) concurrently in infancy and early childhood as in a bilingual environment?
2. Should ASL be taught as a first language to all deaf students with English taught as a second language?
3. Should English be taught as a second language only to students who know ASL as a first language or to all deaf students?
4. If ASL is taught as the first language, at what grade or age level should English be introduced?
5. When both ASL and English are used, how much exposure should be allotted to each language?

Despite the importance of this issue, there is little empirical research available (e.g., see discussions in Paul & Quigley, 1994a, 1994b). In addition, several proposed bilingual programs, especially their instructional plans for developing English literacy, do not have strong theoretical and research foundations. It has also been suggested that the main impetus for these programs might be the attainment of sociopolitical objectives (e.g., Stuckless, 1991).

The major focus of Chapter 6 is on the acquisition of second-language literacy, that is, the reading and writing of English as a second language. Much of what we know about second-language literacy has been influenced by the theoretical and research literature on first-language literacy (e.g., see discussions in Grabe, 1988, 1991; McLaughlin, 1984, 1985, 1987). Despite this influence, it is important to study second-language learning also as an entity unto itself (e.g., see discussion in Bernhardt, 1991).

Several issues relevant to deafness and second-language literacy are examined. First, it is necessary to provide a broad overview on bilingualism and second-language learning with hearing students. Due to limited research data on students who are deaf, the information in this type of synthesis (and others) is critical for establishing sound bilingual and/or ESL educational programs for deaf students. Specifically, this background should help understand the task of teaching English to students who either have limited use of a first language (English or another language) or know a first language for which there is no written language form (e.g., American Sign Language).

The second major issue is the question of whether similarities and/or differences exist between first- and second-language acquisition of English. In other words, the emphasis is on whether the development of English by second-language students is qualitatively similar (i.e., in manner) to that of first-language users of English (i.e., native users). There are two salient aspects to this issue. One, it raises the question of whether English (or any language) can be or should be *taught* at all. It is also related to the ongoing debate on the teachability/learnability dichotomy in *conversational* language development—the development of the primary form (speech and/or sign) of a language.

The second major aspect of the qualitative similarity issue has to do with instructional and curricular practices. For example, if it is found that there are general similarities in first- and second-language development of English, a case can be made for utilizing principles, methods, and materials in second-language instruction that are similar to those employed in first-language instruction. If there are differences, then there might be a need for developing other types of methods and materials.

Finally, related to the second aspect is the notion of *best method*. The notion of best method is discussed briefly in Chapter 6 and is mentioned in both chapters on instruction (7 and 8). It should be clear that this concept is pervasively affected by one's views on the dichotomy of reductionism versus constructivism and the corresponding research methods associated with these views. For example, reductionists generally use quantitative research methods, and constructivists generally use qualitative research methods (for in-depth discussions of research methods, see Borg & Gall, 1983; Lincoln & Guba, 1985). Quantitative researchers might delineate the specific aspect of a best method via group comparisons or via single-subject designs. On the other hand, qualitative researchers might argue that the notion of best method is, at best, misguided because of the complex interactions between instructors and students. This complex set of interactions defies the traditional sense of method as separate from the interactions themselves. This debate is similar to the one discussed previously regarding the separation of the subject (i.e., observer) and object (i.e., entity being studied) as in traditional scientific paradigms.

The last section of Chapter 6 contains a synthesis of a representative sample of research on bilingual educational models developed for hearing students. It is argued that any bilingual program for deaf students needs to address or consider these tenets of models for hearing students.

Two World Views for Theorizing, Research, and Instruction

Relative to literacy, another dichotomy to discuss briefly is reductionism versus constructivism. It is shown that theories, research, and theory-driven practices can be or have been categorized into one of these two areas. As with other dichotomies, this is construed as an either-or situation. It should be clear to the reader that setting this up as an either-or situation is also based on a metatheory (that is, it must be construed as either-or, there is no middle ground, etc.).

Reductionism and Literacy

Historically, much of the research on literacy, particularly reading, has been influenced by the scientific paradigm (e.g., Kamil, 1984; Venezky, 1984). This is also true for much of educational research (Travers, 1978). Although descriptions of the scientific method vary, certain terms that characterize this approach include empirical, experimental, positivism, quantitative, and reductionism. An adequate, albeit not exhaustive, understanding of this theoretical persuasion can be obtained via a discussion of reductionism and literacy.

One description of reductionism can be found in a dictionary of psychology:

> reductionism: the point of view which holds that the correct method to employ in the understanding of phenomena is to analyze them or reduce them to their component parts. (Chaplin, 1975, p. 447)

Influenced by the philosophical description by Immanuel Kant (e.g., see discussions in Copleston, 1985; Shuy, 1981), this point of view asserts that complex behavior can only be understood by reducing it into smaller parts and combining the parts again. In addition, this behavior can be understood in isolation, that is, it is not dependent on contextual information.

A discussion of the prominent reading theories that are purportedly based on this perspective can be found elsewhere (e.g., Douglas, 1989; McCarthey & Raphael, 1992; Rosenblatt, 1989). It is possible to categorize nearly all of the bottom-up and interactive theories in the reading-comprehension framework as reductionist and passive. Instructional methods based on this view focus on the explicit teaching of reading skills (e.g., word identification skills and comprehension skills) and support the view that learning to read is essentially a synthetic process. There is also a heavy reliance on external forms of motivation, particularly in relation to a specific instructional lesson. The prototypical example of this situation can be seen in the use of applied behavior analysis in research and instruction—particularly precision teaching techniques (e.g., see discussion in Cooper, Heron & Heward, 1987).

Not all interactive theories can be labeled strictly as reductionist; some evidence has been presented previously in the discussion of interactive models and phenomenology (see also McCormick, 1988). It can also be shown that reductionism has advanced our knowledge of the literacy process; however, it has not, and probably cannot, be used to paint the complete picture. Nevertheless, the intent of the foregoing discussion was to provide a snapshot of the scientific approach to the study and teaching of reading/writing. Within this purview, some examples of instructional activities that might be labeled reductionist are illustrated in Table 1-3.

Constructivism and Literacy

If reductionism represents a point at one end of the continuum, its bipolar opposite point is constructivism. This notion has been influenced by the work of Piaget (e.g., 1980; see also Flavell, 1985) on cognitive development. It has been used to describe the development of language, which is argued to be part of the overall cognitive development of an individual (cf., Chomsky, 1975, 1988). Other important influences come from the work of Vygotsky (e.g., 1962) on the thought/language process and the work of others on the development of pragmatics in the language development of children (Bates, 1976; Bloom & Lahey, 1978; Searle, 1976).

TABLE 1-3   Examples of reductionist instructional activities

Programming Exercises (Self-Instructing, Self-Correcting)

In the sample exercise below, the student reads the sentences and fills in the blanks. He covers the answers on the side and checks his answers as he proceeds.

Answers

flood	1. The high water *inundated* the countryside. High waters often cause a fl_____.
flooded	The countryside was probably f_____d.
flooded	Inundated means f_____.
	2. The Chinese worshipped in an ancient *pagoda*.
temple	A pagoda is probably like a church or a t_____e.

Now the student is asked to match column A with column B to further test his understanding of these words out of context.

Answers	A	B
1. c	1. culpable	a. relieved
2. e	2. ephemeral	b. commanding
3. h	3. pentagon	c. guilty
4. j	4. dirge	d. of trees
5. g	5. intransigent	e. not lasting
6. k	6. pugnacious	f. reluctant
7. d	7. arboreal	g. uncompromising
8. b	8. imperious	h. five-angled
9. n	9. captious	i. doubtful
10. l	10. irrefutable	j. funeral song

Here the student chooses the conjunction that expresses a difference or contrast between ideas.

Answers

a   1. It was eight o'clock in the evening, _____ there was still some light in the sky.
a. but   b. thus   c. because   d. besides

c   2. The children enjoyed eating the large birthday cake. _____, many of them woke up the next morning with a stomach ache.
a. But also   b. Thus   c. However   d. Otherwise

b   3. It was a difficult tune to play. _____ Howard played it without making any mistakes.
a. Besides   b. Nevertheless   c. Consequently   d. So

a   4. Edward had had a good night's sleep. _____ he was very tired in the morning.
a. Still   b. And   c. Since   d. Otherwise

c   5. Aunt Mary gave the baby his bottle, _____ he continued to cry.
a. therefore   b. so   c. yet   d. besides

a   6. There were many happy people in the stadium enjoying the game.
_____ there were also many sad fans outside who had not been able to get in.
a. On the other hand   b. For instance   c. Otherwise   d. Besides

Source: Dale & O'Rourke (1971; pp. 39, 41, and 47)

Constructivism has also been used to represent the manner in which individuals learn academic subjects, particularly language and reading. As in theories of language development, the constructivist view maintains the importance of the social milieu on the learning process. This view also maintains that the focus must be on transmitting the *whole* of literacy, not on the various parts, which purportedly leads to the whole. Within this framework, the emphasis is on naturalistic or experiential approaches to the teaching of literacy and on social-constructionist views of literacy. As noted by Douglas, "the holistic or constructivist view is one in which the whole is equal to more than the sum of its parts" (1989, p. 35).

The role of the teacher in this approach can be described as one of *facilitator* or *catalyst*. The use of direct or precision teaching methods is avoided or kept to a minimum. In addition, there is no need for external forms of motivational techniques. In other words, it is the reader/writer that is in control of the literacy process. The student is actively seeking or creating meaning, which is heavily dependent upon what is already in the reader's head. Literacy skills are developed or refined during this meaning-seeking/creating process of the student. Seeking or creating meaning is a major impetus for the continuing process of literacy acquisition. In other words, the reader/writer is internally motivated to continue; there is no real need for external or extrinsic motivational rewards. According to Piaget (1971, 1977; see also, Flavell, 1985), the intrinsic motivational process is critical for the development of self-autonomy and self-reliance. In Piaget's eyes, the excessive use of external rewards leads to what is called external locus of control (e.g., learned helplessness) in which individuals possess no self-confidence or self-initiative or no desire to strive for success (e.g., for an in-depth discussion, see Weiner, 1974).

Douglass (1989) implies that top-down models of literacy reflect predominantly the constructivist position. Specifically, Douglass asserts that Goodman's work on the notion of a psycholinguistic guessing game is the most widely known constructivist model of reading. Another well-known constructivist in this area is Frank Smith (1975, 1978). In the field of deafness, the whole language approach to literacy, along with the constructivist approach to teaching, has become a widely used, albeit debatable, framework (e.g., see discussions in Dolman, 1992; Paul & Quigley, 1994a).

A description of the constructivist view of reality has been presented by Douglas, who also cites the work of Magoon (in Douglas, 1989):

> Although the constructivist view of reality is usually attributed to eighteenth-century philosopher Immanuel Kant (1724-1804), with credit for its more modern interpretation given to twentieth-century thinker Ludwig Wittgenstein (1889-1951), its origins can be traced to Aristotle, and perhaps before. To the constructivist, learning consists of acquiring knowledge and skills largely through personal experiencing, and not as a consequence of association in response to external stimuli largely out of the control of the learner. In language learning—in all its forms, including the learning of a second language—this means one gains knowledge and skill primarily through reading, speaking, writing, and listening. One quite literally learns to read by reading; one "constructs" knowledge and skill about the process almost exclusively, if not entirely, through one's own individual efforts. Thus, one's purpose, one's desire to create meaning, and the context in which language behavior is learned are all critical. (1989, p. 40)

Discussion of Deafness

A discussion of deafness is undertaken in this section because it is important to (1) relate the perspectives on deafness with those on literacy and (2) provide a framework for discussing the findings of theoretical and research studies, which are synthesized throughout the text. For example, it is suggested that any description of literacy should incorporate an understanding of the tenets and functions of members of the Deaf culture (e.g., Padden & Ramsey, 1993). It has been argued also that theories of literacy can be interpreted as *positive* or *negative* relative to the perspectives on deafness (e.g., Lemley, 1993). In essence, a better understanding of the theoretical and research literature is dependent upon, in part, the descriptive framework of the sample under study. In other words, the manner in which deafness is defined in a particular study is important for interpreting the results of the research investigations.

In the field of deafness, it is possible to identify two broad dichotomous paradigms or perspectives: clinical and cultural (e.g., Baker & Cokely, 1980; Moores, 1987; Paul & Jackson, 1993; Reagan, 1990). This dichotomy is the impetus for the ongoing debate on several issues, for example, whether (1) there is a psychology of deafness, (2) deafness should be defined as a disability or a natural condition, and (3) English or ASL should be the first language for most deaf students (e.g., see discussions in Lane, 1988; Paul, 1994a, 1995a, 1995b; Paul & Jackson, 1993). As with other controversial issues, this issue is often construed as an either-or situation, in which one position is right or positive and the other is wrong or negative.

Some scholars have maintained that a specific position must be selected and adhered to consistently (e.g., Crittenden, 1993; Reagan, 1990), even with respect to the teaching or researching of reading and writing (e.g., Lemley, 1993). The present writer has argued that these perspectives are similar to the notions of paradigms or metatheories, and thus, it is not possible to label them as positive or negative (e.g., Paul, 1994a; Paul & Jackson, 1993; Paul & Quigley, 1994a). If these perspectives are viewed as either-or choices, then educators must make a choice; any choice that is made will have pervasive implications for theorizing, research, and instructional practices.

Clinical View of Deafness

Much of the research on language, literacy, and deafness has been influenced by the clinical perspective (Moores, 1987; Paul & Jackson, 1993; Paul & Quigley, 1994a). In addition, this perspective has been used to characterize the major tenets of both oral and total-communication programs (e.g., Reagan, 1990). For some educators and researchers, the clinical perspective is viewed as negative because of its focus on remedying the deficiencies of individuals with disabilities or other individuals who deviate from the standards or norms in achievement or ability areas. Within this purview, synonymous terms for this concept include medical or pathological.

Consider the following example relative to the condition of deafness. Suppose that a 5-year-old child receives an audiological examination. The results reveal a hearing impairment that is severe; that is, in the better unaided ear, the pure-tone average is 75 decibels (dB) (for a good discussion of hearing impairment and hearing testing, see Davis, 1978; Meyerhoff, 1986). It is suspected that this child incurred the hearing loss postlingually, that is, after the age of two years, relative to the development of spoken language. Thus, it can be stated that this child has a postlingual, severe hearing impairment.

This hypothetical child has had much difficulty with spoken and/or signed communication with her parents and teachers. The child is in a total-communication program with a planned program to improve speech, the use of residual hearing, and speech reading skills. The parents also want the child to learn to read and write and to interact with typical hearing children as much as possible. The parents are currently evaluating the possibilities of a cochlear implant for their child (a surgical procedure to improve the perception of sounds in the auditory cortex).

The scenario above is an example of the application of the clinical perspective. This perspective describes the hearing acuity of children according to two major criteria: degree of hearing impairment and age at onset. Other important descriptive factors include the hearing status of parents and siblings, etiology (cause) of hearing impairment, and type of hearing impairment (e.g., conductive, sensorineural, etc.; see Davis, 1978; Meyerhoff, 1986). Other factors important for the general population, such as intelligence (IQ) and socioeconomic status (SES), are also provided, especially in research studies. The crux here is that demographic and psychoeducational characteristics are presented and compared with those for typical children or with typical standards and norms.

It can be argued that reading-comprehension theories represent a clinical view of the literacy process because of their focus on improving and understanding the literacy process of children. In fact, Lemley (1993) has argued that most reading-comprehension theories are based on the deficiency view; that is, there is an identification of deficient skills (e.g., either bottom-up, top-down, or both) for remediation purposes. Lemley argues for more positive views of literacy and deafness, such as those expressed in literary critical theories. As discussed previously, literary critical theories attempt to explain the uses of literacy within social contexts. There is no attempt to teach reading and writing; rather, the focus is on understanding such skills, especially within a broader context of literate thought. Lemley's views can also be seen in the work of Padden and Ramsey (1993), also mentioned previously.

On one hand, the clinical perspective is viewed as negative or pathological because of the focus on preventing or curing the condition of deafness (e.g., Crittenden, 1993). Deafness is viewed as a disabling condition that should be remedied. The goal is to enable the person who is deaf to function like a hearing person in mainstream society.

On the other hand, it is also possible to assert that the clinical view is a positive one because it might lead to an improvement in the life of the child with a hearing impairment, relative to the use of spoken language or the development of reading and writing skills. It is clear that the clinical perspective is a mainstream view; however, this writer maintains that the view is neither positive or negative. It is a simply a viewpoint, which happens to be widely accepted by many theorists, researchers, and educators. Nevertheless, this does not mean that the view does not have negative consequences with respect to speech, English language, and English literacy development. The prevalence of these negative consequences—for example, impoverished development of English language and literary skills— has provided substantial support for an opposing viewpoint, the cultural perspective.

Cultural View of Deafness

An emerging, but rapidly growing, viewpoint has been labeled the cultural perspective (e.g., Baker & Cokely, 1980; Padden, 1980; Padden & Ramsey, 1993; Reagan, 1990). The growth of the cultural perspective occurred in tandem with the legitimacy of American Sign Language as a bona fide language and a movement to depathologize deafness (e.g., Reagan, 1985, 1990). In short, within this paradigm, deafness is viewed as a natural condition, not as a disease or disability. It is considered wrong or narrow to describe deafness relative to the factors of degree of hearing impairment and age at onset.

Within this perspective, the role model for students who are deaf is said to be the typical Deaf adult who is a member of the Deaf culture. This Deaf adult is one who is proficient in and prefers to communicate via the use of American Sign Language. This individual is also a graduate of a residential school, which is considered the bastion of Deaf culture (e.g., Gannon, 1981).

In essence, this view (Paul & Quigley, 1990, pp. 6-7):

1. Emphasizes differences rather than deficiencies.
2. Maintains that communication is important, primarily by using signing, preferably American Sign Language.
3. Maintains that the most appropriate education for most deaf students is in residential schools; favors the use of special instructional materials and practices.
4. Argues that a well-adjusted, well-balanced deaf person is one who can communicate and express needs; that the ability to read and write are important but not highly valued; and that literacy is more important than well-developed oral-communication skills.
5. Maintains that it is both a hearing and a deaf world, with only limited interaction between the two; deaf individuals may work in a hearing world, but they live in a deaf world.

With respect to literacy, there seem to be two strong lines of thought. One approach focuses on the development of ASL/English bilingual programs; however, even within this purview, there are strong differences about the manner in which English should be taught as a second language (e.g., see discussion in Paul & Quigley, 1994b). Differences aside, there seems to be some consensus that English literacy skills might only be feasible for some students who are deaf (i.e., students with severe to profound hearing impairment). For many students who are deaf, ASL should be taught or used as the first language and English should be taught, if possible, as the second language. The most important issue is the development of a first language at as early an age as possible, particularly for the development of literate thought.

The second major approach is related to the notion of literate thought and is pervasively influenced by literary critical theories. This line of thought focuses on the manner in which literacy is used by people who are deaf and are members of the Deaf culture (e.g., Padden & Ramsey, 1993). From another perspective, it is asserted that there is a need to understand how children who are deaf approach and deal with print-related information such as literature and other genres (e.g., Lemley, 1993; Williams, 1994, Williams & McLean, 1996). That is, the focus should be on the manner in which deaf readers/writers construct meaning, rather than on comparing their efforts and levels with hearing counterparts. This focus also assumes that meaning is not in the text; it is only in the individual's head. In addition, there is no right meaning; the construction of meaning is an interpretative, subjective, and personally and socially constructed phenomenon.

It should be emphasized that one major assertion of the cultural perspective is the need for Deaf theorists and researchers (e.g., Lane, 1988). That is, there is a need for developing deafness theories and models in order to understand the manner in which students who are deaf learn, particularly how they learn to deal with literacy. Within this view, it is considered inappropriate to develop instructional strategies and techniques that are based upon our understanding of the literacy process of hearing individuals. It is argued that mainstream theories cannot be applied fully to individuals who are deaf (for an in-depth analysis of this notion, see Gliedman & Roth, 1980). One possible implication of this focus is that any method of literacy that attempts to teach the sound system of English (e.g., via phonics) is considered to be inappropriate.

Overview of Literacy Achievement and Deafness

Much of what is known about the reading and writing achievement of students with severe to profound hearing impairment has been obtained via the use of norm-referenced or criterion-referenced tests (see Chapter 9 on assessment). Prior to the 1970s, most of the assessments were normed on students with typical hearing ability. The accuracy of these results was questioned (e.g., see discussion in Quigley & Paul, 1986); these arguments led to the development of special tests for students with hearing impairment in the 1970s and 1980s (Allen, 1986; Quigley, Power, Steinkamp, & Jones, 1978; Trybus & Karchmer, 1977).

Reading Achievement

Relative to reading, the discussion here is based on the scores of students who have taken the adapted versions of the Stanford Achievement Test (e.g., see Allen, 1986; CADS, 1991) and the Test of Syntactic Abilities (Quigley, Steinkamp, Power, & Jones, 1978). The Stanford Achievement Test-Hearing Impaired Version is the most commonly used standardized assessment in special-educational programs for students with hearing impairment. Via the use of the TSA, syntax is the most researched area of language structure and deafness (e.g., see review in Paul & Quigley, 1994a).

As discussed in Chapter 3, it is well documented that most students with severe to profound hearing impairment do not read as well as their hearing counterparts upon graduation (Allen, 1986; CADS, 1991; King & Quigley, 1985; Quigley & Paul, 1989). The recent findings on the SATs are similar to those reported for the unadapted versions of achievement tests in the early 1900s (e.g., see research review in Quigley & Paul, 1986). Two general findings can be stated. One, the results consistently reveal that average 18- to 19-year-old students with hearing impairment are reading no better than average 9- or 10-year-old students with typical hearing. Two, the results show an annual growth rate of only 0.3 reading grade level per year with a leveling off or plateau occurring at the third- or fourth-grade reading level. There is also some agreement that these general achievement batteries might be overestimating the reading ability of students with hearing impairment (Davey, LaSasso, & Macready, 1983; Moores, 1987). Thus, the true reading achievement levels of most students in special-education programs may be even lower than the levels reported.

Much of the research on students with hearing impairment has been conducted within the purview of reading-comprehension theories (King & Quigley, 1985; Quigley & Paul, 1989). Although the whole-language movement (i.e., within top-down models) seems to be prevalent, there is some question about the relevancy and research support for these approaches (Dolman, 1992; Paul, 1993a, 1993b). One of the major points stated in Chapter 3 is that reading approaches should not be construed as either-or situations, that is, word identification or comprehension. It is argued that this is not supported by research on hearing students (e.g., Adams, 1990a, 1990b).

Research on the literacy development of students within literary critical frameworks is in its infancy (e.g., Lemley, 1993; Padden & Ramsey, 1993). As discussed in greater detail in Chapter 5, there is a great deal of merit in using this framework to investigate the literacy development of students with hearing impairment. One of the implications of these theories is that the focus should be on the development of the ability to think creatively, reflectively, and critically.

Writing Achievement

Relative to writing achievement levels, Moores (1987, p. 281) has remarked that "The evidence suggests that the problems deaf children face in mastering written English are more formidable than those they face in developing reading skills." This is true if it is accepted that writing involves much more than the knowledge and use of reading skills. In addition, much of what is known about writing and deafness has been influenced predominantly by investigations that focused on the products of writing, that is, written language samples.

If poor readers are invariably poor writers, then it is not surprising that the findings of research on the written language productions of students with hearing impairment reveal low levels of achievement similar to those reported for reading levels. Students with hearing impairment are struggling with both lower-level (e.g., mechanics) and higher-level (e.g., organization, purpose) skills in writing. Even more distressing is the fact that these students cannot benefit from the reciprocal, beneficial relationship between reading and writing. That is, typically, students can increase their reading skills through writing activities and can improve their writing skills via reading activities. Because students with severe to profound hearing impairment have not developed an internal representation of English, they receive limited benefits from the two major reciprocal relationships: between the conversational and written forms of a language (i.e., speech and/or print) and between the reading and written forms (i.e., the reading-writing connection).

In Chapter 4, it is asserted that there needs to be additional research on the writing development of students within the emerging conceptual framework of writing as a process approach. Based on this research thrust, there has been some recent research on students with hearing impairment (e.g., Gormley & Sarachan-Deily, 1987; Livingston, 1989; Sarachan-

Deily, 1982, 1985). In essence, some investigators have used analyses that proceed beyond the sentence level (e.g., Yoshinaga-Itano & Snyder, 1985), and others have suggested that writing and reading should be taught as a whole-language process, that is, as a literacy process, not as a process that should be separated into components as in instruction based on reductionist principles.

Nevertheless, the debate on writing, similar to the debate on reading, has also been construed as an either–or situation—in this case, product or process. It should be underscored that this dichotomy is not supported substantially by theory and research. Even more important is the understanding that poor writers, like poor readers, might benefit from direct or precision teaching, especially in the beginning stages. This line of thinking has provided some support for research and instructional methods based on reductionist principles, discussed previously. As will be argued in Chapters 3 and 4, a combination (i.e., creative synthesis) of both reductionism and constructivism, in the areas of theory, research, and practice, might be necessary to enable students with hearing impairment to become independent readers and writers.

A Final Word

The main objective of this introduction was to provide an overview and background on the major topics discussed in the rest of this text. This necessitated a discussion of several terms important for understanding the traditional and emerging perspectives on literacy and deafness. This chapter also provided a brief description of the major underpinnings of terms to assist readers with the interpretations of theories, research, and practice.

In light of the historical view of literacy achievement and deafness, it should be inquired and addressed whether text-based literacy is a realistic goal for the majority of students with severe to profound hearing impairment. The impetus for this inquiry is the emerging paradigm of literary critical theory, which has also influenced the development of second-language or bilingual programs for students who are deaf. If text-based literacy is indeed a viable goal, then additional pertinent research is needed within the framework of reading-comprehension theories. Reading-comprehension theory and hearing students are the focus of the next chapter.

Further Readings

HEGEL, G. (1967). *The phenomenology of mind* (J. Baillie, trans.). New York: Harper & Row.

LANG, H., & MEATH-LANG, B. (1995). *Deaf persons in the arts and sciences: A biographical dictionary.* Westport, CT: Greenwood Press.

PADDEN, C., & HUMPHRIES, T. (1988). *Deaf in America: Voices from a culture.* Cambridge, MA: Harvard University Press.

RUSSELL, B. (1972). *A history of western philosophy.* New York: Simon & Schuster.

SMITH, T., & GRENE, M. (Eds.). (1940). *Berkeley, Hume, and Kant: Philosophers speak for themselves.* Chicago, IL: The University of Chicago Press.

WINEFIELD, R. (1987). *Never the twain shall meet: Bell, Gallaudet, and the communications debate.* Washington, DC: Gallaudet University Press.

Reading-Comprehension Perspective: Theories and Research on Hearing Students

Word recognition is the foundation of the reading process. . . . To be sure, there is much more to reading than word recognition. The reader who would understand an aphorism, such as the following, must do much more than recognize 11 words.

A woman needs a man like a fish needs a bicycle. (Gough, 1984, p. 225)

Whether we are aware of it or not, it is this interaction of new information with old knowledge that we mean when we use the term comprehension. To say that one has comprehended a text is to say that she has found a mental "home" for the information in the text, or else that she has modified an existing mental home in order to accommodate that new information. (Anderson & Pearson, 1984, p. 255)

Research indicates that the most critical factor beneath fluent word reading is the ability to recognize letters, spelling patterns, and whole words, effortlessly, automatically, and visually. The central goal of all reading instruction—comprehension—depends critically on this ability. (Adams, 1990a, p. 54)

This chapter is concerned with reading-comprehension theories and research on hearing students who are learning to read English as a first language. Reflecting on the previous passages, it can be inferred that these theories are differentiated by their treatment of two concepts: word recognition (or word identification) and comprehension. The more promising models have attempted to describe the relationship between word recognition and comprehension. In essence, it is argued that word recognition facilitates comprehension and comprehension facilitates word recognition. Nevertheless, it still can be argued that "word recognition is the foundation of the reading process."

The major objective of this chapter is to describe what is meant by the reading-comprehension framework. This framework is discussed relative to three broad groups of models: bottom-up (or text-based), top-down (or reader-based), and interactive (or parallel-processing). Each group of models is discussed and implications for instruction and curricula are presented. It should be kept in mind that these are cognitive models, which have been influenced by information-processing theories (McCarthey & Raphael, 1992; Samuels & Kamil, 1984). The other two groups of models, naturalism and social-constructivism, are discussed in Chapter 4 on writing; however, a few brief remarks are stated in this chapter.

After discussing the reading-comprehension models, the chapter focuses on research with hearing students. This research covers two broad areas: word identification and comprehension. *Note:* comprehension also includes word knowledge or vocabulary. Task-based variables are discussed in Chapter 9 on assessment. The intent of this chapter is to emphasize the reciprocal, facilitative relationship between word identification and comprehension.

Reading-Comprehension Framework: The Notion of Models

Prior to discussing the three groups of models, it is important to present some brief remarks on the notion of models. What is the purpose of models? What are their underpinnings? Is modeling really necessary? Is there a relationship between models and instructional practices? Contentious debates notwithstanding, the term model is considered synonymous with the term theory in this text.

A model is a schematic map or representation of the manner in which a particular entity functions or operates. It attempts to describe the parts, delineate their relationships to each other and to the entire entity itself. Models might be comprehensive (e.g., the entire reading process) or cover a small, albeit critical, area (e.g., letter or word recognition). They might be expressed via the use of formal logic or mathematical language (e.g., see discussion in Massaro, 1984) or through the use of prose, as indicated in more recent literature (e.g., see discussion in Kamil, 1984). "A reading model is a theoretical representation of reading processes" (Harris & Hodges, 1981, p. 200).

The development, assessment, and even understanding of a particular model need to be undertaken within a scientific framework, which is typically a metatheoretical framework (Massaro, 1984). Chapter 1 of this text presented some examples of metatheoretical frameworks (namely, reductionism/constructivism; positivism/relativism). In addition, the more comprehensive the model (e.g., the whole reading process), the more difficult it is to proceed from theory to practice. This is also the case for models of specific processes of literacy. For example, Massaro (1984, p. 112) remarked that "These models of reading processes are usually developed and tested within the framework of laboratory experiments, and their exact relationship to normal reading is necessarily indirect."

Relative to models, one common framework often used is the one described by Popper (1959, 1972). In essence, Popper argued that the building and testing of models should be based on the use of deductive, rather than inductive, methods. A general conclusion induced from specific instances might turn out to be false. For example, if we observed that many swans are white, it would be an error to conclude that all swans are white. Consequently, experiments can "falsify" a theory, but they cannot "verify" it. If experiments falsify conclusions based on a theory, then it is necessary to modify or even reject the theory.

Popper's falsification principle is not universally accepted; in fact, it might be rejected by most educational researchers, including those interested in literacy. For example, Bronowski (1977) argued that most scientists/researchers are interested in *what works* or in true statements, rather than in false statements. This is certainly the case for most educators, including those interested in teaching reading and writing.

There are alternatives to model building and testing. It has been suggested that developing a single model of the reading process is not possible because there is no single reading process (Gibson & Levin, 1975). One approach to take might be the proffering of principles. Kamil (1984) has offered another perspective:

> An alternative to the use of theory is a reliance on descriptive data collection. In this approach, for educational research, the emphasis is on the description of educational practice, not validation. A goal might be to identify "successful" or "nonsuccessful" instructional components, methods, or environments. Subsequent efforts may or may not involve validation of the findings. These techniques may have real advantages over methods based in incomplete theory, given the argument over assumptions. While descriptive techniques are not necessarily nontheoretical, they may approach that state . . . (1984, p. 44)

Despite the shortcomings of models (e.g., oversimplification of the process), it is argued that they do provide some insights about the process (e.g., Mitchell, 1982; Samuels & Kamil, 1984). The advantages of models over the proffering of general principles have been established (e.g., Coltheart, 1977; Massaro, 1976). Instead of multiple models, one can develop a model that accounts for different kinds of reading and that specifies the conditions under which each particular kind occurs. This model would also take into account the individual differences of various readers by specifying conditions for mature reading processes.

Perhaps the best approach might be to build and test models along with the use of descriptive data collection, especially if such data collection becomes nontheoretical. The problem for metatheorists is to bridge this seemingly *either–or* situation. As stated previously, the assumption that two opposing positions can be bridged is itself a metatheoretical position.

In the ensuing sections on models, the approach taken by the present writer is to describe the basic tenets of the group of models. Instead of flow charts and diagrams, a discussion of key points and assumptions of certain prototypical models is undertaken, for example, those of Gough (1972), Goodman (e.g., 1985), and Rumelhart (e.g., 1977, 1980). Contributions of other models, especially in the interactive category, are also acknowledged (e.g., Perfetti, 1985; Stanovich, 1980). The critique of each group also includes a discussion of disadvantages or problems that need to be solved. A more formal, detailed critique of these models can be found elsewhere (e.g., Mitchell, 1982; Nicholson, 1993; Samuels & Kamil, 1984).

Bottom-Up Models

Much of the essence of bottom-up (or text-based) models of reading can be garnered from the work of Gough's (1972) one second of reading model. However, it is possible to see the influences of the works of Holmes' (1953) substrata factor theory and the early LaBerge and Samuels' (1974) automatic information-processing model. As is shown later, these models have enhanced our understanding of the importance of the phonological and morphological processes in literacy (e.g., see discussions in Brady & Shankweiler, 1991; Gough, Ehri, & Treiman, 1992; Shankweiler & Liberman, 1989). Even more striking is the relationship of phonological processes to short-term working memory and the limited role of context in rapid, automatic, fluent reading.

As noted in Chapter 1, three words that characterize bottom-up models are empiricism, linearity, and hierarchy. The focus here is on linearity and hierarchy, which are used to describe the acquisition of subskills from the smallest element to the largest. Any bottom-up model exemplifies reductionism because there is the tendency to deal with (e.g., teach) the *parts* of reading in a systematic manner. Within this view, the whole is equal to the sum of the parts.

Bottom-up, or text-based, models refer to the directions of the process of reading, that is, from the print on the page to meaning in the reader's head. The process begins at the bottom with the text and proceeds upward through various levels of higher analyses to the top level, which is meaning. Thus, the reader must begin with the smallest units of analysis (letters and letter clusters) to the next largest (syllables) on to the largest (textual meaning).

In bottom-up models, much of the attention is placed on the identification of letters and words, that is, the decoding process. Comprehension receives some attention; however, it is purportedly accounted for by the procession through the various levels of analyses, the sum of which adds up to meaning. The reader cannot move to the next higher level without mastery of the lower level. Within this perspective, it is argued that meaning is in the text, and it is the reader's job to extract that meaning via the use of decoding skills.

Consider a prototypical bottom-up model with the text at the bottom and the reader's comprehension at the top. In this view, information flows from the text to the reader via analyses such as perceptual, lexical, syntactic, and semantic (Mitchell, 1982; Nicholson, 1993; Samuels & Kamil, 1984). As aptly stated by Lipson and Wixson (1991):

> The visual input from the text is processed through a series of analyses that proceed in a step-by-step manner. The first level of processing is the *perceptual* analysis of the visual features of the text into distinctive features, letters, letter clusters, and/or words. Many models also include the recoding of visual information into phonological or sound codes that corresponds to the visual units. . . . At the second level of processing, the visual or sound units that result from the perceptual analysis are analyzed according to word entries in the internal dictionary, or *lexicon*. At the third level, strings of identified words are analyzed according to rules of grammar, or *syntax*. For example, in analyzing a string of words such as *the, cow, barn, the, chased, dog, the,* our knowledge of grammar tells us that something chased something into something. However, there are still a number of syntactically acceptable possibilities for what chased what

into what (e.g., "The dog chased the cow into the barn"; "The cow chased the dog into the barn."). It is these types of possibilities that are considered at the final level of analysis when words, phrases, and sentences are analyzed in terms of *semantic* knowledge about events, feelings, and ideas. Therefore, it is our semantic knowledge about cows, dogs, and barns that make "The dog chased the cow into the barn" the most likely interpretation of this string of words. (pp. 7–8)

Implications for Instruction

The major implication of bottom-up models is a skills-based approach to instruction. It is argued that skills must be taught early in the reading process, preferably in first to third grades. The early acquisition and comprehensive mastery of these skills are critical for the development of higher-level reading skills.

The most common skills associated with word identification are phonics, structural analyses, and contextual analyses (e.g., Durkin, 1989; Johnson & Pearson, 1984). There is no *best* phonics or structural analysis program (Adams, 1990a). In addition, there does not seem to be strong research supporting the use of structural or contextual analyses, at least not conclusively (e.g., see review in Johnson & Baumann, 1984; Nagy, Winsor, Osborn, & O'Flahavan, 1994). Nevertheless, good programs aim to enable children to obtain a fairly deep understanding of the phonological and morphological processes. In addition, these programs also help children to learn about the alphabet principle, the system on which the written language of English is based.

Relative to phonics instruction (and any other type of language instruction), it should be remembered that the phonics rules resemble, in a cursory manner, the deep, underlying rules that a reader knows about the morphophonological system of English (e.g., see discussions in Adams, 1990a, 1994; Gough & Hillinger, 1980). Phonics rules are explicit and conscious whereas the rules readers use are implicit and unconscious (see also, an analogical discussion relative to syntax in Chomsky, 1975). The goal is to enable readers to use their deep knowledge of the sound system to generate pronunciations, not to state the phonics rules explicitly. In any case, it is assumed that phonics can help readers use their intuitive knowledge to learn about the alphabet system, or the relations between letters and sounds.

Examples of lessons containing phonics and structural analyses are presented below. According to Johnson and Pearson (1984, p. 116), the major objectives of using phonics are to teach:

1. The patterns of letter-sound relationships
2. The generalization that describes the patterns
3. The strategies for using both patterns and rules so that unrecognized printed words may be sounded out and pronounced

The following serves as an example for the three major concepts: pattern, generalization, and strategy (Johnson & Pearson, 1984, pp. 116–117).

Pattern :	The letter *c* nearly always represents the sound of /k/ as in *cup* or /s/ as in *nice.* (An exception is *cello.*)
Generalization:	The letter *c* is pronounced /s/ before *e, i,* or *y,* as in *cent, cider, cycle.* The letter *c* is pronounced /k/ before other letters, as in *candy, cotton, cupid, success.*
Strategy :	One instructional *strategy* is to teach the children several words with the letter *c* in them. Then the children are asked to look carefully at the words to discover the pattern and the rule (for example, *c* is /s/ before *e, i, y* in *cell, city, cyst*). A different instructional strategy is to teach the rule directly and have children use it to pronounce unfamiliar words containing *c* (*cyclops, cemetery, cipher*).

Structural analysis involves an understanding of morphemes, the smallest unit of meaning in the English language (Matthews, 1991; Nagy et al., 1994). From one perspective, it is possible to classify morphemes as *free* and *bound.* Examples of free morphemes are, typically, words; in any case, they can stand alone as in *bat, cat,* and *dog.* Bound morphemes need to be attached to other morphemes as in *-s, -ed,* and *un -.* In addition to affixes (e.g., prefix, suffix, inflection), bound morphemes can be a root part of a word as "*vis* (*revision, provision*), *pon* (*component, exponent*), *mit* (*admit, transmit, intermittent*), *scribe* (*prescribe, subscribe*) . . . "(Johnson & Pearson, 1984, p. 128).

In essence, structural analysis refers to a set of procedures that readers apply to examine meaningful elements within words. Children might be familiar with a word such as *ice* and a prefix such as *re -;* however, they might be perplexed at encountering a word such as *reice.* By analyzing the structure of this longer word and recognizing the familiar morphemes (free and bound), children might be able to identify the unfamiliar word.

One of the most interesting examples provided by Johnson and Pearson (1984, pp. 133–134) concerns the use of compound words. These researchers provided examples of compound words in several categories. The approach they recommended follows:

1. Ask students questions like, "What would you call a woman who scrubs, a truck that tows, a bean that jumps, and so on?" Work with one category at a time.
2. Then reverse the process. Ask questions like, "If a scrubwoman is a woman who scrubs, then how would you define a loan officer, a tow truck, a race car?"
3. Then, ask questions like those in 1 and 2 across the six categories of compound words.
4. Finally, . . . it is advisable to have the students use several of these compound words in sentences. Have the students construct their own sentences, or else give them modified cloze activities in which they have to select one of the compounds to fit the context in the sentences you provide.

An example of a cloze activity, mentioned in the example above, is as follows: Mary sat on the river_____ (bank, noon, sand).

These instructional activities and others are discussed further in Chapter 7 and Chapter 8, dealing with instruction in first- and second-language literacy. An in-depth discussion of structural analysis, including research in this area, can be found in Nagy et al. (1994).

Critique of Bottom-Up Models

The work of Gough (1972) is the major impetus for several bottom-up models of reading. This section provides some major criticisms of this model and other bottom-up models in general. Finally, despite these criticisms, it is shown that research generated by bottom-up models has provided important information about the reading process.

The criticisms of Gough and other bottom-up models are based on assumptions that have been generally refuted by research and these are still contentious issues (Adams, 1990a, 1990b; Gough, 1985). Three major assumptions are listed and discussed here: (1) readers read words letter by letter from left to right; (2) word recognition is mediated by phonological recoding; and (3) reading is primarily visual (see Gough, 1985). Other areas of criticism can be found elsewhere (e.g., Mitchell, 1982; Nicholson, 1993).

In critiquing his own model (Gough, 1972), Gough (1985) acknowledges that the model is limited (or in his words, <u>wrong</u>). He argues that research has shown that readers do not read words letter by letter from left to right. Nevertheless, Gough adheres to the view that the letter mediates word recognition. There might be some truth to Gough's view on the letter. In fact, it seems to be clear that readers are processing all the letters of the words and, at the same time, these skilled readers are recognizing words as whole units (Adams, 1990a, 1990b). In the words of Adams (1994, p. 9):

> Ultimately, readers come to look and feel like they recognize words holistically because they have acquired a deep, richly interconnected, and ready knowledge of their spellings, sounds, and meanings. However, to the extent that readers make a habit of skipping, glossing, or guessing at unfamiliar words, there can be no opportunity for such knowledge to develop. Skillful readers automatically and quite thoroughly process the component letters of text because their visual knowledge of words is built from memories of the sequences of letters of which the words are comprised. Conversely, because they do so, their orthographic knowledge is reinforced and enriched with each word they read.

The second assumption, purportedly erroneous, is Gough's claim that word recognition is mediated by phonological recoding (also called phonological coding). It is more correct to say that this assumption has been refined. It is suspected that skilled readers have direct (visual) access to some words, particularly those that are of high frequency or those that do not conform to letter-to-sound generalization principles, such as foreign words (e.g., *soiree*) and other types of words (e.g., *was, one*).

Nevertheless, the vast majority of words do not appear frequently in print and do conform to letter-sound correspondence rules. For these words, it is argued that skilled readers engage in phonological coding (see additional discussion in a later section on Word Identification in this chapter). It should be stressed that there is little doubt that skilled readers, both hearing and deaf, engage in the use of a phonological code beyond the word level (e.g., Shankweiler & Liberman, 1989; Hanson, 1989, 1991). As discussed elsewhere (e.g., Hanson, 1989, 1991; Paul & Quigley, 1994a), the use of a phonological code in short-term memory is most efficient for sentence comprehension because of the development of rapid, automatic, and fluent word identification skills. This ability to identify words rapidly and fluently enables readers to have and expend more energy on the important top-down comprehension processes.

The third claim—reading is primarily visual—has also been refined. It is true that readers need to pay attention to the letters and words on the page and to use their knowledge of letter-sound correspondence in this process. However, knowledge of letter-sound correspondence is not sufficient. That is, the ability to recognize words rapidly and fluently, albeit critical, is not enough to become a proficient reader. Reading demands other skills, as indicated by both top-down and interactive models to be discussed later.

The ability to recognize letters and words quickly and effortlessly should not be underemphasized. In addition, research has shown that readers do not use context in a conscious, deliberate manner to anticipate upcoming words or to preselect the meanings of multimeaning words (Adams, 1990a, 1990b, 1994). Word identification is, indeed, the foundation of the literacy process. As aptly stated by Gough (1985, p. 688):

> The hallmark of the skilled reader is the ability to recognize, accurately, easily, and swiftly, isolated words (and, even more so, pseudowords). . . . this skill can only be attributed to the ability to decode, for while highly predictive context can and does facilitate word recognition, proving a strictly "bottom-up" model like mine wrong, most words are not predictable and so can only be read bottom-up. A successful model of reading must account for this ability.

A synopsis of the major tenets and criticisms of bottom-up models is presented in Table 2-1.

TABLE 2-1   Major points and criticisms of bottom-up models

Points

- Most of the models are based on the work of Gough (1972)
- Models have enhanced our understanding of the phonological and morphological processes in literacy
- Much of the attention is placed on the identification of letters and words
- Reader's task is to extract meaning from text via the use of decoding skills

Criticisms

- Readers do not read words letter by letter from left to right; however, they do process all the letters of words
- Word recognition is mediated by phonological recoding; this has been refined to mean that readers can access some words via a visual route, but need to use a phonological recoding strategy for many other words
- Ability to recognize letters and words effortlessly is important; however, it is not sufficient for reading comprehension

---

Top-Down Models

As pointed out in Chapter 1, four broad terms characterize top-down models: linearity, hierarchy, rationalism, and constructivism. It might be that these labels are most often associated with the works of Goodman (e.g., 1985) and Smith (1971, 1978). However, the influence of other top-down theorists (e.g., Kintsch & van Dijk, 1978) should also be noted.

In general, *pure* top-down models emphasize comprehension to the virtual exclusion of word recognition, or word identification, skills. In essence, word identification is taken care of through the use of comprehension strategies and skills. The bias toward comprehension is based on the notion that meaning is in the reader's head. Thus, as a linear and hierarchical process, the reading process begins at the top with the information in the readers' heads and proceeds downward to the bottom, that is, the words in the text, for lower-level processing. The information in the text is used as necessary to confirm hypotheses and predictions. Only samples of the text are processed; the reader does not need to fixate on every letter of every word. Lipson and Wixson (1991) have characterized this as *whole-to-part* processing in which readers begin with the largest units (i.e., meaning) and proceed downward to the smallest units (letters and words).

In a prominent top-down model, reading is considered to be a transactional-psycholinguistic process (Goodman, 1985). As a psycholinguistic process, reading is said to be similar to the language-learning process. Goodman was heavily influenced by the work of Chomsky (e.g., 1975) on language development. Thus, like language, Goodman argued that it is not necessary to teach reading and writing. Children just need ample opportunities and exposure to reading and writing activities. Goodman was also influenced by Rosenblatt's view of literacy as a transactional process rather than as a cognitive-interactive process and by Piaget's work on cognitive development (e.g., Piaget, 1971, 1977, 1980). In addition, Goodman borrowed concepts from speech-act theory, particularly the work of Searle (1976, 1992). Considering these concepts together, it can be seen that the transactional-psycholinguistic model is the epitome of rationalism (knowledge in the reader's head) and constructivism within a naturalistic perspective (i.e., knowledge is constructed *individually* rather than *taught* as in reductionist techniques such as direct or precision teaching).

The following passage is reflective of Goodman's view of reading as a transactional-psycholinguistic process (Goodman, 1985, p. 814):

> Rosenblatt has drawn on Dewey's view that both the knower and the known are changed in the course of knowing. In a transactional view, the writer constructs a text through transactions with the developing text and the meaning being expressed. The text is transformed in the process and so are the writer's schemata (ways of organizing knowledge). The reader also constructs a text during reading through transactions with the published text and the reader's schemata are also transformed in the process through the assimilation and accommodation Piaget has described.
>
> In a transactional view, reading is seen as receptive written language, one of four language processes in literate societies. In the productive generative processes (speaking and writing), a text is generated (constructed) to represent the meaning. In the receptive processes (listening and reading), meaning is constructed through transactions

with the text and indirectly through the text with the writer. Both generative and receptive processes are constructive, active, and transactional.

Implications for Instruction

Relative to implications for instruction, it is safe to conclude that top-down models have spawned an array of approaches to reading instruction that can be labeled *whole language* and *language experience* (e.g., see discussion in Lipson & Wixson, 1991). These approaches seem to be quite common in the field of deafness (Dolman, 1992; Kelly, 1995). The main intent of this section is to illustrate some examples of these approaches. However, it should be kept in mind that even these examples should be accepted with caution. An understanding of this situation has been described aptly by Schirmer (1994, p. 108):

> Defining whole language is akin to eating spaghetti with a knife. You think you've got it. No, you don't. Now you've got it. Carefully, carefully. No, it slipped again. One of the problems is that the terminology used to define whole language tends to be as ambiguous as "whole language." Another problem is that whole language is conceptualized in a number of ways, from a movement to a philosophy, a set of principles to a learning theory, types of materials to teaching strategies, and a curriculum focus to a political perspective.

It is important to remember that, within the framework of whole language, reading is considered essentially a naturalistic language-learning process. Many activities have been influenced also by Halliday's (1984) three types of learning with language, that is, learning language, learning through language, and learning about language. Some of the major principles of whole language have been proffered. For example, according to Stoodt (1989, p. 273):

> Whole-language instruction is characterized by the following factors:
>
> 1. Curriculum that is meaningful for students, based on their interests, strengths, and needs.
> 2. Incorporation of children's literature in the literacy program. Teachers should read or tell stories and poetry *every* day.
> 3. Students must participate in authentic writing *every* day.
> 4. Students read literature *every* day.
> 5. Students learn to reflect on and control their own reading and writing processes (metacognition).
> 6. Cooperative learning, which promotes literacy, through such activities as paired reading, peer tutoring, peer writing conferences, team activities, and the like.

Whole-language classrooms tend to use the following methods and materials, although nothing in this philosophy dictates these particular methods.

> 1. Literature (in significant amounts).
> 2. Language-experience instruction.
> 3. Writing.

4. USSR or DEAR (uninterrupted sustained silent reading; drop everything and read).
5. Paired reading.
6. Interest inventories.
7. Directed-Reading-Thinking-Activity (DRTA).
8. Metacognitive skills (monitoring one's own learning and or understanding).
9. Discovery learning.

One of the most popular activities, especially with students who are deaf, is the language-experience approach (McAnally, Rose & Quigley, 1994). This approach has been in existence since prior to the emergent label of whole language; nevertheless, it is considered a common whole-language approach. The language-experience approach is often utilized as a natural language-learning approach for students who are deaf (McAnally et al., 1994). The experiences of children from field trips and other activities are expressed in the children's language, and this becomes their reading material. This approach is presumed to be relatively free of difficulties for beginning readers because both the language and experiences are familiar to the children. More important, it integrates receptive and expressive behaviors, that is, thinking, listening, speaking, reading, and writing. This approach can be individualized or used with a whole group.

A language-experience approach used with a group of children might contain the following steps (Gunning, 1992, pp. 377–378):

Day 1

Step 1. The students have an experience that they share as a group and that they can write about. It could be a field trip, the growing of a plant, the acquisition of a pet for the classroom, the baking of bread, or a similar experience.

Step 2. The students think over their experience and talk about it. During the discussion, the teacher helps them organize the experience. In discussing a visit to the circus, the teacher might ask them to tell what they liked best so that they don't get lost in details. If they baked bread, the teacher would pose questions in such a way that the children would tell the steps in order.

Step 3. The children dictate the story. The teacher writes it on large lined paper, an overhead transparency, or on the board, or might even type it on a computer, if it has an attachment that magnifies the input and projects it on a screen. The teacher reads aloud what she is writing so that the children can see the spoken words being written. She reads each sentence to make sure it is what the child who volunteered the sentence wanted to say. As she reads, she sweeps her hand under the print so that students can see where each word begins and ends and that reading is done from left to right. For students just learning to read, each sentence is written on a separate line when possible.

Step 4. After the whole story has been written, the teacher reads it aloud once more. The children listen to see that the story says what they want it to say. They are invited to make changes.

Step 5. The teacher reads the story, running her hand under each word as she reads it. The children read along with her.

Step 6. Volunteers are asked to read sentences or words that they know. The teacher notes which children are learning words and phrases and which are just getting a sense of what reading is all about.

Day 2

Step 1. The story is read by the teacher. The children read along. They might be able to read some familiar words or phrases.

Step 2. The teacher has duplicated the story and cut it into strips. The teacher points to a line in the master story. The children find the duplicated strip that matches. A volunteer reads the strip. The teacher helps out as necessary.

Critique of Top-Down Models

Similar to the arguments against bottom-up models, one of the major criticisms of top-down models is their linearity (e.g., see Samuels & Kamil, 1984). Although there have been a number of critiques concerning the prominent top-down models of Goodman (e.g., 1985) and Smith (e.g., 1978) (see critiques in Mitchell, 1982; Nicholson, 1993; Samuels & Kamil, 1984), this section focuses on the general problems with top-down models, rather than on a specific critique of one or two models.

There are four general areas that will be discussed: beginning readers, comprehension breakdowns of good readers, the sampling of text, and the use of context cues. This is not an exhaustive list of major areas; however, the discussion of these issues should convey the gist of critical concerns with pure top-down reading models.

The top-down model does not account for the behaviors of young children learning to read, either in a first language (e.g., Samuels & Kamil, 1984) or in a second language (e.g., Bernhardt, 1991; Grabe, 1988). When beginning readers are unfamiliar with the topic of the passage and with text features, it can be shown that their reading behavior is primarily text driven. There is research indicating that beginning readers can and do derive the meaning of text within this text-driven system (e.g., see research reviews in Adams, 1990a; Lipson & Wixson, 1991; Stanovich, 1992). It should be emphasized that, as readers mature, they can and do rely on well-developed, top-down processes to construct a model of what the text means.

Top-down models also fail to describe adequately what skilled readers do whenever there is a comprehension breakdown. The cause of the breakdown might be either difficult or inappropriate text features (e.g., difficult words) or reader-based features (e.g., difficult topics). When skilled readers need to devote conscious attention to the problem, it has been shown that they will resort to the use of bottom-up skills (e.g., word identification skills). Of course, it should be stressed that skilled readers have the skills to engage in a text-driven process even if this is not their preferred mode.

One of the most interesting rebuttals has emerged in the research on the use of context cues, relative to two areas: sampling of text and deriving meanings of words from the use of context. In general, top-down models seem to indicate that readers can skip over words and focus on the more important words in the text. The notion is that reading is not a precise process; readers can sample the text and proffer tentative hypotheses. These hypotheses are either confirmed or refined after further analysis of other samplings of text. Thus, because of contextual constraints (or contextual redundancies), the readers can reduce the amount of information to use from a given page or passage.

To address this area, the research synthesis work of Adams (1990a) is illustrative. Adams (1990a, pp. 100–101) posed a set of questions and then provided answers to the questions.

- Do skilled readers skip over any significant number of words in meaningful text?

  Not really. Normal adult readers fixate most of the words of a text, regardless of its difficulty. When they do skip, they almost never skip more than one single word, and skipped words tend to be very short . . . many function words and the vast majority of content words receive the reader's direct gaze.
- Do skilled readers spend more time on the "important" words of a text?

  Sort of, but apparently not because they are investing more effort in graphemic processing. The strongest determinant of the amount of time for which a reader fixates on a word is its length in letters, and this seems directly due to the visual labor required to recognize it. A second determinant of fixation durations is the word's familiarity, but this effect seems due to the time required to access its meaning. When consideration is shifted from individual words to larger units of text, such as phrases and clauses, people do tend to spend more time gazing at thematically important material than at details, but again this effect seems owed, not to closer visual attention, but to nonvisual processes involved in thinking about its meaning. Even if skilled readers look at every word, they might not process every word in equal detail.
- Do skilled readers sample the visual features of predictable text less thoroughly?

  No. Regardless of semantic, syntactic, or orthographic predictability, the eye seems to process individual letters. Whether or not graphemic details are consciously noticed, they seem quite reliably to be processed by the eye. Disruptions in adult readers' eye movements indicate that the visual system tends to catch the slightest misspellings, involving a visually similar letter and buried in the very middle (and thus least informative) part of long words that are highly predictable by the preceding context.

The second major issue relative to context is that good readers use context cues consciously to figure out or derive meanings of words. That is, good readers use context cues to anticipate the meanings of words, and this process facilitates the speed of their reading. Of course, one implication is that poor readers need instruction in the use of context cues. More interesting are the predictions of this issue, most often associated with Goodman's model (1976, 1985). One, readers would read words better (i.e., faster and more accurately) in context than in a list, and two, good readers would make better use of context than poor readers.

The responses to these issues have been dealt with eloquently in at least three sources/reviews (Adams, 1990a; Nicholson, 1993; Stanovich, 1992). Adams argued that relevant context does not accelerate the recognition of words nor does it speed up the derivation of word meanings. In fact, she averred that research shows that "for skilled readers

TABLE 2-2   Major points and criticisms of top-down models

Points

- Most widely recognized model is that of Goodman, the basis for the Whole Language approach
- Emphasis is on comprehension almost to the exclusion of word identification skills
- Readers do not fixate on every letter of every word
- Models are similar to those developed for language acquisition

Criticisms

- Does not account for the behavior of young children learning to read
- Fails to adequately describe what skilled readers do in the event of a breakdown in comprehension
- Relevant context does not accelerate the recognition of words nor does it speed up the derivation of word meanings
- Difficulties in using context cues during connected reading for word recognition purposes is not strongly related to reading comprehension problems

. . . it seems to do so only after they have quite thoroughly identified the word—both visually and semantically" (1990a, p. 102). Her examples include ambiguous words in sentences such as They all *rose* (p. 103) and John saw several spiders, roaches, and *bugs* (p. 103). The possible meanings of the ambiguous words are activated and quickly resolved by context. It should be emphasized that this is a very fast process, one of which the reader is rarely aware. In fact, research by Mason, Kniseley, and Kendall (1979) and others (see Adams, 1990a) showed that the selection of inappropriate meanings occurs if such meanings are prevalent in the minds of the readers for whatever reasons. Even more interesting, the speed at which real words are recognized in an isolated list is a good predictor of reading comprehension skills, that is, of connected reading ability.

Despite the so-called facilitative effects of context, Nicholson (1993) asserted that poor readers do not have the necessary skills to access text-based information adequately, or rather, they are less skilled in this ability. Poor readers tend to rely heavily on the top-down use of syntactic and semantic information. "On the other hand, good readers are less reliant on syntactic and semantic information than poor readers, and are more proficient in using graphic information" (Nicholson, 1993; see also, research review in Stanovich, 1992). In essence, Stanovich (1992) argued that difficulties in using context cues during connected reading for word recognition purposes is not strongly related to reading comprehension problems; this is not even "a major determinant of variability in reading achievement" (p. 308).

The major tenets and criticisms of top-down models are presented in Table 2-2.

Interactive Models

As discussed in Chapter 1, most interactive models seem to reflect some elements of several concepts, notably reductionism and constructivism, empiricism and rationalism, or from another perspective, phenomenology, and finally, the notion of parallel processing (also known as parallel distributed processing). The focus in this section is on parallel processing because it is this feature that distinguishes the potential of these models for explaining the reading process and for deriving effective instructional practices and materials (cf., McCarthey & Raphael, 1992, for an opposing view on this issue). Parallel processing is considered to have advantages over (and a reaction to) the linearity of the other two groups of models (e.g., Samuels & Kamil, 1984).

There are several interactive models. Two models that have received considerable attention are Rumelhart's Schema-Interactive Model (Rumelhart, 1977, 1980), which has evolved into a parallel distributed processing cognitive model (Rumelhart, McClelland, and the PDP Group, 1986), and Stanovich's Interactive-Compensatory Model (Stanovich, 1980), which is considered a derivative of Rumelhart's model. Another model that should be mentioned is Perfetti's Verbal-Efficiency Model (Perfetti, 1985), which places a great deal of emphasis on word recognition and only recently has become an interactive model due to the addition of a feedback loop.

Despite these differences across models, the notion of parallel processing is considered to be more accurate in explaining the behaviors of both beginning and mature readers (e.g., Nicholson, 1993; Samuels & Kamil, 1984). More importantly, this notion does a better job of describing the reciprocal relationship between word identification (or recognition) and comprehension (e.g., Adams, 1990a). This reciprocal relationship is present at several levels of analyses, for example, lexical, syntactic, semantic, schematic, and interpretative. As indicated by the passage by Adams (1990a) at the beginning of this chapter, this is not an either-or situation. That is, the emphasis is not on either word identification or comprehension.

Within the framework of interactive models, it is possible to state that beginning reading is primarily text-driven and mature reading is primarily reader-driven. This statement, at least, acknowledges that both bottom-up and top-down skills should be developed simultaneously during literacy instruction. In other words, reading is an interactive process involving the text, reader, and the reading context. The reader's goal is to construct a model of what the text means by using information from the text and the information in his or her head and by considering the context of reading. It is also important to develop reading and writing simultaneously because of the reciprocal relations of these two entities (e.g., see research review in Adams, 1990a). More importantly, it should be emphasized that writing develops in tandem with reading, and children might actually engage in beginning writing activities prior to beginning formal reading activities.

The notion of parallel processing encompasses what is considered a balanced view of literacy, especially for children with hearing impairment (King & Quigley, 1985; Paul & Quigley, 1994a). Why poor readers, including those who are deaf, rely heavily on top-down skills, relative to the use of context cues, can be explained adequately by focusing on some tenets of Stanovich's model. Stanovich averred that:

> The compensatory assumption states that a deficit in any knowledge source results in a heavier reliance on other knowledge sources, regardless of their level in the processing hierarchy. Thus, according to the interactive-compensatory model, the poor reader who has deficient word analysis skills might possibly show a greater *reliance* on contextual factors. In fact, several studies have shown this to be the case. (1980, p. 63)

Perhaps the most important point to underscore is that interactive models also apply to children with hearing impairment and to other children who have reading difficulties (Hanson, 1989; Lipson & Wixson, 1991; Paul & Quigley, 1994a). Reviewing and synthesizing the research literature, Paul and his collaborators (e.g., Paul, 1993a, 1993b, 1994a; Paul & O'Rourke, 1988; Paul & Quigley, 1994a, 1994b) have concluded that the reading process of children with hearing impairment, including children who are deaf, is qualitatively similar to that of children with typical hearing abilities. As is discussed in the chapters on instruction (Chapters 7 and 8), this has important implications for the teaching of literacy skills.

Implications for Instruction

In this section, a few examples of instructional activities based on interactive models are presented. A more detailed discussion is presented in the subsequent chapters on instruction (Chapters 7 and 8). The focus is on the development of both word identification and comprehension skills. Examples of word identification skills have been presented previously (e.g., Johnson & Pearson, 1984); here, the main tenets of teaching such skills, especially via the use of phonics, are described briefly. The new instructional examples concern those associated with comprehension, particularly the concepts of prior knowledge and metacognition.

Interactive models of literacy emphasize both word identification and comprehension instruction. Although there is value in the variety of word identification approaches, one of the most critical aspects is for young or emergent readers to appreciate and understand the relationships between sounds and letters. There is continuing debate over whether it is feasible to develop these relationships in isolation and/or context (Adams, 1990a; Copeland, Winsor, & Osborn, 1994; Strickland & Cullinan, 1990). For example, is it necessary to proceed with direct instruction of phonics (Adams, 1990a) or can phonics be learned in the context of reading and writing (e.g., Strickland & Cullinan, 1990)? In later chapters, we will explore whether students who are deaf and who do not read widely can learn adequately about the sound-letter system via reading and writing. How does one teach students who cannot hear about the *sound* system and its relations to letters? Do we need to do this? For readers who are deaf, and other poor readers, direct instruction might be very important.

Despite the controversies regarding the *teaching* of phonics, most educators would agree that ". . . deep and thorough knowledge of letters, spelling patterns, and words, and of the phonological translations of all three, are of inescapable importance to both skillful reading and its acquisition" (Adams, 1990a, p. 416). Those who favor direct instruction would agree that ". . . instruction designed to develop children's sensitivity to spellings and their relations to pronunciations should be of paramount importance in the development of reading skills. This is, of course, precisely what is intended in good phonic instruction" (Adams, 1990a, p. 416).

In my view, one of the most important instructional implications of interactive theories is that *phonics* should be taught or rather learned as early as possible so as to facilitate the use of the more important top-down (or comprehension) skills of literacy. Or, to put it another way, one major role of phonics is to enable students to continue their development of and to use phonemic awareness during reading. Phonemic awareness seems to enhance children's ability to internalize orthographic patterns, and it plays a role in the learning of sound-symbol correspondences.

Perhaps the most interesting and far-reaching instructional implication of interactive theories is that instruction should be designed to enrich and activate the prior knowledge and background of the reader (e.g., Lipson & Wixson, 1991; Mason & Au, 1986; Pearson &

Johnson, 1978). Prior knowledge refers to the wealth of experiences, knowledge, and background the student brings to the task of reading and writing. This knowledge might include, but not be limited to, knowledge of the language of print, metacognitive skills (thinking about knowledge and applying it), and knowledge about the topic of the passage and related knowledge. As is discussed later in this chapter, there are strong relations between prior knowledge and its application (i.e., metacognition) and reading comprehension ability.

There are a number of instructional activities that have been developed to capitalize on the importance of activating and applying prior knowledge (e.g., see Mason & Au, 1986; Nagy, 1988; Pearson & Johnson, 1978). These activities relate to the teaching of vocabulary and the judicious use of asking questions. For example, a number of research educators have argued that vocabulary instruction should focus on depth of knowledge of a few words rather than breadth of a number of words that are often difficult to remember. The most common techniques are the use of semantic elaboration and integration techniques such as semantic maps, semantic feature analysis, and word maps (e.g., see discussions in Heimlich & Pittelman, 1986; Nagy, 1988; Paul, 1989; Paul & O'Rourke, 1988). Two examples of a word map are illustrated in Figure 2-1.

One of the most popular techniques is the use of semantic maps. There are several purposes for the use of this technique. For example, students should be able to learn important vocabulary words and identify the main points of a story. This technique should also aid in organizing information for either studying or remembering purposes or for producing a written report. In some cases, students might improve their skill in outlining information from a story. Two examples of a semantic map are illustrated in Figure 2-2. Specific details

---

Example 1: bat

What is it?   What is it like?

animal, mammal   furry, flies like a bird,

bat

What are some examples?

brown bat, vampire bat, fruit bat

Example 2: bat

What else is it?   What else is it like?

stick, club, baseball's tool   made of wood, aluminum

bat

What are some examples?

Mickey Mantle, Henry Aaron, Louisville slugger

Figure 2-1   Two examples of a word map.

Source: Based on examples in Mason & Au (1986).

Example 1: Sea Otters

Description	Live in water a lot
brownish black fur	dive deep for food
long body	

Sea Otters

Play a lot	Float on back a lot
jump in air; flip around	put rocks on stomach
throw and catch rocks	to sleep

Example 2: Washington, DC: A Great City

History	Capitol Buildings	White House
built in forest	near park	President's home
by two rivers	white dome	Pennsylvania Ave.
	statue on top	white pillars

Washington, DC: A Great City

Many Monuments	Other Things to See
Jefferson Memorial	Supreme Court building
Lincoln Memorial	Smithsonian Institution
Arlington Cemetery	Library of Congress
George Washington Monument	

Figure 2-2   Two examples of a semantic map.

Source: Based on examples in Heimlich & Pittelman (1986, pp. 14, 18).

on how to use word maps and semantic maps during literacy instruction are discussed in Chapters 7 and 8.

In the area of questions, Pearson and Johnson (1978) have discussed several critical aspects that have spawned a number of research projects (e.g., see discussions in King & Quigley, 1985; Paul & Quigley, 1990). Prereading questions should enrich and activate the prior knowledge of students. In essence, such questions should get the students ready for the story and even focus on the purpose for reading the story. For example, suppose the students are preparing to read a story (mostly expository) about bats. Some possible examples of prereading questions include the following:

1. Has anyone ever seen a bat? Tell us about it? How big was it? What color was it? Where did you see this bat?
2. Here are pictures of some bats. You are going to read a story about bats. Look at the title of the story. What do you think the story will tell us? Do you think we will find out where bats live? What bats eat? How bats can find their food?
3. Are all bats small? How do you know? When do most bats hunt for food?
4. How are bats similar to birds? How are they different?
5. Do you know what a mammal is? Are bats mammals?
6. Are bats dangerous to humans? Why or why not?

The answers to some of these questions can be found, explicitly or implicitly, in the story. However, the answers to other questions depend on the prior knowledge of the students.

Pearson and Johnson (1978) have also proposed a taxonomy of questions, actually question-answer relationships, which have been subjected to research, particularly by Raphael and her colleagues (see discussion in Raphael & Pearson, 1985). The three broad categories proposed are text-explicit, text-implicit, and script-implicit questions. Text-explicit (TE) are the typical literal questions, and both text-implicit (TI) and script-implicit (SI) are inferential questions. Typically, these questions are asked at the end of the story (i.e., postreading) as one method for checking the reading comprehension of the students (other methods include retelling the story, summarizing certain aspects, and so on). It should be noted that making inferences is a metacognitive skill, which is especially needed for answering TI and SI questions. Examples of TE, TI, and SI question-answer relationships follow.

Additional examples of these types of instructional activities are discussed in detail in the chapters on instruction (Chapters 7 and 8).

Question-Answer Relationships

Story

Peter and Paul always bowled on Friday nights. They were very competitive. Each person wanted to beat the other one badly. Peter was the better bowler. His average (175) was almost 20 points higher than Paul's. He had beaten Paul the last five Fridays.

Paul was becoming desperate. So, one Thursday night he put chewing gum in Peter's bowling ball. This made Peter very angry. It took him two hours to clean the holes of his ball.

After the bowling game on Friday night, Paul had a big smile on his face. He looked forward to the next game.

Questions and Answers

The answers to TE questions are right in the story. They are easy to find. The words used for creating the question and the answer can be found in the passage. A <u>wh</u>- substitution for some words is permissible. Frequently, a cloze format is used for this type of question (i.e., a word is omitted and replaced with a line).

Examples of TE questions

1. Peter and Paul always bowl on _____ nights.
2. When do Peter and Paul bowl?
3. Who was becoming desperate?

The answers to TI questions are in the story, but they require an inference. The words used to create questions and answers might be found in two different places, that is, two different phrases, sentences, and paragraphs. The use of pronouns is an example of an inferential-type question.

Examples of TI questions

1. Who had beaten Paul the last five Fridays?
2. Whose average was 175 points?
3. What made Peter very angry?

The answers to SI questions are not in the story. The questions are motivated by the story, but the answers must come from the readers' heads. These are also known as application-type questions.

Examples of SI questions

1. What was Paul's bowling average (score)?
2. Why was Paul becoming desperate?
3. Who won the last bowling game?

Critique of Interactive Models

Because there are several interactive models, it is difficult to present common criticisms of these models and their instructional implications. In addition, there might be a need to separate criticisms of the models from criticisms of instructional implications. In any case, despite their improvement over linear bottom-up and top-down models, interactive models are certainly not above criticism (e.g., see Carnine, Silbert, & Kameenui, 1990; Mitchell, 1982; Rosenblatt, 1989; Samuels & Kamil, 1984). Only a few of the salient problems are noted in this section.

Relative to the modeling aspects, several points have been made. Interactive theorists, particularly Rumelhart (1980), have emphasized the importance and effects of schemata (i.e., prior knowledge structures) on reading comprehension ability. Nevertheless, it is still not clear how a schema develops initially and what are the precise relations between and among schemata. Additional research is needed on the precise interactions or contributions of certain schemata to the comprehension of text material.

Interactive theories, especially schema-interactive models, have done better than previous models in explaining the role and effects of context cues. However, it should not be considered a comprehensive model of the reading process. For example, some theorists do not perceive literacy as an interactive process, but rather as a transactional process (e.g., see Rosenblatt, 1989; see also Chapter 1 of this text). In addition, there are still some unanswered problems (associated with Rumelhart's model) as noted by Mitchell (1982, p. 136) that are still applicable:

> It says nothing about the basis on which the various kinds of hypotheses are generated and it does not specify the relative importance of the contribution from each knowledge source. Nor does it indicate how the influence of each source varies with the reader's strategy and with the reading conditions. It has little to offer on issues such as the control of eye movements, the use of a phonological route and other back-up strategies in word recognition and problems in comprehension beyond the level of sentences.

Several criticisms have also been made relative to the instructional implications. Some of these have already been stated in previous sections (e.g., the teaching of phonics). Despite the importance of prior knowledge to reading comprehension, some research educators argue that it is still necessary to teach specialized knowledge in school because such knowledge is not part of the everyday knowledge of the students. Such knowledge includes the areas of science and social studies as well as other content areas (e.g., Carnine et al., 1990).

As stated previously, any of the contentious remarks concern the direct teaching of reading skills, both word identification and comprehension. This is, admittedly, fueled by a philosophy of instruction discussed previously as constructivism. The emphasis here is on the teaching of phonics. To stress this issue, two passages from Strickland and Cullinan are used:

> ... let us say that we *do* believe in phonics; that is, we believe in providing opportunities for children to learn about letter-sound correspondences. We do *not* believe, how-

TABLE 2-3   Major points and criticisms of interactive models

Points

- Represents a balanced approach to the teaching and understanding of the reading process
- Argues for a reciprocal relationship between word identification and comprehension skills
- Asserts that beginning reading is text-driven and mature reading is reader-driven
- Avers that the reader's goal is to construct a model of what the text means by using the information in the text and the information in the head

Criticisms

- Not clear how a schema develops initially; no precise relations between and among schemata described
- Not clear how certain schemata contribute to the understanding of a text
- Does not address adequately additional word-recognition strategies or problems in comprehension beyond the sentence level

ever, that phonics should be taught in isolation from other aspects of a child's literacy development or that it is a precursor to reading development. [This narrow focus ignores] the way phonics instruction fits into a broader framework of language learning. (1990, pp. 426, 428)

Current naturalistic research strongly suggests that phonics is best learned in the context of reading and writing. If learning is to occur, we must give children good stories that intrigue and engage them; we must give them poetry that sings with the beauty of language; we must enchant them with language play; and we must give them opportunities to write. In short, we must surround them with literature that helps them understand their world and their ability to create meaning. . . . In countless demonstrations of story reading and experimentation with writing, children develop the knowledge of the way print works. (1990, pp. 426, 428)

The major tenets and criticisms of interactive theories of literacy are delineated in Table 2-3.

Research on Reading Comprehension and Hearing Students: A Summary

In this section, a brief discussion of relevant hypotheses and a representative sample of research on selected aspects of two major components are discussed and synthesized: word identification and comprehension (for in-depth discussions of research, see Adams, 1990a; Balota, Flores d'Arcais & Rayner, 1990; Barr, Kamil, Mosenthal & Pearson, 1991; Lehr & Osborn, 1994; Pearson, Barr, Kamil, & Mosenthal, 1984; Singer & Ruddell, 1985). The research on word identification includes findings in areas such as lexical access, the use of phonics, structural analyses, contextual analyses, and the notion of isolated, contextual, or integrated approaches to teaching these skills. Comprehension is a broad entity referring to vocabulary knowledge, prior knowledge, and metacognitive knowledge.

The goal of the following sections is to briefly describe the issues of word identification and comprehension and present summaries of the results of studies. The reader is reminded that interpreting the results depends on which *model glasses* an individual researcher wears. For example, bottom-up theorists might be consumed with the process of word identification (specifically, lexical access) and argue that this is the essence of reading comprehension. Other theorists, notably interactive theorists, might argue that word identification is only one process, albeit an important one, for the overall goal of comprehension. In addition, it is possible to have different interpretations of the same results. The absence of a broad consensus on a particular theory is not necessarily problematic for research syntheses or for translative researchers (e.g., deriving practices based on theories). That is, it is still permissible to provide educators with usable guidelines that pertain to several models as opposed to those that are limited to one model. Furthermore, using a metatheoretical approach, it should be possible to develop guidelines that combine the common tenets across models.

Word Identification

At least three major questions can be identified for discussion purposes: (1) What is word identification? (2) What process is involved in accessing a word? (3) What does research offer relative to instruction? These three major questions are not exhaustive; rather, in my view, they hold the most promise for offering implications for instruction.

The term word identification has been known by other labels that can be found in the literature: word recognition, word attack, word analysis, and decoding (e.g., Adams, 1990a, 1990b; Gough, 1984, 1985; Johnson & Baumann, 1984; Johnson & Pearson, 1984). Johnson and Pearson (1984) have provided arguments for the use of the term word identification; however, other researchers (e.g., Gough, 1984, 1985) have used the term word recognition. This text uses word identification and word recognition interchangeably. Nevertheless, what we are interested in is how good readers develop the ability to read words automatically, rapidly, and efficiently (e.g., see discussion in Ehri, 1991).

Relative to word identification, the focus is on "the various graphophonic, morphemic, syntactic, and semantic generalizations and strategies readers employ independently to expand their reading vocabulary and comprehend printed discourse" (Johnson & Pearson, 1984, p. 112). In accordance with Johnson and Pearson (1984), the three major word identification skills that require instruction are phonics, structural analysis, and contextual analysis. Examples of these areas were presented previously in the section on implications relative to bottom-up models of literacy. Although some researchers argue that one of the three skills (notably, phonics) is most important (e.g., see discussions Adams, 1990a; Chall, 1983; Gough, 1984), Johnson and Pearson (1984) have suggested that all three areas are important for expanding children's reading vocabulary knowledge. In addition, because of the either-or situation of phonics versus whole words, researchers have overlooked the contributions of knowledge of letter-sound relations (e.g., the alphabetic system) to understanding and improving sight word vocabulary (e.g., the orthographic system) (Adams, 1990a; Ehri, 1991). For example, it has been shown that it is possible to see the influence of letter-sound knowledge on reading sight words if children have understood letters (i.e., names and sounds) and can read some words in isolation (e.g., Ehri & Wilce, 1985).

The processing of words (i.e., lexical access) seems to be one of the most interesting lines of current research. One aspect of this research is the importance of the role, if any, of phonological awareness or, from another perspective, of the use of a phonological code (e.g., see discussions in Adams, 1990a; Gough, 1984, 1985; Leybaert, 1993). During reading, the individual needs to access words from memory based on the written forms. This is what is meant by word identification. As aptly described by Ehri:

> Speakers of a language possess a *lexicon*—that is, a store of words held in memory. When people read words by sight or lexical access, they utilize information that is remembered about the words from previous experiences reading these words. Upon seeing the spellings, readers access the identities of the words in memory. These identities include the word's pronunciation, its meaning, its syntactic identity (i.e., its typical grammatical role in sentences), and its orthographic identity (i.e., information remembered about its conventional spelling) . . . (1991, p. 384)

Theorists and researchers disagree about the nature of the retrieval routes for accessing words from memory (e.g., see discussions in Adams, 1990a; Ehri, 1991). A number of hypotheses have been proffered, for example, the phonological access, morphological access, semantic access, visual access, dual access, and hypotheses associated with either the modularity model (Fodor, 1983) or the parallel distributed processing model (Rumelhart, McClelland, and the PDP Research Group, 1986) (see also, Balota, Flores d'Arcais, & Rayner, 1990, for example, Besner, 1990; Seidenberg, 1990).

It is beyond the scope of this text to explicate the major hypotheses pertaining to lexical access. It is becoming clear that none of the hypotheses is completely right nor is any of the hypotheses completely wrong. Research is important here because it can shed light on the predictive power of phonological awareness for later success in reading, the difficulty of poor readers in decoding pseudowords, and, most important, the relative merits of the various instructional programs that emphasize phonics (e.g., see discussion in Adams, 1990a, 1994; Copeland et al., 1994).

Relative to a summary of the research on lexical access, the following statements by Adams (1990a, p. 105) are representative: "The emerging view is that skillful word recognition involves both direct visual processing and phonological translation. However, these two routes stand, not as independent alternatives to one another, but as synergistic parts of the same process." These statements by Adams also address the *great debate* issues researched by Chall (e.g., 1967, 1983), that is, the whole word (look-say) versus phonics (code-emphasis) controversy. In addition, it has been argued that when readers use one method (e.g., sight word), this does not mean that they are not using or are not influenced by another strategy (e.g., letter-sound relationships). For example, synthesizing research, including her own research, led Ehri (1991, p. 383) to remark: ". . . sight word reading is not necessarily a rote memorization process that ignores letter-sound relations." In fact, ". . . evidence suggests that phonological recoding skill is not a mere facilitator but a necessity for reading words by sight" (Ehri, 1991, p. 402).

The questions now become: Do word identification skills need to be taught and is it possible to develop these skills during the process of reading? As might be expected, the answers is *yes* and *no,* depending on the skills and ages of the readers. Perspectives on these questions can be found in several reviews of the literature (e.g., Adams, 1990a; Ehri, 1991; Johnson & Baumann, 1984; cf., Strickland & Cullinan, 1990). Two assertions should be underscored here: (1) Adequate word identification skills do not automatically lead to adequate reading comprehension skills (e.g., see discussions in Adams, 1990a, Stanovich, 1991); and (2) good readers rely less on context cues than poorer and beginning readers mainly because the latter two groups have not developed proficient levels of word identification skills (e.g., Stanovich, 1986, 1992).

As discussed in the research on word knowledge (presented in the next section), it is possible for younger and poorer readers to learn some aspects of word identification during the process of reading. However, there is considerable evidence that this is not a very efficient way for these types of readers to learn about word identification, word knowledge, and reading comprehension because they do not and will not attempt to read widely (e.g., see discussions in Johnson & Pearson, 1984; Lipson & Wixson, 1991; Paul & O'Rourke, 1988). In some cases, it might be important for good, young readers to be reinforced by what it is they know about the important words in the selection. That is, can they identify (e.g., pronounce, etc.) these words? Do they know anything about the words?

If instruction is important, should the words be isolated, presented in context, or introduced via some kind of integrated approach? By now, the reader can see that the isolation versus context issue is another one of the either-or situations so prevalent in the field of literacy. Rapid and automatic word identification skills might require an integrated approach, especially for younger and poorer readers (e.g., see discussion in Lipson & Wixson, 1991). In an integrated approach, all three conditions are used depending on the skills of the readers. In some cases, the context approach should be initially used for readers who are having difficulty.

Despite the type of approach used, it needs to be emphasized that phonics (or knowledge of letter-sound relations) cannot be ignored (Adams, 1990a, 1994; Copeland et al., 1994; Ehri, 1991; Johnson & Baumann, 1984). Several comprehensive reviews of this issue conclude that programs that emphasize early, reasonably intensive phonics instruction seem to result in better word identification skills than those that are focused on meaning only (e.g., whole word, sight word, etc.) (Adams, 1990a, 1994; Johnson & Baumann, 1984). However, it should be recalled that the sight word approach also involves the use of knowledge of letter-sound relations (e.g., Ehri, 1991). In any case, the development and use of letter-sound knowledge is a problematic issue for students who are deaf and for many other poor readers in special education programs. Ignoring phonics is related to the either-or condition, which I have argued against so far.

A good summary of research on structural analyses and contextual analyses can be found in Johnson and Baumann (1984) and Nagy et al. (1994) with some related issues presented in Adams (1990a), for example, on the use of context cues. The crux of the issue is the contribution of these skills to the development of rapid, automatic word identification (recognition) skills. The value of structural analysis has been emphasized by Nagy et al. in the analysis of words seen/read by students in a year.

Nagy et al. argued that the average fifth grader reads about one million words per year, 10,000 of which the student will see or read only once. An in-depth analysis of the possible 10,000 words revealed that only about a 1000 are truly new words. That is, these 1000 words are not directly related to words that might be more familiar to the students. In essence, a substantial number of the 10,000 words are related to other familiar words via the use of structural units such as prefixes or suffixes. For example, *wanted* is related to *want* and *unhappy* is related to *happy*.

Students do have the ability to use structural knowledge in figuring out meanings of words (e.g., Nagy & Scott, 1990; Sternberg & Powell, 1983; Tyler & Nagy, 1989). In fact, there are three general uses of structural analysis: (1) to identify familiar words in a more efficient manner, (2) to remember the spellings and meanings of known, familiar words, and (3) to figure out the meanings and pronunciations of new words (Nagy et al., 1994). Nagy et al. also provided some guiding principles (five) for teaching students about structural analysis. These are listed below with only some elaboration.

1. Provide explicit explanations. . . . students often need to be told explicitly *why* they are doing some particular activity. In the case of structural analysis, it is important to make clear both the immediate purpose—determining the meaning and pronunciation of an unfamiliar word—and the ultimate purpose—to construct a coherent meaning for the text.

2. Rely on examples more than abstract rules, principles, or definitions. . . . concepts such as prefix, suffix, and compounds must be taught as part of instruction in structural analysis. However these concepts are more abstract and potentially difficult for students than may be apparent, and they need to be illustrated with numerous examples.

3. Recognize the diversity of English word structure. Instruction in structural analysis must deal with the diverse types of word parts. We cannot assume that the instruction that is best for prefixes will necessarily be the best for suffixes, or vice versa. The differences between prefixes and suffixes involves more than just their position with respect to the stem. [Additional discussion involved the use of compounds and affixes, etc. (words added)].

4. Make the limitations of structural analysis clear. Part of giving explicit instruction in structural analysis is letting students know its limitations—about how often structural analysis may give incomplete or misleading information, or no information and what to do in such cases.

5. Use extended text in opportunities for application. Instruction in structural analysis is unlikely to transfer automatically to reading. Instruction in structural analysis must target specifically the kinds of application we expect students to make; therefore, opportunities for applying structural analysis to extended text are an indispensable part of structural analysis instruction. (pp. 53–56)

To reiterate the importance of word identification skills, we end this section with the following passage from Stanovich (1991):

. . . skill at word recognition is so central to the total reading process that it can serve as a proxy diagnostic for instructional methods. That is, while it is possible for adequate word recognition skill to be accompanied by poor comprehension abilities, the converse virtually never occurs. It has never been empirically demonstrated, nor is it theoretically expected, that some instructional innovation could result in good reading comprehension without the presence of at least adequate word recognition ability. Since word recognition skill will be a by-product of any successful approach to developing reading ability—whether or not the approach specifically targets word recognition—lack of skill at recognizing words is always a reasonable predictor of difficulties in developing reading comprehension ability. (p. 418)

Comprehension: Word Knowledge

There seems to be some consensus that vocabulary knowledge is important for developing reading comprehension ability (e.g., Anderson & Freebody, 1979, 1985; Stahl, 1986). Some scholars have argued that it is either *one* of the most important variables or *the* most important variable; that is, good readers are independent word learners (Becker, 1977; Dale & O'Rourke, 1986; Devine, 1986; Johnson & Pearson, 1984; Paul, 1996; Paul & O'Rourke, 1988). The importance of vocabulary can also be seen in a number of available instructional texts (e.g., Dale & O'Rourke, 1986; Johnson & Pearson, 1984; Nagy, 1988; O'Rourke, 1974).

It might be surprising to state that there is little agreement on why vocabulary knowledge is so important for reading comprehension. It seems obvious that good readers know many words, and also that they have a deep understanding (e.g., multiple meanings, nuances) of the words that they do know. But the question still remains, Why is this knowledge important? In addition, it is not always apparent what good readers know about words and how they acquire this knowledge. These issues are also made even more complex in light of debates on questions such as, What is a word? What is a meaning? What does it mean to know a meaning? What does it mean to know a word? (See discussions in Anderson & Nagy, 1991; Beck & McKeown, 1991.)

Beck and McKeown (1991) offer an interesting perspective on the question of what it means to know a word:

> The question of what it means to know a word draws two kinds of responses: One pertains to how information about word meanings is represented in memory. The other response involves the extent or dimensions of knowledge that people may have about individual words. (p. 791)

The latter response has been the focus of Beck and McKeown (1991) and others because of the implications for understanding the notion and value of vocabulary instruction.

At least three major hypotheses have been proffered to explain readers' knowledge of words (e.g., see discussion in Anderson & Freebody, 1979, 1985; Paul, 1996; Paul & O'Rourke, 1988). These hypotheses are labeled instrumentalist, aptitude, and knowledge-based. A fourth position, termed the access hypothesis (e.g., Mezynski, 1983), has also been discussed. However, the access hypothesis can be argued to be a part of any hypothesis dealing with vocabulary acquisition; therefore, it should not be considered separately from the major positions. In fact, the access notion is strongly related to word identification processes discussed previously.

Proponents of the instrumentalist position aver that individuals with a high score on vocabulary tests will also score well on reading comprehension measures. Thus, the more words an individual knows the easier it is for that person to comprehend reading materials. This suggests a causal relation between vocabulary knowledge and reading comprehension. That is, vocabulary knowledge causes reading comprehension. Instrumentalists have not explained how this knowledge is acquired; they only focus on the effects of having this type of knowledge. Instrumentalists place a great deal of emphasis on environmental factors (e.g., the effects of direct teaching, exposure to words, etc.). It is also possible to see the relationship of the instrumentalist position to bottom-up theories of reading. For example, the accumulation of vocabulary words adds up to an increase in reading comprehension ability.

The implications of this position can be observed in several avenues. One popular rendition can be seen in magazines such as *Readers' Digest* (e.g., It Pays to Increase Your Word Power) and others that provide vocabulary tasks or tests. Typically, there is a list of 20 or so unrelated words and readers are required to select the best meanings. This activity is not different from that which can be found in some reading series. Teachers might be asked to introduce a list of prereading vocabulary words, typically about 10 to 20 words, that are deemed important for the story to be read. What is often overlooked in all these avenues and activities is the fact that it is difficult—maybe downright impossible—for anyone to learn 10 to 20 new words in a short period of time. Learn, in this sense, refers to what can be called a dictionary knowledge of words.

Proponents of the second position, the aptitude hypothesis, are not really interested in vocabulary instruction. Indeed, they might argue that such instruction is futile. In the aptitude position, it is averred that individuals with large vocabularies possess excellent mental agility, and this, in turn, aids in the comprehension of reading materials. The influence of this position can be seen in what used to be a predominant practice: using vocabulary knowledge as a measure of intelligence (e.g., see discussion in Anderson & Freebody, 1985). Relative to the notion of instruction, there is some connection between the aptitude hypothesis and top-down theories of reading. For example, there seems to be an emphasis on what is in the readers' heads.

Aptitude proponents are likely to favor the effects of genetics over those from the environment. That is, individuals who have large vocabularies and good reading comprehension ability are said to have good, sharp minds. A large vocabulary is reflective of a high verbal ability. Again, the source of this ability is not explicitly stated; there seems to be an appeal to *a priori* tendencies. A good description of the tenets of this position has been provided by Anderson and Freebody (1985), who also maintained that this position is the most fully developed of all hypotheses:

A person who scores high on such a test has a quick mind. With the same amount of exposure to the culture, this individual has learned more word meanings. He or she also comprehends discourse more readily than the person who scores low on a vocabulary test. The essential claim of the aptitude hypothesis is that persons with large vocabularies are better at discourse comprehension because they possess superior mental agility. A large vocabulary is not conceived to be involved in a direct way in better text understanding in this model. Rather vocabulary test performance is merely another reflection of verbal ability and it is verbal ability that mainly determines whether text will be understood. (p. 346)

The third position, the knowledge-based hypothesis, has been influenced by interactive theories of reading, particularly schema-interactive models (e.g., see discussions in Anderson & Freebody, 1985; Johnson & Pearson, 1984; Mason & Au, 1986; Paul, 1996; Paul & O'Rourke, 1988). Proponents of this position aver that vocabulary knowledge is reflective of knowledge of specific topics or areas, or even knowledge of the general culture. For example, if a student understands a word like *touchdown,* it is likely that he or she has an extensive knowledge of the game of football (*Note:* Of course, this might not be the case). The major instructional implication of this position is that students need to possess depth of vocabulary knowledge, not simply to know the meanings of numerous isolated words. This requires teachers to select fewer words and spend more time on these words using techniques such as semantic maps, semantic features analyses, and word maps (e.g., Heimlich & Pittelman, 1986; Johnson & Pearson, 1984; Nagy, 1988; Paul, 1996; Paul & O'Rourke, 1988). Several examples of these techniques are illustrated in Chapters 7 and 8.

It should be underscored that there is no substantial evidence for the superiority of any of the above vocabulary hypotheses in explaining the relationship between vocabulary knowledge and reading comprehension. Word learning is an extremely complex process. Knowledge of a word is not an all-or-nothing phenomenon. In addition, understanding and use of a word changes with the experiences of an individual. A particular method of vocabulary instruction might increase a reader's knowledge of some aspects of a word, but not others or all aspects of a word.

A summary of the main tenets of the three models of vocabulary acquisition is presented in Table 2-4.

TABLE 2-4   Major tenets of the three models of vocabulary acquisition

Instrumental Hypothesis

- Individuals with a high score on vocabulary tests will also score well on reading achievement tests
- Vocabulary knowledge causes reading comprehension
- A great deal of emphasis on environmental factors such as teaching techniques and instructional materials

Aptitude Hypothesis

- Favors the effects of genetics over those from the environment
- Large vocabulary is reflective of a high verbal ability
- Implies that vocabulary tests are a good measure of intelligence (IQ)

Knowledge Hypothesis

- Influenced by interactive theories of literacy, particularly schema-interactive models
- Vocabulary knowledge is reflective of knowledge of specific topics or areas
- Emphasis placed on depth of vocabulary knowledge such as multiple meanings, nuances, and figurative usage

One of the most controversial issues in vocabulary and reading is the tension between vocabulary instruction proponents and the learning from context proponents (e.g., see discussions in Beck & McKeown, 1991; Paul, 1996; Paul & O'Rourke, 1988). Vocabulary instruction has been influenced by the acquisition theories discussed previously. It should be noted that at least two general kinds of learning from context have been identified: deliberate and incidental (e.g., Jenkins, Stein, & Wysocki, 1984; Nagy, Herman, & Anderson, 1985). Deliberate learning refers to an individual reader's skill in deriving meaning from context when required to performed the task. Incidental learning refers to the learning of words and meanings during normal or typical independent reading. The debate has centered on the relative merits of different types of vocabulary instruction versus different types of learning from context.

One problem with this debate is that it can be construed as an either-or situation with proponents lining up on either side arguing for instruction or context. In the ensuing paragraphs, it should become clear that vocabulary learning is so complex that research on neither instruction nor context alone can account for what readers know about words (see also the discussions in Beck & McKeown, 1991; Paul, 1996; Paul & O'Rourke, 1988). In addition, it might be that theorists and researchers have overestimated vocabulary growth and have underestimated the influence of word learning in oral or speaking contexts (e.g., Beck & McKeown, 1991). Relative to the latter point, several scholars have emphasized the importance of classroom discussions of words along with either vocabulary instruction or reading (e.g., Dale & O'Rourke, 1986; Devine, 1986; O'Rourke, 1974; Paul & O'Rourke, 1988). It is difficult to capture the relative merits of these discussions, although there needs to be additional research in this area (Beck & McKeown, 1991).

There have been several studies on the learning of words during reading (i.e., context) either by deliberate learning (e.g., Beck, McKeown, & McCaslin, 1983; Schatz & Baldwin, 1986) or by incidental learning (e.g., Herman, Anderson, Pearson, & Nagy, 1987; Nagy, Herman, & Anderson, 1985). It has been argued that incidental learning of words from context is more effective than any type of vocabulary instruction (e.g., Nagy & Anderson, 1984; Nagy, Herman, & Anderson, 1985).

Results suggested that learning words from context does occur and occurs in small increments. However, there is a contentious debate regarding the power of contextual effects, which results in different interpretations of the same data (e.g., Beck & McKeown, 1991). If learning from context does occur, it is more evident for good readers than for poor readers, who are not likely to engage in wide reading, a condition necessary for the beneficial effects of context. Furthermore, as noted by Schatz and Baldwin (1986), it is not easy to learn difficult words during natural reading because much of the context does not provide sufficient insights into the meanings of these words.

As stated previously, vocabulary instruction might not produce powerful effects either. This includes instruction that focuses on teaching students how to use context to derive meanings of words or instruction that focuses on the direct teaching of word meanings (e.g., see discussions in Beck & McKeown, 1991; Paul, 1996; Paul & O'Rourke, 1988). There seems to be accruing evidence that there is no best method for teaching vocabulary. Based on several research syntheses, a few remarks can be made about vocabulary instruction (e.g., see Graves, 1986; Paul, 1996; Paul & O'Rourke, 1988; Stahl & Fairbanks,

1986). For some readers, especially poor readers, some instruction is better than no instruction. Vocabulary instruction should not be viewed as an all-encompassing entity; its beneficial effects might be most noticeable when it is combined with either deliberate or incidental learning from context. The focus of instruction should be on deep processing of words and related concepts as evident in semantic elaboration techniques such as semantic maps, word maps, and semantic feature analysis (e.g., Heimlich & Pittelman, 1986; Johnson & Pearson, 1984; Nagy, 1988; Paul, 1989; Paul & O'Rourke, 1988).

One of the goals of future research on vocabulary instruction should be to provide guidelines for improving techniques, developing more powerful techniques, and showing when and why certain techniques are more useful or beneficial than others. The search for the best or ultimate technique is as elusive as the search for the best semantic model for how words are stored in the mind (e.g., Aitchison, 1994; Anderson & Nagy, 1991).

A considerable portion of research on hearing students in this chapter has been devoted to word identification and word learning. Aside from the importance of these variables to reading comprehension, there is another important reason: In my view, these variables, along with other text-based variables such as orthography and grammar (notably, syntax), are the major reasons for the reading difficulty of students with severe to profound hearing impairment. These factors are related to the acquisition of English language variables, particularly via the conversational (i.e., spoken or primary) form. There is no question that literacy is much more than language development; nevertheless, the difficulty that students who are deaf have in accessing phonology and morphology of English might explain their tremendous deficits noted in the areas of word identification and word knowledge as discussed in the next chapter. In fact, this difficulty (with phonology and morphology) is so pronounced that it has been argued that this supports the notion of a *psychology of deafness* (e.g., Paul, 1995a, 1995b; Paul & Quigley, 1990, 1994a). That is, it calls into question whether high levels of reading and writing (i.e., beyond functional literacy) are realistic goals for many students with severe to profound hearing impairment. In any case, word recognition and word knowledge do not constitute the whole story. It is important also to consider the influences of higher-order knowledge as discussed in the next section.

Comprehension: The Use of Higher-Order Skills

In general, the higher-order skills associated with comprehension entail the use of prior knowledge and metacognition. In this section, only a brief summary of the research on comprehension is presented. The reader is referred to other sources, notably the chapters by Anderson and Armbruster; Baker and Brown; Rosenshine and Stevens; and Tierney and Cunningham in Pearson, Barr, Kamil, and Mosenthal (1984) and the chapters by Alvermann and Moore; Chall and Squire; Roehler and Duffy; and Sulzby and Teale in Barr, Kamil, Mosenthal, and Pearson (1991). Other readable accounts of comprehension and comprehension instruction can be found in Lipson and Wixson (1991) and Mason and Au (1986).

As mentioned previously, prior knowledge refers to the stock of background experiences individuals bring to the task of reading. In addition to world knowledge, this stock refers to passage-specific and topic-specific knowledge (e.g., see Mason & Au, 1986). Passage-specific knowledge involves knowledge of information in the text such as that relating to the topic, the genre, and all text features such as vocabulary, grammar, and items such as parentheses and headings. Topic-specific knowledge refers to the general knowledge associated with the topic that proceeds beyond the information in the text.

Using the traditional description by Baker and Brown (1984, p. 353), metacognition involves "knowledge about cognition and regulation of cognition." Knowledge about cognition

> . . . is concerned with a person's knowledge about his or her own cognitive resources and the compatibility between the person as a learner and the learning situation. Prototypical of this category are questionnaire studies and confrontation experiments, the main purpose of which is to find out how much children know about certain pertinent features of thinking, including themselves as thinkers.

The regulation of cognition:

> . . . consists of the self-regulatory mechanisms used by an active learner during an ongoing attempt to solve problems. These indexes of metacognition include *checking* the outcome of any attempt to solve the problem, *planning* one's next move, *monitoring* the effectiveness of any attempted action, and *testing*, *revising*, and *evaluating* one's strategies for learning. (p. 354)

The beneficial effects of higher-order skills such as prior knowledge and metacognition can be understood via the number of research syntheses on comprehension instruction, especially by Pearson and his collaborators (e.g., Pearson, 1986; Pearson & Dole, 1987; Pearson & Fielding, 1991; Pearson & Gallagher, 1983) and others (Levin & Pressley, 1981; Pressley, Goodchild, Fleet, Zajchowski, & Evans, 1989; Tierney & Cunningham, 1984). Research has focused on improving the student's comprehension of the text (i.e., text comprehension) and on improving the student's ability to comprehend the text (i.e., comprehension ability). This is related to the issue of whether it is possible to teach comprehension.

The debate on the teachability of comprehension is similar to the either-or debate discussed previously on whether word identification skills can or should be taught. This debate is also related to specific *teaching* views as discussed in Chapter 1. That is, direct teaching proponents often adhere to the concept of reductionism whereas those who describe the teacher as one who facilitates or is a catalyst favor the notion of constructionism. The review by Tierney and Cunningham (1984) proffered some cautionary remarks relative to the prevalence of systematic, direct, precision instructional strategies often described and advocated in instructional research. They suspected that the *mechanistic* character of this type of instruction might be undermining the *aesthetic* nature of reading, which might be lost to students who are labeled as poor readers.

Relative to improving student's comprehension of the text, one of the most important variables that has had a pervasive influence on comprehension instruction is prior knowledge (Anderson, 1985; Anderson & Pearson, 1984). In essence, readers need to fill in text gaps with inferences drawn from their prior knowledge (particularly topic-specific). Texts are not explicitly written and probably would be extremely boring if they were, because one of the major goals of reading is and should be the making of inferences. Comprehending, learning, and remembering information during reading are markedly influenced by prior knowledge of topics that readers bring to the text (e.g., Anderson, 1985; Anderson & Pearson, 1984; Pearson & Fielding, 1991). For example, having knowledge about the game of football enables readers to interpret and remember information from a passage on this topic.

Results of reading research on students with typical or normal hearing indicate that prior knowledge of a topic increases the amount of information that children recall from the text on that topic (e.g., see reviews in Anderson & Pearson, 1984; Pearson & Fielding, 1991). Prior knowledge in many of the studies refers to general knowledge of the story structure (e.g., story grammar) and knowledge and experiences about topics and themes in stories. For comprehension to occur, readers must relate information in the text to knowledge characteristics that exist in their own memory structures (i.e., schemata). Readers with high prior knowledge are able to answer more questions correctly than readers with low prior knowledge in that subject area. This is especially true for inferential questions discussed previously (e.g., text-implicit and script-implicit).

There are several effects of this research on comprehension instruction (see Chapter 7 for detailed descriptions of activities). Almost any type of attempt to help children understand text structure, including the various techniques authors use to put ideas together and to express major themes, has been found to be beneficial. In addition, teachers are encouraged to allot additional time for pre-story discussion. Pre-story questions should be based on important information in the story (e.g., main story ideas) so that these inquiries assist children in building models of what the text means. There is also an emphasis on asking prediction and inferential questions about the main aspects of the story. Both of these types of questions should require children to apply what it is they have understood or will have understood about the story. Finally, children should be able to provide several interpretations of a story. This requires the use of unedited stories and the use of broad, open-ended questions to encourage different points of views.

What have we learned from research on *summarizing* (another important area of comprehension)? Despite the lack of positive effects in earlier studies, the more recent studies have shown that summarizing texts leads to a higher level of comprehension and recall (e.g., see research review in Pearson & Fielding, 1991). Earlier studies might have underestimated the intent of summarization training and the actual outcomes desired (i.e., what the students were expected to remember). More important, the improvements in this area might be due to the stronger emphasis on metacognitive activities, or in the words of Pearson and Fielding (1991, p. 835) the: " 'metacognitive' underpinnings of the instruction: the *what, how, why,* and *when*."

Metacognition is concerned with strategies readers use to monitor and repair their comprehension of written texts (e.g., see reviews in Baker & Brown, 1984; Paris, Wasik, & Turner, 1991). Brown (1975) asserts that metacognition is *knowing about knowing* and *knowing how to know*. It is also important to know *when* and *why* to use a particular strategy (Cross & Paris, 1988). In one stance, metacognitive instruction deals with improving students' *ability* to comprehend (e.g., see discussion in Pearson & Fielding, 1991).

Studies on metacognition have focused on several areas. For example, the relation between metacognition and reading comprehension has been studied. The effects of metacognitive training relative to answering questions is another important area of inquiry. Also of interest are instructional studies that attempt to enable students to become involved in their own learning and to engage students and teachers in cooperative activities in the classroom.

It has been argued that metacognitive activity is related to children's reading comprehension (e.g., Baker & Brown, 1984; Brown, Armbruster, & Baker, 1986). In addition, metacognitive status has been shown to vary with age and with reading level (e.g., Paris, Cross, & Lipson, 1984; Paris & Jacobs, 1984). Older and skilled readers know more about reading strategies, detect errors more often during reading, and have better recall of text information.

Perhaps the most interesting studies on metacognition are those that show the effects of students *monitoring their own comprehension activities*. For example, the work of Miller and her associates is illustrative (Miller, 1985, 1987; Miller, Giovenco & Rentiers, 1987). Based on research with average and below-average readers, these researchers were able to show that these students can learn to monitor their comprehension activities. It is important to inform students on how a specific strategy can be used to improve comprehension ability (similar to the finding expressed in Cross & Paris, 1988). In addition, encouraging students to self-verbalize might be beneficial.

For the second and final example, the work of Raphael and her collaborators is illustrative (Raphael, 1984; Raphael & McKinney, 1983; Raphael & Pearson, 1985; Raphael & Wonnacut, 1985). These investigators were interested in improving reading comprehension by increasing children's awareness and use of strategies to answer questions, especially inferential questions (see previous examples of text-implicit and script-implicit questions). In general, it was found that trained students performed better than untrained students at evaluating types of questions and at providing correct answers. Raphael concluded that, compared to untrained students, trained students who understood question-answer relationships were better able to monitor their comprehension and were better able to comprehend materials read independently. Examples of metacognitive activities are presented in the chapters on instruction (Chapters 7 and 8).

A Final Word

The main intent of this chapter was to present a summary of reading-comprehension theories and research on students with typical or normal hearing. The two major areas were word identification and comprehension. It was emphasized that word identification facilitates comprehension and comprehension facilitates word identification. Research syntheses do not support an either-or dichotomy relative to these two variables.

A portion of the chapter was devoted to word identification and to one comprehension factor, word knowledge. It was argued that these variables are critical for understanding the difficulty that students who are deaf have with reading. Rapid, automatic word identification skills are necessary for facilitating the use of mature, top-down or comprehension strategies. As discussed in the next chapter, students who are deaf have problems with both bottom-up and top-down processing.

Further Readings

BARTLETT, F. (1932). *Remembering.* Cambridge: Cambridge University Press.

DAVIS, F. (Ed.). (1971). *The literature of research in reading with emphasis on models.* New Brunswick, NJ: Graduate School of Education, Rutgers University.

FOUCAULT, M. (1972). *The archaeology of knowledge.* London: Travistock.

KAVANAGH, J., & MATTINGLY, I. (1972). *Language by ear and by eye.* Cambridge, MA: MIT Press.

KINTSCH, W. (1974). *The representation of meaning in memory.* Hillsdale, NJ: Erlbaum.

SULLIVAN, J. (1972). *Classifying and interpreting educational research studies.* New York: American Book.

Chapter 3

Reading-Comprehension Perspective: Research on Students Who Are Deaf

"Is reading different for deaf individuals?" The answer appears to be both yes and no. Clearly the answer is yes in the sense that deaf readers will bring to the task of reading very different sets of language experiences than the hearing child. These differences will require special instruction. But the answer is also no. The evidence indicates that skilled deaf readers use their knowledge of the structure of English when reading. Although sign coding, in theory, might be used as an alternative to phonological coding for deaf signers, the research using various short-term memory and reading tasks has found little evidence that words are processed with references to sign by the better deaf readers. Rather, the better deaf readers, like the better hearing readers, have learned to abstract phonological information from the orthography, despite congenital and profound hearing impairment (Hanson, 1989, p. 85).

The answer to the question posed by Hanson (1989) in the above passage has pervasive implications for the instruction and assessment of reading (and writing) for students with severe to profound hearing impairment, at least from a cognitive information-processing perspective. It is important to emphasize the dual nature of her answer—yes *and* no. This dual nature encourages research scholars and educators to strive for a better understanding of the similarities and differences between readers who are deaf and readers who are hearing. In my view, this response is much better or more productive than the *either–or* answer, yes *or* no.

Proponents who argue that the answer is only *yes* are bound to favor the development of theories, models, and instructional programs for students who are deaf that are different from those available for hearing students. In essence, these proponents argue that mainstream theories and research are not applicable to students who are deaf and, thus, should be indiscriminately rejected. They support their assertions by citing the long-standing low literacy achievement levels in cases in which instructional methods for these students have been based mostly on the research on hearing students. As discussed in Chapters 5 and 6, this seems to be one of the underlying themes for developing bilingual programs for students with severe to profound hearing impairment.

Within this domain, there also exists the possibility that reading and writing are unrealistic goals for many students who are deaf (see Paul & Quigley, 1994a; Chapter 6 of this text). That is, the answer is *yes,* reading is different; however, it is so qualitatively different that we might need to question whether or not it is reasonable or feasible to develop these skills. As is discussed later in this chapter, this is a likely response from individuals, such as myself, who adhere predominantly to a cognitive-processing point of view. It might not be shared, necessarily, by others who ascribe to a naturalistic or social-constructionist perspective. Obviously, if this is the case, then it becomes necessary to construct or use alternative methods for developing literate thought in persons with severe to profound hearing impairment.

Proponents who argue that the answer is only *no* tend to overemphasize the similarities to the exclusion of the differences. There is an emphasis on citing research that shows that phonics or the use of a phonological code *only* is critical for the development of high-level literacy skills. This leads to the assumption that for students who are deaf an improvement of accessibility to the sound system results in the automatic acquisition of the alphabetic system—the deep relationships between letters and sounds. These proponents are also likely to argue that, due to limited time and resources, the implementation of a bilingual program (i.e., ASL/English) is bound to be counterproductive.

Much of the research in this chapter seems to support mostly the *no* answer to Hanson's question and has been influenced mainly by the cognitive information-processing paradigm. In one sense, the answer is similar to that of the research on the English language development of students who are deaf reported by Quigley and his collaborators (e.g., see reviews in Paul & Quigley, 1994a; Quigley & Paul, 1990). The predominant conclusion has been that the English language development of deaf students is qualitatively similar (in manner of acquisition) to, albeit quantitatively slower than (i.e., rate), that of students with typical hearing. Even though the literacy development of students who are deaf might be qualitatively similar to that of hearing students, this does not preclude the development of bilingual education programs for some students who are deaf. However, it might be that the literacy instructional aspects of bilingual programs need to be based on *mainstream* theories and models, especially those related to second-language learning, as discussed in Chapter 6.

From a cognitive information-processing perspective, it is the *no* answer to Hanson's question that is most critical to explore, relative to the development of literate thought— the ability to think reflectively and critically, as mentioned previously. For example, the literacy development of students who are deaf might be qualitatively similar to that of hearing students, but it is so quantitatively delayed that it impacts access to the school curriculum and, subsequently, all areas of educational achievement. (This is somewhat similar to an aspect of the *yes* answer, discussed previously). In addition, if English literacy, in conjunction with the use of English language skills, becomes the only or predominant way to acquire knowledge and critical thinking skills, this might have detrimental effects on the educational development of most students with severe to profound hearing impairment who, as discussed in Chapter 1, do not reach a high literate level by the time their formal education is completed. Thus, educators are faced with the possibility that most deaf students will not only be functionally illiterate, but also will not have acquired adequately a first language, which is necessary for the development of literate thought.

The major intent of this chapter is to present and synthesize research on literacy and deafness within the framework of reading-comprehension models, particularly cognitive information-processing models. The limited research related to the naturalistic model is presented in Chapter 4 on writing, especially on the process of writing. Initially, the reading comprehension achievement of students who are deaf since the beginning of the use of formal tests is discussed. This provides a historical background on the magnitude of the difficulty and a precursor to *explanatory adequacy* relative to literacy development (i.e., why these students have reading problems). Subsequently, a summary of results is discussed relative to two categories: text-based variables and reader-based variables. The relevant information on task-based variables is described in Chapter 9 on assessment. After the discussion of the research, some directions for further instruction and investigation are proffered. Finally, the chapter ends with an in-depth discussion of Hanson's question, and a tentative answer is provided relative to the interpretation of the research literature.

Perspectives on Reading Achievement and Deafness

Prior to the 1970s, at least three observations could be made about the nature of reading research and deafness. One, much of what was known was based on achievement and other formal tests normed on students with typical or normal hearing ability. The subsequent development and use of assessments normed on students who are deaf were due mainly to the inappropriateness of and biases associated with the other types of tests, which led to unreliable and invalid results (e.g., see discussion in Babbini & Quigley, 1970). Two, it could be argued that almost all reading research on deafness was influenced by the clinical perspective (see Chapter 1). In essence, the reading ability of students who are deaf was compared to that of their hearing counterparts, and the interpretation of the findings was influenced markedly by the *language-dominate-cognition* hypothesis, which stated that language was the fundamental quality (see discussions of this view in Paul & Jackson, 1993; Paul & Quigley, 1990, 1994a). Indeed, it was suspected that for students who are deaf much of their difficulty with reading was due mainly (perhaps solely) to their inadequate development of the English language. So pervasive was this view that it was common then, and still is somewhat common today, to hear that many teachers of students who are deaf considered themselves to be *language teachers*. The third major observation that could be made is that almost all assessments ascribed to what can now be called precursors to bottom-up theories of reading (see Chapter 2). There was a heavy reliance on a hierarchy of subskills (i.e., proceeding from letters to syllables to words and so on), and this was reflected in the nature of the assessment used.

The research on reading and deafness is presented relative to two major periods: (1) from Pintner to the 1970s and (2) from the 1970s to the present. During the first period, the work of Pintner is examined along with the results of general achievement tests, including the Stanford Achievement Test (SAT). The interpretations of the findings were influenced by the views of both Pintner and Myklebust, both of whom espoused an *internalization principle* (for an in-depth treatment, see Paul & Jackson, 1993). The early part of the second period is dominated by the results of the SAT (adapted versions) administered and interpreted by the Center for Assessment and Demographic Studies (CADS), housed in Gallaudet University. Another line of research, especially on syntax, was conducted by Quigley and his collaborators (e.g., see review in Paul & Quigley, 1994a). The latter part of the second period has been influenced by the work of several individuals in the area of *phonological coding* (e.g., Conrad, 1979; Hanson, 1989; Leybaert, 1993). Some interpretations of the reading ability of students who are deaf have been influenced also by the cultural perspective (see Chapter 1), especially the work of literary critical theorists (this is explored in depth in Chapter 5). The works of Quigley and those of other individuals interested in short-term memory research (e.g., phonological coding) are discussed in the section in this chapter dealing with reader variables.

From Pintner to the 1970s

During the time of Pintner, language comprehension was considered to be the basis for literacy development. Thus, Pintner and his collaborators assessed reading via the use of language tests (e.g., Pintner, 1918, 1927; Pintner & Paterson, 1916, 1917). The Trabue Language Completion Tests were administered to both students who are deaf and students who are hearing. Examples of items included sentences such as:

1. We like good boys _____ girls.
2. The _____ is barking at the car.

This activity, now known as a cloze procedure, was a common task used by teachers of students who are deaf during their teaching of language skills. Students were required to write the correct words on the blank lines.

Pintner also used the Woodworth and Wells' Direction Tests (e.g., Pintner & Paterson, 1917). This test was designed to assess the students' ability to understand the printed language of the test. Examples included:

1. How many ears has a cat?
2. Put a question mark after this sentence

The deaf subjects for Pintner's studies were drawn from residential schools in midwestern United States. They were enrolled in both oral and manual (similar to total communication) classes, and some students had completed almost 12 to 13 years of schooling. The findings were compared with those for hearing counterparts. A summary of Pintner's major findings are presented here:

1. The majority of students who are deaf were reading at or below the fourth-grade level in one study (e.g., Pintner & Paterson, 1916).
2. Students in oral classes performed significantly better than those in manual classes, and the differences between the two groups were most obvious for age 14 and older. [*Note:* The highest average reading grade of the oral students was 4.5 whereas that of the manual group was 3.6 (Pintner & Paterson, 1916). In another study (Pintner & Paterson, 1917), the median grade level ranged from six to nine for the 15- to 18-year-old oral students.]
3. Based on the results of a national study (Pintner, 1927), Pintner reported that the educational level of typical 18- to 19-year-old students who are deaf, regardless of educational environment, was equivalent to that of typical 8- or 9-year-old hearing students.
4. Pintner concluded that certain language tests, for example, the Trabue tests, were not sufficiently sensitive to measure small gains in achievement.

It is remarkable that the findings of Pintner have not changed substantially since the dates of the published studies. More interesting, Pintner attributed the superior performance of oral students to two major variables: higher intelligence and greater emphasis on language training in the classroom. The factor of higher intelligence has been untenable (see discussions in Paul & Quigley, 1990, 1994a). From another perspective, it is not the greater emphasis on language training, but rather, it is the inaccessibility of this English language training by *manual* students. This has been interpreted to mean that manual students had difficulty internalizing the principles of a spoken language such as English. As noted by Paul and Jackson (1993):

> Probably, the most interesting findings resulted from Pintner's use of the Digit-Symbol and Symbol-Digit tests. The results of these tests indicated that children with severe hearing impairment had difficulty with symbolic, verbal learning. This can be interpreted to mean that deaf students had difficulty in internalizing a spoken (i.e., verbal) language. This does not mean, of course, that the students had not internalized any language (e.g., a sign language) or did not have an internalized, idiosyncratic symbol system. (p. 87)

Another common way to assess the reading ability of students who are deaf was the use of standardized achievement tests, particularly the Metropolitan and Stanford tests. As indicated previously, these tests were normed on students with typical or normal hearing ability. Typically, the reading score was the combined score associated with two subtests: *Word Meaning* and *Paragraph Meaning*. Again, the findings indicated that the mean reading grade level was around the fourth or fifth grade (e.g., Balow, Fulton & Peploe, 1971; Pugh, 1946; Wrightstone, Aronow & Moskowitz, 1963).

Goetzinger and Rousey (1959), for example, analyzed the scores of residential deaf students, aged 14 to 21 years, on the SAT. Focusing on students with at least 12 years of instruction, the researchers reported a mean grade of 4.5 years (*Paragraph Meaning* subtest). They also found that the gap between students who are deaf and those who are hearing widens as the students become older.

Using the *Elementary Reading Test* of the Metropolitan Achievement Test, Wrightstone et al. (1963) conducted a national study on deaf students between the ages of 10 and
16 years, inclusive. The mean degree of hearing impairment of the whole sample was 84
dB (in the better unaided ear), even though there were some students with average impairment better than the mean (i.e., less than 84 dB). The researchers developed a single set of
norms for the whole sample.

The results of the Wrightstone et al. study was analyzed in depth by Furth (1966), who
was interested in comparing the norms to those of hearing children. Furth (e.g., 1966,
1973) has proffered a language and experiential hypothesis to explain the low reading
scores of students who are deaf. He reported that less than 25% between age 14 years, 6
months and 16 years, 6 months reached a mean level of fifth grade or higher. Furth concluded that most students in the Wrightstone et al. study could be classified as functionally
illiterate (assuming that fifth grade is a functionally literate level).

Quigley (1969) and Babbini and Quigley (1970) studied the educational achievement
of students who are deaf across a five-year period. Of interest here are the scores on the language and reading subtests of the SAT. Babbini and Quigley (1970) reanalyzed the data
from Quigley's (1969) study and documented an increase of *one-third grade per year* on the
subtests. The means of the language and reading subtests are illustrated in Table 3-1.

The most important and far-reaching finding of the Babbini and Quigley study was the
observation of high intercorrelations among all subtests of the SAT. This led the researchers to argue that the SAT was measuring only one general ability, namely, the English language ability of students who are deaf. Based on this assumption, Babbini and
Quigley argued for the development of tests normed on students with hearing impairment.

1970s to the Present

Since the 1960s, the Center for Assessment and Demographic Studies (CADS) has conducted several investigations on the academic achievement of a national sample of students
with hearing impairment who are in special programs in the United States (e.g., Allen,
1986; CADS, 1991; DiFrancesca, 1972; Gentile & DiFrancesca, 1969; Trybus & Karchmer, 1977). Gentile and DiFrancesca (1969) reported on the results of about 12,000 stu-

**TABLE 3-1   Means of language and reading subtests on the Stanford Achievement
Test in Babbini & Quigley (1970)**

	Years					
Subtest	1	2	3	4	5	Gain
Combined Reading	3.3	3.6	4.0	4.3	4.6	1.3
Language	3.9	4.5	5.0	5.7	6.2	2.9

Source: Based on information in Babbini & Quigley (1970).

dents between the ages of 7 and 19 years. Of relevance here are the results of students whose hearing impairment was 60 dB or greater and whose ages ranged from 16 to 19 years old. The grade equivalent means for the subtests of *Language, Paragraph Reading,* and *Total Reading* are given in Table 3-2.

The researchers reported that about 80% of the students taking the SAT were reading at a grade level of 4.5 or lower.

DiFrancesca (1972) reported even lower scores for the national sample of 17,000 students between the ages of 6 and 21 years. These scores were deemed to be more accurate because of improvements in the screening procedures (i.e., assigning a student to a specific test battery). DiFrancesca reported that most students with severe to profound hearing impairment were reading at a fourth-grade level or lower. The mean grade scores of the 16- to 19-year-old students on the Paragraph Reading subtest of the Advanced Battery (i.e., the highest group) were 7.4, 7.5, 7.6, and 6.9, respectively.

Trybus and Karchmer (1977) analyzed the scores of the first special edition of the SAT for students with hearing impairment (i.e., normed on students with hearing impairment). The scores, however, were not much different from the other test administrations. The researchers reported that the mean reading grade level for the whole sample was 4.5. In addition, they noted that only 10% of the students in the best reading group were reading at the eighth-grade level or better. Finally, considering results across a three-year period, it was found that the overall growth in reading was less than one year (0.8).

These findings are not different from the more recent surveys (see discussions in Kelly, 1995; Paul & Quigley, 1994a). For example, Allen (1986) argued that the median reading scores of the 1983 sample were significantly higher than those for the 1974 sample at every age compared, based on statistical conversion methods. Nevertheless, the median grade level of most students with severe to profound impairment is still below the fourth grade (see also, Kelly, 1995).

TABLE 3-2   Means for selected subtests on Intermediate II Battery and the Advanced Battery of the Stanford Achievement Test in Gentile & DiFrancesca (1969)

	Age of Students				
	16 Years Old		17 Years Old		18 Years Old
	Intermediate Battery II	Advanced Battery	Intermediate II	Advanced	Advanced
Subtests					
Spelling	6.08	7.38	5.64	7.60	7.93
Language	4.57	5.82	4.40	6.02	6.15
Total Reading	4.17	—	4.02	—	—
Paragraph Meaning	—	5.77	—	5.90	5.79

Source: Based on information in Gentile & DiFrancesca (1969).

Select Subgroups

The findings of national surveys should be interpreted with caution because they tend to obscure the performances of *select* subgroups within the population of students with hearing impairment. For example, students in some exemplary Total Communication programs (e.g., Luetke-Stahlman, 1988a; 1988b) and Oral programs (e.g., Lane & Baker, 1974) or in mainstream settings (e.g., Geers & Moog, 1989) tend to have significantly higher scores than the norms associated with the CADS surveys. In addition, a large number of these students are performing on grade level when compared with their hearing peers.

What contributes to the superior performance of these students? Several factors have been proffered: quality of language input, type of language/communication input, parental participation, oral communication skills, and access to the phonological and morphological components of English (e.g., Brasel & Quigley, 1977; Delaney, Stuckless, & Walter, 1984; Geers & Moog, 1989; Hanson, 1989; Leybaert, 1993; Luetke-Stahlman, 1988a, 1988b). Geers and Moog (1989) attributed the high literacy skills of oral subjects in their study specifically to competence in the primary oral form of English.

The most promising interpretation, from an information-processing, interactive theoretical perspective, is that these students have good bottom-up and top-down processing skills, which were discussed in Chapter 2 (e.g., see discussions in Kelly, 1995; Paul, 1993a, 1993b, 1994a; Paul & Quigley, 1994a). This interpretation leads us to a discussion of text-based and reader-based variables. It should be kept in mind that the use of terms such as text-based or reader-based is an arbitrary decision. It is difficult to separate text-based problems from reader-based ones. For example, if the text contains difficult syntax (text-based), this might present processing problems (reader-based) for students who are deaf. Or, the problems with syntax in the text (text-based) might be one of knowledge (reader-based); that is, children and adolescents who are deaf do not understand (or possess competency in) the syntactic structures of English. Finally, the concept of processing has two aspects: difficulty with understanding age-inappropriate materials and structures, and difficulty with understanding age-appropriate materials and structures.

Research on Selected Text-Based Variables

Much of the research on students who are deaf has been conducted on what can be labeled text-based variables (e.g., see research reviews in King & Quigley, 1985; Myklebust, 1960, 1964; Paul & Quigley, 1994a). Text-based variables refer to features associated with text or print such as the structure of words, orthography, vocabulary, syntax, connected discourse, and figurative language. Earlier studies focus almost exclusively on demonstrating quantitative differences between students who are deaf and those who are hearing (e.g., see review in Myklebust, 1960, 1964); these findings continue to be documented by recent national surveys (e.g., Center for Demographic and Assessment Studies [CAD]; e.g., DiFrancesca, 1972; Trybus & Karchmer, 1977; CADS, 1991). The more recent studies also provide evidence for qualitative similarities and strong correlations among variables such as vocabulary (LaSasso & Davey, 1987; Paul, 1984, 1996; Paul & Gustafson, 1991), syntax (see research review in Paul & Quigley, 1994a) and reading comprehension.

A better understanding of these relationships requires a discussion of internal coding strategies (see the section on reader-based variables). More light can be shed if researchers consider investigating the word identification skills of students who are deaf in light of what is known about the use of a phonological code and knowledge of the alphabet system. Some of these issues are examined in this chapter. It is important to keep in mind that much of the interpretation of the research is influenced by the present author's bias toward interactive theories of literacy. However, it is also possible to make a similar case by focusing on similarities across the three broad groups of reading-comprehension theories: bottom-up, top-down, and interactive.

Word Identification

Studies on students who are deaf have focused more on their knowledge of words than on their word identification skills. As discussed in Chapter 2, word identification skills depend on a working command of the phonological and morphological components of the language of print as well as on the development of top-down (comprehension) skills. Thus, one indirect way to assess students' word identification skills is to focus on their understanding of phonology and morphology. The reader is reminded that, although a working conscious knowledge of the sounds (phonology) and parts (morphology) of words is important for word identification, it is not sufficient for developing high-level reading comprehension skills.

There is little research on deaf students' understanding and use of word identification skills, particularly if one uses the descriptions provided in Chapter 2: phonics, structural analysis, and contextual analysis. The limited research on contextual analysis, especially the use of context skills, relative to vocabulary and syntax is discussed later. Compared to the research on hearing children, the research on deaf children's use of phonics and structural analysis is extremely limited. One reason for this is the difficulty of conducting these types of research with students with impaired hearing. For example, it has been difficult to assess the knowledge of these structures using the conversational form (speech and/or sign) of the language (for an in-depth discussion of these problems, see Kretschmer & Kretschmer, 1978; Paul & Quigley, 1994a).

Thus, our understanding of structural analysis (e.g., morphology) has been the result of the research on written language (see Chapter 4) or the use of tests such as The Berko Morphology Test (Berko, 1958; see also, Cooper, 1967; Raffin, 1976). For example, Cooper (1967) found that children who are deaf had more difficulty with derivational morphology (e.g., *deaf* to *deafness* or *ice* to *reice*) than with inflectional morphology (e.g., *slow* to *slowly* or *see* to *sees*). Several investigators have focused on the acquisition and use of morphemes via exposure to a particular sign system (e.g., Gilman, Davis, & Raffin, 1980; Looney & Rose, 1979; Raffin, 1976; Raffin, Davis, & Gilman, 1978). In these studies, the value of systematic instruction was demonstrated. In addition, the researchers concluded that, relative to inflectional morphology, the order of acquisition was qualitatively similar to that of students with typical hearing. Nevertheless, children who are deaf and adolescent had difficulty acquiring morphological knowledge, and the gap between students who are deaf and those who are hearing typically increased with the advancing age of the students.

Documenting differences between students who are deaf and those who are hearing relative to word identification skills might not be terribly interesting to teachers of these children and adolescents. Future research needs to address the following questions, at least:

1. Are word identification skills important for the acquisition of reading comprehension skills?
2. What types of skills are important or even critical: phonics, structural analysis, or others?
3. Do word identification skills need to be taught, as in direct or precision instruction programs, or are they best learned by the use of natural reading materials (with little or no instruction)?
4. Is the use of word identification skills related to the type of processing in short-term working memory?
5. Is the relationship between word identification and reading for hearing students similar to that for students who are deaf?

It seems that we have some tentative answers relative to hearing children and youths (see Chapter 2). Whether we have clear answers relative to students who are deaf is an open debate. As is discussed later in the text, these answers are also important for teaching English literacy to second-language students, including students who are deaf and who know American Sign Language as a first language.

Word Knowledge

Word knowledge has two aspects: knowledge of the words and word meanings stored in the mind, and the ability to derive this knowledge from either incidental or deliberate contexts (see Chapter 2 for details). There has been very little research on how words and their meanings are organized and stored in the minds of students with severe to profound hearing impairment. Much of the research on hearing individuals has been influenced by models based on the cognitive information-processing paradigm.

There have been several studies on students who are deaf regarding their knowledge of words and word meanings (e.g., LaSasso & Davey, 1987; Paul, 1984; Paul & Gustafson, 1991, Walter, 1978). At least three major thrusts of this research can be identified: (1) to determine the breadth and depth of vocabulary knowledge (e.g., Paul & Gustafson, 1991; Silverman-Dresner & Guilfoyle, 1972), (2) to show the relationship of this knowledge to reading comprehension (e.g., LaSasso & Davey, 1987; Paul & Gustafson, 1991), and (3) to evaluate the ability to derive word meanings from the use of context cues (e.g., deVilliers & Pomerantz, 1992). The findings of these lines of research have important implications for the teaching of vocabulary to students with hearing impairment, especially for students who have poor literacy skills. It seems that part of the difficulty in reading is due to the difficulty of words and their meanings. As is discussed later, there are, at least, two major reasons for this problem: (1) students who are deaf do not know the meanings of words, especially words with multiple meanings, and (2) the reciprocal relationship between word identification and comprehension is deficient due to their inadequate word identification skills.

There have been several studies that sought to determine the breadth and depth of vocabulary knowledge of students who are deaf (e.g., see research reviews in Paul, 1984, 1996). The general finding has been that students with severe to profound hearing impairment at all age levels comprehend fewer words from print than peers who have typical hearing (e.g., Myklebust, 1960, 1964; Schulze, 1965; see also reviews in King & Quigley, 1985; Paul & Quigley, 1994a). The vocabulary knowledge of these students also seems to reflect their use of words in written language (discussed in Chapter 4). That is, students with severe to profound hearing impairment use more nouns and verbs than adverbs and conjunctions. In addition, due to their limited range of vocabulary words, their written language productions reflect a style that is direct or stilted, almost devoid of imaginative and idiomatic expressions (see written language examples in Chapter 4).

One of the most extensive studies on breadth of vocabulary knowledge was conducted by Silverman-Dresner and Guilfoyle (1972). Accessing vocabulary word lists (Dale & Chall, 1948; Dale & Eicholtz, 1960), the researchers eventually constructed definitions for a list of 7300 words. Their goal was to develop a set of age-graded vocabulary lists that reflected the actual reading vocabulary level of students who are deaf at various ages. This source would be similar to that produced for hearing students from grade 4 to college age (e.g., Dale & O'Rourke, 1981). Using a computer, the researchers created 73 sets of 100 randomly selected words, which became vocabulary tests. They administered two tests per student to approximately 13,000 students between the ages of 7 and 17 years in 89 schools for students who are deaf.

The criterion for knowing a word for each age group was 62 percent correct responses or 50 percent when corrected for guessing. The researchers assessed knowledge of only one meaning of the words. They reported that girls knew more words than boys and that the older students knew more words than the younger ones. A summary of all the words known by each age group, based on the criterion, was listed.

As is typical of early studies on vocabulary knowledge, Balow, Fulton, and Peploe (1971) reported low vocabulary scores and low reading achievement scores on the Metropolitan Achievement Test. The researchers studied 157 students with hearing impairment between the ages of 13 and 21 years. The students were divided into three groups based on degree of hearing impairment in the better unaided ear across the speech frequencies. Students in one group had hearing impairment ranging from 40 to 60 decibels (dB). In a second group, the range of hearing impairment was from 65 to 95 dB, and the hearing impairment for the third group was 100 plus decibels.

The mean score for this sample was reported to be 4.5 grade level for vocabulary. The mean score was inflated by the high performance of the students with hearing impairment ranging from 40 to 60 dB. Students in this group had a mean score that was more than one grade level above the mean score for the total sample. In addition to the insights into vocabulary knowledge, this study underscored the importance of providing complete descriptions of the characteristics of students with hearing impairment when conducting group studies. One of the most important variables is degree of hearing impairment, aided or unaided.

Although the main focus of the work of Quigley and his collaborators (e.g., see research review in Paul & Quigley, 1994a) was on the syntactic development of students who are deaf, these researchers also documented the results of the Stanford Achievement Test, normed on hearing students (e.g., Quigley, Steinkamp, Power, & Jones, 1978). Of interest here are the results on the *Word Meaning* subtest for students with profound hearing impairment from age 10 to 19 years old. The students in this study were assigned to one of three age groups: 10 to 12 years old, 13 to 15 years old, and 16 to 18 years old, inclusive. The gain score for the nine-year period was 1.1 grade. The SAT grade equivalent means for the three age groups were 2.5, 2.9, and 3.6, respectively.

Despite the adaptations and norms developed for the Stanford Achievement Test—Hearing Impaired Version, these low vocabulary scores persisted in the 1970s, 1980s, and into the 1990s (Allen, 1986; CADS, 1991; DiFrancesca, 1972; Kelly, 1995; Paul, 1996; Trybus & Karchmer, 1977). A number of investigators conducted analyses on students with hearing impairment in special elementary and secondary education programs in the United States. In these investigations, it was also speculated that there was a strong relationship between low vocabulary scores and low reading achievement scores.

Although the vocabulary scores are low, there is some research indicating that these estimates might be spuriously high. For example, Walter (1978) investigated the vocabulary knowledge of both students who are deaf and those who are hearing. The researcher was interested in the relationship between vocabulary knowledge and frequency level of the word. Frequency level refers to the number of times a particular word appears in print within a corpus of a certain number of words (e.g., a million words). The students with hearing impairment were between the ages of 10 and 14 years, inclusive, and were selected from 17 programs across the United States. Their scores were compared to hearing age-peers in a suburban Detroit parochial school. Walter administered the Frequency Based Test of Vocabulary (Walter, 1976), which consisted of 90 sentences, each with one word omitted. The students had to select the correct word from five alternatives. The frequency level of the words ranged from 100 to about 26,000 (Carroll, Davies, & Richman, 1971). Only one meaning of the words was assessed.

Walter (1978) reported that the oldest hearing impaired group performed significantly poorer than the youngest hearing group. As expected, the differences between the two overall groups (hearing and deaf) widened as the frequency of words decreased (i.e., became less frequent in print and thus more difficult). The researcher speculated that differences between the two groups would be even greater if additional meanings of words were evaluated, especially multimeaning words that appear infrequently in print.

There have been several studies that focus on the knowledge of multiple meanings of words. For example, in an early study, MacGinitie (1969) assessed the skills of both students who are deaf and those who are hearing. He was interested in the students' ability to shift in their knowledge of word meanings based on the context that was provided. Consider the following four test items:

(1) BEAR   forest   wild   paw   animal
(2) BEAR   forest   wild   paw   carry
(3) BEAR   burden   weight   land   carry
(4) BEAR   burden   weight   land   animal

In these examples, the two common meanings of bear are <u>animal</u> and <u>carry</u>. MacGinitie hypothesized that the students might most likely recognize <u>carry</u> as one meaning in a supportive context as in item *3* rather than in item *2*. The context of the second item should persuade the students to select a meaning that is different from the present one. Thus, the researcher compared the number of correct responses to items with misleading contexts to the number of correct responses to items with supportive contexts.

The students for the study were oral deaf students between the ages of 9 and 20 years, inclusive. The mean degree of hearing impairment for the entire sample was 88 dB, and none of the students had a mean hearing impairment that was less than 65 dB. The performances of these students were compared to those of a group of students with typical hearing in grades four through eight.

Results indicated that item context had no significant effect on the performance of the students who are deaf. On the other hand, the scores of the hearing students were depressed by the misleading contexts. Nevertheless, the hearing students knew more words than the deaf students in both supportive and misleading contexts.

In another early study, Letourneau (1972) evaluated the effects of two instructional methods for teaching words with multiple meanings. The effectiveness of the methods was related to the subsequent effects on reading comprehension. Eighty students with hearing impairment in grades four through six served as subjects. The students needed to possess a degree of hearing impairment of at least 70 dB in the better unaided ear for inclusion in the study. Students were selected from one oral school and three schools that used simultaneous communication (i.e., speaking and signing simultaneously).

Students and instructors were randomly assigned to one of six experimental or control groups. Students in the experimental groups were provided with specific instructions and exercises on the words with multiple meanings that appeared in their reading selections. Students in the control group also read the same materials containing these words; however, they were not provided with any special instructions or exercises. The multimeaning words were simply presented *casually* to the students.

The researcher found that instruction of multimeaning words had a positive effect on the students' ability to comprehend the passages containing the words. It was also remarked that these students with hearing impairment could learn words with multiple meanings; however, they needed numerous experiences and exercises in dealing with these words. Finally, it was stated that reading achievement was positively correlated with the students' ability to comprehend multimeaning words in a reading context.

The relationship between vocabulary knowledge and reading comprehension was explored further in several more recent studies in the 1980s and 1990s. Indirectly, this was the assumption of early studies (e.g., Balow et al., 1971; Quigley et al., 1978) and the various CAD studies (e.g., Allen, 1986; DiFrancesca, 1972; Trybus & Karchmer, 1977). That is, one could inspect the scores on the vocabulary and paragraph meaning subtests (reading comprehension) and conclude that low vocabulary scores are, more often than not, associated with low reading achievement scores. Thus, part of the reason for low reading achievement could be attributed to inadequate vocabulary knowledge.

What is meant by inadequate vocabulary knowledge is still not clear. Should students know only one meaning of many words? Is it necessary to know several meanings of many multimeaning words? What about the conceptual fields surrounding a particular word, as indicated by the knowledge hypothesis in Chapter 2? In essence, what should a student know about a word that seems to be critical for reading comprehension? Some perspectives on these questions were discussed in Chapter 2 in the section on word knowledge.

If low reading achievement is due, in part, to poor vocabulary knowledge, does the teaching of vocabulary lead to an improvement in reading achievement per se? Earlier studies failed to find positive effects of vocabulary instruction on reading achievement level. An illustrative example is the investigation by Robbins and Hatcher (1981). These researchers administered reading comprehension tests to 36 students whose hearing impairment ranged from severe to profound and whose ages ranged from 9 to 12 years. One half of the students consisted of the experimental group in which vocabulary instructional training was provided. This training focused on the use of words in sentences or what is often called the definition-and-sentence approach or the definition-and-context approach (Nagy, 1988; Paul & Gustafson, 1991). The other half consisted of a control group which received no specific vocabulary training. The researchers concluded that the reading comprehension scores of the group that received training did not significantly improve. No specific reason for this lack of improvement was proffered.

More recent studies have provided additional insights into the relationship between vocabulary knowledge and reading comprehension. For example, LaSasso and Davey (1987) argued that the negative results from the study by Robbins and Hatcher (1981) were due to the small sample size and to the reading comprehension task used, that is, "single, unrelated sentences" (p. 212). In addition, LaSasso and Davey (1987) investigated the vocabulary and reading comprehension relationship in 50 students with a profound hearing impairment (85+ dB ISO average in the better unaided ear) and between the ages of 10 and 18 years. Subjects incurred their hearing losses prior to the age of 2 years and had no additional handicapping conditions. The measures used were the vocabulary subtest of the Gates-MacGinitie Reading Tests, 1972 edition, and the reading comprehension subtests of the Stanford Achievement Test, the 1973 norms. The tasks included a cloze procedure and four question answering conditions—multiple choice, free response, lookback condition (i.e., subjects could read the passage as often as necessary), and no lookback condition (i.e., subjects could not read the passage more than once).

LaSasso and Davey (1987) found that the vocabulary scores correlated strongly with reading comprehension scores. In fact, vocabulary knowledge was said to be a strong predictor of reading comprehension ability. Vocabulary knowledge was a stronger predictor than SAT scores for the cloze tests, free response tasks, and questions with a no lookback condition. One of their conclusions was stated as follows:

> Practitioners should be aware that there appears to be more of a relationship between lexical knowledge and reading comprehension for hearing-impaired students than previously empirically established. Although this relationship has yet to be established as causal, practitioners should not ignore the lexical abilities of their students. (p. 218)

The findings by LaSasso and Davey (1987) have been corroborated and elaborated upon by the work of Paul and his collaborators (Paul, 1984, 1987; Paul & Gustafson, 1991; see also the research review in Paul, 1996). For example, Paul and Gustafson (1991) studied both hearing and hearing-impaired students' (90+ dB average in the better unaided ear) comprehension of words with multiple meanings on a picture vocabulary test. They were interested in the groups' performance on words with one meaning and those with two meanings. The researchers were also interested in whether vocabulary knowledge increased with age and the relationship between vocabulary knowledge and reading comprehension (i.e., scores on a standardized reading achievement test, SAT).

As expected, the hearing subjects significantly outperformed the subjects with hearing impairment in selecting one meaning and two meanings of words. Both groups selected the primary (most common) meanings more often than the secondary meanings. Surprisingly, the scores for selecting two meanings of words did not improve with age. The researchers also found a strong correlation between vocabulary knowledge and reading comprehension. Because of the prevalence of multimeaning words in reading materials, the researchers argued for direct instruction of common multimeaning words within a knowledge-based framework (see discussion of this concept relative to vocabulary in Chapter 2).

As discussed in Chapter 2, there is much debate on whether vocabulary knowledge should be taught or whether students should simply read widely in order to improve their knowledge of words. Although it might be necessary to encourage both activities, it is suspected that direct instruction might be critically important for poor readers, especially because these readers are not likely to read widely either inside or outside school. In addition, reading widely depends on the ability to use context cues to derive the meaning of words. The question here is how well can students who are deaf derive word meanings from context? As discussed in Chapter 2, this has two parts: (1) the use of context on an automatic, unconscious basis (i.e., natural contextual learning) and (2) the use of context as a strategy for deriving word meanings (i.e., deliberate contextual learning). There is little research on students' ability to use context cues, either unconsciously (natural contextual situations) or consciously (deliberate contextual learning) (e.g., see reviews in Davey & King, 1990; Paul, 1996; Paul & O'Rourke, 1988; Paul & Quigley, 1994a).

Only one empirical study was found in this area (de Villiers & Pomerantz, 1992). These researchers examined students with prelingual hearing impairment (range was 71 to 120 dB). The students were between the ages of 10 years and 18 years, inclusive (10 years, 11 months to 18 years, 7 months).

For the first study, thirty students were selected from an upper level (i.e., high school) of an oral school. The unaided hearing loss varied from 72 to 117 dB (mean was 97.2 dB). The reading comprehension (SAT-HI) grade level of this group ranged from 2.8 to 12.4 (mean = 5.7).

For the second study, there were two kinds of students. Twenty-one students were oral and were selected from a middle level of an oral school. The unaided hearing level ranged from 80 to 120 dB, and the mean was 100.8 dB. The reading grade level ranged from 1.6 to 3.9 (mean = 2.8). The other 15 students in this group were selected from a Total-Communication program. Their mean hearing loss was 94.8 dB, and the range of hearing impairment was from 71 to 110 dB. The reading grade level of this group varied from 2.2 to 4.8 (mean = 3.1). No differences were found between oral and TC students with respect to the above characteristics.

Our interest here is in the results of the abilities of students to infer both lexical (i.e., word meanings) and syntactic (e.g., form class, correct usage) information in a deliberate contextual situation (i.e., contrived passages). The contextual situation had three conditions: lean, rich, and explicit. The lean context provided little information whereas the rich context provided substantial information. The explicit condition provided "a clear contrast or equivalence statement" (1992, p. 414). Examples of these conditions for the middle-school are as follows:

Study 2—Middle School - Eerie

<u>Lean</u>

The boy painted a picture of an *eerie* house in his art class. He took it home to show his mother and father.

<u>Rich</u>

The old house on the hill was an *eerie* place. It was dark and it had broken windows, and it looked like ghosts lived in it.

<u>Explicit</u>

In the daytime the woods look safe and friendly, but at night they can be an *eerie* place. The trees look strange and scary in the dark. (1992, p. 415)

In general, the results indicated that students with hearing impairment can benefit from contexts that are highly informative, that is, rich or explicit, to derive a partial meaning of words. As expected, the ability to derive word meanings was strongly related to reading ability. Good readers significantly outperformed poor readers. More interesting, it was reported that the poor readers had much difficulty with the explicit contextual condition. The researchers hypothesized that this finding might be due either to the inability of poor readers to understand the syntax of the sentence or to their use of an inappropriate reading strategy (e.g., locating and matching key words or phrases). The use of inappropriate reading strategies by poor readers who are deaf has been well documented (e.g., see discussion in King & Quigley, 1985).

It is clear that poor readers who are deaf have problems that are similar to other poor readers, especially poor hearing readers. deVilliers and Pomerantz (1992) remarked that:

> There is, therefore, little relationship between the ability to identify grammatical features for a word based on the immediate syntactic frame in which it is used and the ability to derive a meaning for that word based on the integration of semantic cues across the passage. The latter, meaning-making skill is more closely related to the students' overall reading comprehension. Many hearing-impaired students are caught in a vicious circle: their impoverished vocabularies limit their reading comprehension, and poor reading strategies and skills limit their ability to acquire adequate vocabulary knowledge from context. (p. 428)

Syntax

One of the most extensively researched variables in the field of deafness is syntax. There are several reasons for this phenomenon. Individuals might have knowledge of words and still not be able to comprehend phrases and sentences due to problems with syntax. This explains why it is possible to increase vocabulary knowledge but not improve reading comprehension levels (e.g., see discussion in King & Quigley, 1985; Paul & Quigley 1994a). For students who are deaf and possibly for second-language learners, syntactic knowledge is a good index of reading skill because it requires the ability to integrate information across linguistic units such as words, phrases, and sentences. This integration is dependent on both bottom-up and top-down skills relative to interactive models of literacy. Finally, there is a growing consensus that working memory has an important role in reading comprehension and that the effects of this entity can be seen most readily on both intrasentential and intersentential levels. Even more interesting is the assumption that the use of a phonological code in working memory is critical in order to make processing more efficient, especially for a temporal-sequential phonetic language such as English.

Research on syntax has provided insights and debates on a number of issues; only a few major issues are examined here. One major issue concerns the comparison of the syntax comprehension abilities of individuals, both deaf and hearing. This comparison allows researchers to make assertions about the rate and manner of syntactic development. The debate here focuses on comprehension on the sentential level (e.g., the work of Quigley, see review in Russell, Quigley, & Power, 1976) and comprehension beyond the sentential level (e.g., Ewoldt, 1981; McGill-Franzen & Gormley, 1980; Nolen & Wilbur, 1985).

The second major issue revolves around the explanations for difficulty that students who are deaf have with syntax. The two aspects are knowledge and processing. That is, early researchers have argued that these students have problems with syntax because they simply lack the knowledge (e.g., the work of Quigley; see review in Paul & Quigley, 1994a). Other researchers have argued for a processing problem related mainly to the use of a phonological code in short-term working memory (e.g., see reviews in Hanson, 1989; Lillo-Martin, Hanson, & Smith, 1991, 1992). Both of these interpretations have been influenced by the work of Chomsky (1957, 1975), particularly the notion of Universal Grammar.

Still other researchers have proffered additional views. For example, Wilbur, Goodhart, and Fuller (1989) have shown that a syntactic explanation only is not sufficient. In addition, within an interactive theoretical framework, Paul and his collaborators (e.g., Paul, 1993a, 1993b; Paul & O'Rourke, 1988; Paul & Quigley, 1994a) have argued that it is both a knowledge and processing issue.

Much of the recent debate on syntax cannot be fully understood or appreciated without a good rendition of the early investigations by Quigley and his collaborators (e.g., Quigley, Power, & Steinkamp, 1977; Quigley, Smith, & Wilbur, 1974; Quigley, Wilbur, & Montanelli, 1974, 1976; see also the reviews in Paul & Quigley, 1994a and Russell, Quigley, & Power, 1976). First, the work of Quigley and his collaborators is synthesized and presented. Then, the major conclusions relative to quantitative and qualitative development of syntax by children and adolescents who are deaf are discussed. Finally, the findings of later studies relative to these issues and the explanatory adequacy issue are provided.

Quigley and his associates developed a standardized and criterion-referenced syntax test, the Test of Syntactic Abilities (TSA; Quigley, Steinkamp, Power, & Jones, 1978). This test was administered to a representative sample of hearing students between the ages of 8 and 10 years, inclusive, and to a national, stratified random sample of students with hearing impairment between the ages of 10 and 19 years, inclusive. In addition to the age variable, other important characteristics of these students were (Quigley et al., 1978; p. 1):

- IQ of 80 or higher on the performance scales of the Wechsler Intelligence Scale for Children (WISC), the Wechsler Adult Intelligence Scale (WAIS), or comparable tests;
- Hearing Threshold Level (Better Ear Average) of 90 dB or higher (ISO) at 500, 1000, or 2000 Hz;
- Age at onset of hearing impairment of 24 months or younger; and
- No apparent disabilities in addition to hearing impairment other than corrected visual defects.

Quigley and his associates focus on nine major syntactic structures; some examples of these structures are illustrated below.

Structures	*Examples*
Negation	The girl will not read the journal.
	The boy did not do his homework.
Conjunction	I like basketball and hockey.
	She caught and punished the cat.
Disjunction and Alternation	I read the paper but not the journal.
	She is either sick or tired.
Question Formation	
Yes/No	Did you do your homework?
Wh-	What is your name?
Tag	Mary married John, didn't she?
Verb Processes	
e.g., Passive	The girl was kissed by the boy.
Truncated	The window was hit.
Pronominalization	
e.g., reflexive	Mother bought herself a car.
Relativization	The boy who kissed the girl ran away.
Complementation	
e.g., that-clause	That John was crazy was obvious to his students.
infinitive	I would like for you to kiss my mother-in-law.

These investigators provided information in two broad areas: (1) the order of difficulty of the various syntactic structures for students, both deaf and hearing, and (2) the frequency of occurrence of each structure in a reading series from Houghton-Mifflin (McKee, Harrison, McCowen, Lehr, & Durr, 1966). The data on order of difficulty are presented in Table 3-3.

Relative to syntactic knowledge, Quigley and his researchers reported that most 18- to 19-year-old students with profound hearing impairment performed inferiorly to the 8- to 9-year-old hearing students on all structures assessed. That is, the syntactic development of students who are deaf was quantitatively slower than that of hearing students. Nevertheless, a perusal of Table 3-3 indicates the other major conclusion: students with profound hearing impairment were learning the structures in a manner similar to that of younger hearing students (i.e., qualitatively similar). That is, the order of difficulty of the structures

TABLE 3-3   Order of difficulty of syntactic structures in Quigley, Wilbur, Power, Montanelli, & Steinkamp (1976)

Structures	Across Ages	Age 10	Age 18	Gain
Negation				
be	79%	60%	86%	26%
modals	78	58	87	29
have	74	57	78	21
do	71	53	82	28
means	76	57	83	26
Conjunction				
deletion	74	59	86	27
conjoining	72	56	86	30
Disjunction &				
Alternation	36	22	59	37
Question Formation				
yes/no	74	48	90	42
wh-	66	44	80	36
tag	57	46	63	17
means	66	46	78	32
Verb Processes				
tense sequencing	63	54	72	18
auxiliaries	54	52	71	19
means	58	53	71	18
Pronominalization				
backward	70	49	85	36
personal	67	51	88	37
possessive adj.	65	42	82	40
reflexives	50	21	73	52
poss. pronouns	48	34	64	30
means	60	39	78	39
Relativization				
processing	68	59	76	17
embedding	53	51	59	8
referents	42	27	56	29
means	54	46	63	18
Complementation				
infinitives & gerunds	55	50	63	13

Source: Based on information in Quigley, Wilbur, Power, Montanelli & Steinkamp (1976). See Quigley et al. (1976) for additional examples and detailed descriptions.

was similar for students, both deaf and hearing. Furthermore, based on the presence of syntactic structures in the written productions of students with profound hearing impairment (see Chapter 4), it was argued that these students (and second-language students) were making errors and using strategies similar to those of hearing students. Thus, the acquisition of syntax, and possibly English, was a developmental process for students who are deaf, similar to the developmental process of hearing students at younger ages. These findings support the notion of a knowledge hypothesis relative to the quantitative and qualitative aspects of syntactic development.

Quigley and his collaborators were also able to document a huge mismatch between the appearance of the specific structures and their understanding by students who are deaf. Given this condition, the researchers argued that the work and time teachers spent on modifying materials were probably of limited value due to the immense task before them. As a result, the researchers have developed language and reading materials (Quigley & King, 1981, 1982, 1983, 1984; Quigley, Paul, McAnally, Rose & Payne, 1990, 1991) specially designed for this group of students who are deaf. The use of specially-designed materials is another area of contentious debate (e.g., see discussions in King & Quigley, 1985; Paul & Quigley, 1994a). This issue is explored in some depth in Chapters 7 and 8, which deal with instruction of reading and writing.

It should be underscored that the work and findings of Quigley and his collaborators focused on syntactic comprehension on a sentential level. Different, and perhaps conflicting, findings have been observed for studies that focused on syntactic comprehension beyond the sentential level. The work of McGill-Franzen and Gormley (1980) is representative of this line of research. These researchers explored the ability of students with profound hearing impairment to understand truncated passive sentences, for example, *The window was broken; The bike was stolen.* McGill-Franzen and Gormley (1980) presented the sentences in isolation (similar to the format of Quigley and collaborators) and in context (e.g., short paragraphs). The researchers found that the subjects with profound hearing impairment obtained significantly superior scores on structures presented in context. It was concluded that these students do not have difficulty with syntax; that is, this difficulty was the result of test artifacts. Finally, the works of McGill-Franzen and Gormley and others (e.g., Ewoldt, 1981) have lent support to the notion that students who are deaf do not overrely on text-based information in attempts to interpret sentences. This seems to suggest that it is possible for the students to by-pass text information as implicated in a pure whole-language approach, specifically a top-down approach (see Chapter 2).

Difficulty with Syntax: The Knowledge and Processing Hypotheses

It is possible to reconcile the differences in the research on sentential and intersentential comprehension of syntax. Two broad hypotheses have been proposed: knowledge and processing (e.g., Lillo-Martin, Hanson, & Smith, 1991, 1992; Paul & Quigley, 1994a). The knowledge hypothesis is discussed here relative to text variables. The processing hypothesis is discussed in the section on reader-based variables.

Relative to the knowledge hypothesis, McGill-Franzen and Gormley (1980) seem to indicate that the problem is mainly one of text or test artifact. That is, students only have problems understanding syntax on a sentential level. In their view, the use of syntax on a sentential level is an inappropriate measure of reading comprehension. With the use of natural stories, their research seems to show that the students could understand the stories despite their difficulty with syntax on a sentential level.

The work of McGill-Franzen and Gormley (1980) has been criticized (e.g., see Robbins & Hatcher, 1981; Paul & Quigley, 1994a). It is argued that, by using highly familiar reading materials, the students with profound hearing impairment did not have to pay close attention to the details of the story; that is, very little knowledge about the story was text dependent. These readers might have been able to respond to questions about the story without reading it or without even understanding the language (vocabulary, syntax) in which the story was written.

That students who are deaf have difficulty with sentence structures (e.g., syntax), as exemplified by the work of Quigley, has also been supported by other research on the use of context. For example, Israelite (1981) found that the use of context did not assist the students' interpretation of sentences. In a study discussed previously (e.g., deVilliers & Pomerantz, 1992), it was hypothesized that students either have difficulty utilizing syntactic information in sentences or utilizing effective reading strategies. deVilliers and Pomerantz (1992) found that students had difficulty with inferring meanings of words and in inferring syntactic information about the words.

Thus far, the evidence indicates that children and adolescents who are deaf have difficulty with knowledge and use (i.e., application) of syntax, either via the use of incidental or deliberate texts. Without an adequate understanding of syntax (and vocabulary), the students are not able to infer effectively information about words and content. This is a partial explanation of the bottom-up and top-down processing problems of students who are deaf (see also, Kelly, 1995; Paul, 1996; Paul & Quigley, 1994a). As noted by Paul (1996):

> ... the inadequate ability to use context cues reflects difficulty in other written language variables, notably, orthography, morphophonology, syntax, and breadth and depth of vocabulary knowledge. (p. 11)

As discussed later in the chapters on first-language and second-language literacy instruction, one of the most important implications of this line of research is that syntax and other language structures need to be taught or learned by both students who are deaf and students for whom English is a second language. That is, these students need to learn about specific structures that appear in the text: vocabulary, syntax, and anaphora, to name a few. How this is to be done from an instructional viewpoint and whether it can be done are among the main topics of those chapters.

From another perspective, it has been argued that the reading problems of students who are deaf are characterized mainly by a processing problem, rather than a knowledge deficit. The processing issue is rather complex and has been influenced by information-processing models, particularly those that focus on the processing in short-term working memory (e.g., Daneman, Nemeth, Stainton, & Huelsmann, in press; Hanson, 1989, 1991; Lillo-Martin et al., 1991, 1992). It is not always obvious that there are educational implications of this line of research. Furthermore, this research thrust presents the strongest evidence that the reading process of readers with hearing impairment is qualitatively similar to that of readers with typical hearing.

Metaphorical Language

Although metaphorical language is discussed here as a text-based issue, it should be clear that this complex aspect involves both text-based and reader-based processing. Perhaps the best example is to use a now famous sentence by Gough (1984): "A woman needs a man like a fish needs a bicycle" (p. 225). In discussing this sentence, Gough (1984) remarks that a good reader must:

> . . . among other things, discern that MAN is a noun, not a verb, and that it is the object of the verb NEEDS, not the subject of that verb; he must, in short, discover the grammatical relations among the words in order to arrive at the meaning of the sentence. If he is to appreciate that meaning, he must draw upon his knowledge of men and women, fishes and bicycles. And if he is to understand its significance, he must integrate it into the discourse of which it is a part. (p. 225)

There are numerous other examples of metaphorical and figurative usage in English. Readers often encounter figures of speech such as simile *(He ran around like a chicken without a head)* and personification *(The sun smiled broadly today)*. Additional examples include figurative expressions such as the following: *It's raining cats and dogs* and *She's driving me up the wall*. In fact, it has been remarked that over two-thirds of the English language contains metaphorical expressions, including figure of speech and the use of words with multimeanings (e.g., Giorcelli, 1982; Paul, 1984; Payne, 1982). Much of the expansion of figurative language in English entails the use of multimeaning words (e.g., *run*, *back*, *check*) and verb-particle phrases (e.g., *look up*, *run into*). Consider the following examples:

1. I could not see the *hands* of the clock.
2. She *ran into* an old friend yesterday.
3. *Look* me *up* when you *get into* town.
4. She was *red with anger*.
5. He has a *green thumb*.

Research on metaphorical expressions and usage is difficult to conduct because of the numerous interactions and influence of text-based and reader-based variables. For example, Conley (1976) reported that students who are deaf had difficulty with figurative expressions; however, some of the expressions were embedded into syntax that has been shown to be complex and difficult for these students, for example, relative clauses, complements, and passive voice (see the information in Table 3-3 presented previously). Even when investigators controlled for vocabulary and syntax, many students who are deaf did not perform as well as hearing peers. Some results can be found in the study by Giorcelli (1982) on figurative expressions (e.g., analogical and syllogistic reasoning), by Payne and Quigley (1987) on verb-particle combinations, and by Paul and Gustafson (1991) on words with multimeaning meanings.

There are several studies that indicate that children and adolescents who are deaf can learn to comprehend some aspects of metaphorical and figurative expressions. To obtain success, it is necessary to control for certain text features such as vocabulary and syntax and to show the students that a literal interpretation of such expressions is not acceptable (e.g., Iran-Nejad, Ortony, & Rittenhouse, 1981). It might also be helpful to provide sufficient contextual information so that the students can figure out the interpretation of the expressions (e.g., Houck, 1982; Page, 1981). This line of research (especially its caveats) is similar to that discussed previously on understanding both vocabulary and syntax via the use of sufficient context cues. In addition, these students might even be able to learn the metaphorical expressions *as a whole*, and vocabulary and syntax do not preclude this endeavor (e.g., Wilbur, Fraser, & Fruchter, 1981). Nevertheless, there seems to be a strong relationship between knowledge and comprehension of figurative language and reading comprehension level (e.g., Fruchter, Wilbur, & Fraser, 1984; Orlando & Shulman, 1989). That is, good readers are able to comprehend figurative language significantly better than poor readers.

Thus, although students who are deaf might have the cognitive ability to learn figurative expressions, they might not possess the independent skills to accomplish this task during extensive reading opportunities. As an analogy, it is possible to teach words and their meanings to the students, but it is much more efficient and effective if the students can become independent word learners. In other words, teachers still need to improve both bottom-up (word identification) and top-down (comprehension) skills of students who are deaf. Otherwise, the teaching of vocabulary, syntax, figurative language, and other text features becomes an isolated, context-specific endeavor.

Research on Selected Reader-Based Variables

There is a growing interest in research on reader-based variables, although this broad line of research is not as extensive as that on selected text-based variables. With respect to hearing students, it is well established that reading comprehension is affected markedly by reader-based factors such as prior knowledge and metacognition (i.e., thinking about your own thinking processes during reading) (e.g., see reviews in Baker & Brown, 1984; Paris, Wasik & Turner, 1991; Pearson & Fielding, 1991). There is some research on the effects of prior knowledge and metacognition in students with severe to profound hearing impairment (e.g., Strassman, 1992; Yamashita, 1992). Relative to students who are deaf, other important reader-based variables are modes of communication (i.e., oralism, signed systems, and American Sign Language) and internal coding strategies in short-term working memory (e.g., phonological-based, sign-based, print-based, or combinations). After synthesizing the research in these areas, some implications for instruction are discussed. These implications provide the background for the information in the chapters on instruction later in this text.

Prior Knowledge and Metacognition

In discussing these two variables, it is important to remember that a reader might have skills in one area but not in the other. For example, some readers might have some prior knowledge about a topic—let's say about *bats*—but might not apply or use this knowledge in making inferences or interpreting aspects of a story about *bats*. Instructional lessons along this line tend to activate prior knowledge and show readers how such knowledge can be used to comprehend or interpret parts of a story (e.g., see discussions in Paris, Wasik, & Turner, 1991; Pearson & Fielding, 1991). This is, in one sense, similar to the notion of understanding the unknown information in the story by relating it to the known (in the readers' heads) or vice versa.

On the other hand, readers might understand the need to apply what they know; however, they might not have sufficient knowledge or background information with which to work. In words, the reader does not have sufficient prior knowledge about a specific topic, and it becomes critical for the teacher to enrich their background in an interactive, meaningful manner (e.g., class discussions, field trips, video tapes, suggested readings, etc.).

It should not be surprising that many readers who are deaf and other poor readers have difficulty with both prior knowledge and metacognitive skills. This affects, for example, their ability to answer inferential questions, that is, questions that require readers to supply missing information or to connect two parts of the text in order to answer the questions. There are some inferential questions that have no explicit answers, for example, application questions. The answers to these questions must come from the readers' heads (i.e., prior knowledge).

The focus on higher-level reading processes has led to the recent argument that reading is a cognitive or reasoning activity. If improvements are made in the thinking or reasoning skills of students who are deaf, there should be concomitant improvements in their reading comprehension. As stated by Erickson:

> The evaluative, inferential reading comprehension act, among other things, is a culturally-loaded, linguistic, metacognitive response to the printed word . . . Inferential and critical reading should be taught as natural extensions of the thinking process. (1987, p. 293)

Erickson's remarks should be interpreted with caution. What is not always stated explicitly is that making inferences during the process of reading also requires fluency with the lower-level word identification skills (e.g., see Kelly, 1995; Paul, 1993a, 1993b; Paul & Quigley, 1994a). To repeat: word identification facilitates comprehension and comprehension facilitates word identification. Thus, it is possible to improve the thinking and reasoning skills of students who are deaf without ever affecting their ability to read and comprehend text-based English materials.

This was alluded to previously in the discussion of the research by Ewoldt (1981) and McGill-Franzen and Gormley (1980). In fact, it is not difficult to find the few studies with evidence that students with severe to profound hearing impairment can use their prior knowledge to comprehend aspects of the text (e.g., Andrews & Mason, 1991; Ewoldt, Israelite, & Dodds, 1992; Kluwin, Getson, & Kluwin, 1980; Yamashita, 1992; see also the reviews in Kelly, 1995; King & Quigley, 1985; Paul & Quigley, 1994a). In addition, some studies have shown that these students' metacognitive skills can be improved with intervention (e.g., Akamatsu, 1988). Nevertheless, many of these students still have inadequate bottom-up or word-identification skills and have attempted to employ a top-down strategy in interpreting or comprehending the text. In most cases, this strong top-down approach can lead students to give misinterpretations of the text or to provide additional, extraneous, irrelevant answers to questions that can typically be answered with an understanding of the information in the text.

Two recent investigations with students who are deaf are synthesized as exemplars of the limited research on the effects of prior knowledge and metacognition on the comprehension of textual information. Strassman (1992) was interested in the metacognitive knowledge of these students relative to school-based reading materials. She studied students with severe to profound hearing impairment between the ages of 14 years and 20 years old. The researcher videotaped her interviews with students, which were conducted on an individual basis. The content of the interview was based on information contained in the Reading Comprehension Interview (Wixson, Bosky, Yochum, & Alvermann, 1984).

Analyses of the videotapes revealed that the students could be labeled as passive readers. Strassman remarked that these students had no clear understanding of expectations or goals for school-based reading activities. Although they learned skills for reading, "they seemed to mechanically employ the techniques that they had been taught" (p. 328). In this case, students who are deaf did not understand the *how, when, why, what* aspects of metacognitive strategies (see discussion in Chapter 2).

In another study, Yamashita (1992) examined the interrelations among prior knowledge, metacognition, and reading comprehension. The researcher defined reading comprehension as the ability to answer questions on different levels (e.g., see Raphael & McKinney, 1983). Subjects in the study had hearing impairment with a range from 36 dB to 120 dB pure-tone average across the speech frequencies in the unaided better ear. Students attended either a middle-school (e.g., age 12) or a high-school program (e.g., age 14 and above) and were enrolled in either an oral or total-communication program. It was not statistically possible to compare oral and total-communication students. However, the researcher found that both prior knowledge and metacognition were significantly related to reading comprehension for the students in this sample. More interesting, it was observed that metacognition has the strongest effects for all measures of reading comprehension, that is, measures involving standardized tests and researcher-developed tests.

English-Based Signed Systems and English Literacy

For students who are deaf, another important reader-based variable is proficiency in the use of sign communication skills, particularly the English-based signed systems. A persistent, controversial issue in the field of deafness has been the effects of the English-based signed systems on the development of English literacy (e.g., see reviews in Moores, 1987; Paul & Quigley, 1990; 1994a; Wilbur, 1987). The intent in this section is threefold. One, a brief synthesis of the major findings with regard to the effects of signed systems is presented. Two, a discussion of the meaning of the so-called relationship between the use of signed systems and the development of English literacy is provided. Finally, the section ends with some directions for future research endeavors.

A review of the literature reveals three major generalizations, at least, on the effects of the English-based signed systems: (1) there is not a substantial amount of data available; (2) it is possible to find successful students who have been exposed to a particular system such as cued speech or signing exact English; and (3) there is no widespread agreement on the best system, and thus, none of the systems, in its entirety, is used widely (e.g., see reviews in Moores, 1987; Paul & Quigley, 1994a; see also another point of view in Luetke-Stahlman & Luckner, 1991). There is some research to suggest that the systems that are most representative of the language of English hold the most promise of success (e.g., see Luetke-Stahlman, 1988a, 1988b; see also the review in Paul & Quigley, 1994a). In essence, this finding refers to the use of systems such as seeing essential English, signing exact English, and cued speech.

The lack of a consensus with regard to research effectiveness certainly contributes to the widespread adoption of a communication mode labeled total communication (as a method) or simultaneous communication (e.g., see discussion in Paul & Quigley, 1990, 1994a). However, it is difficult to describe the signing behaviors of the practitioners of this mode because of the variance in the execution of the signs. In addition, there are no established rules associated with either TC as a method or simultaneous communication. In any case, there are other factors that have influenced the use of TC or simultaneous communication, namely, education and exposure, facility in the use of this mode, and a general dissatisfaction or disillusion on the part of educators toward the idea of a best language/communication method. With a focus on individualized instruction, many educators seem to feel that this notion applies to the use of any instructional method, including a language/communication mode. In other words, any instructional method or mode needs to be individualized to cater to the specific needs of the students.

The lack of a best communication system, however, is really related to the problem of the poorly understood relationship between English-based signing and English literacy skills. In fact, this question is as ambiguous, broad, and complex as the relationship between language and thought (e.g., see research review in Paul & Quigley, 1994a). Much of the current language/thought debate has moved away from the broad, general effects of one entity (e.g., language) on the other one (e.g., thought) because of the difficulty in investigating these effects. The focus now seems to be on the nature of the interactive relationships between these two broad entities. Whether the emphasis should be on holistic variables or on specific variables within each domain is typically influenced by the metatheories of the researchers. More importantly, no one believes that there is a one-to-one relationship between the entity of language and the entity of cognition.

This should shed some light on the problem with previous investigations on the relationships between the signed systems and English literacy skills. To inquire what effects signing exact English has on the development of English, as an example, is simply too broad. How, might it be asked, could an investigator answer the following question, as an example, What effects does spoken English have on the development of English literacy skills? Granted that proficiency in spoken English does have some pervasive effects, there are several other important questions.

1. What does it mean to have proficiency in spoken English? Is knowledge of spoken English the same as knowledge of the conversational form of English, whether in speech or signs?
2. Does the loss of or lack of knowledge of the ability to speak affect the ability to read and write?
3. What does it mean to have proficiency in reading and writing skills?
4. Is knowledge of spoken (or the conversational form of) English sufficient for reading and writing development?
5. What effects, if any, do instructional and curricular variables have on the development of English literacy skills?
6. In addition to cognitive and linguistic variables, are there any effects of social and emotional variables?

If the phrase *spoken English* is replaced with the phrase *signed English,* then my points with regard to the disillusions of practitioners and the language/thought metaphor might make some sense. Just because it is found that some students who are deaf and who are proficient in cued speech or signing exact English have high levels of literacy, this does not mean that cued speech or signing exact English is SOLELY responsible for the development of this high English literacy level as defined by standardized or other formal tests.

There are several directions for future research that could be stated. In fact, some of them have been suggested by an earlier, comprehensive text on reading (e.g., King & Quigley, 1985). In my view, research should be conducted within the three broad categories: empirical (e.g., quantitative), interpretative (e.g., qualitative, ethnographic), and critical (e.g., postmodernist, deconstructionist). One of the most important empirical lines of research is that on the notion of accessibility. It is still not clear what children and adolescents who are deaf are accessing or acquiring when they are exposed to the English-based signed systems. This information seems to be necessary to complement what is known about language acquisition and deafness. In fact, the accessibility issue is one of the major arguments in support of American Sign Language/English bilingual programs (see Chapter 6).

Within the interpretative domain, there is still a great need for understanding teacher-student classroom interactions. This should add to the existing cognitive/linguistic knowledge (i.e., requisites) of what is necessary for becoming highly literate readers and writers. As argued in Chapters 1 and 2, literacy can be construed as a social-cognitive interactive process. Thus, it is critical not only to study the student while reading or writing alone but also to observe the reading and writing activities in a social constructionist environment such as a classroom. Finally, within the literary critical domain, one can explore (1) whether literacy is an oppressive goal for certain members of the population or (2) whether the ability to achieve a high level of literate thought is critically dependent upon the development of reading and writing skills.

It should be reemphasized that all three types of research domains (i.e., empirical, interpretative, and critical) are important, and all three are necessary for handling the myriad of research questions available. In the investigation of the signed systems and English literacy development, there has been a persistent need for more systematic inquiries that proceed beyond studying the overall general effects or relationships. Clearly, there is more to literacy than just having proficiency in the conversational form (i.e., speech and/or signs) of the print.

Internal Mediating Systems

Understanding the link between the phonemes of speech of a phonetic language and the graphemes of print seems to be one critical factor in reading an alphabetic system such as English. In the research discussed previously on syntax, it has been suggested that the lack of this understanding contributes to the processing deficit of poor readers, including poor readers who are deaf. Thus, the foundation of literacy requires an awareness that speech can be segmented into phonemes, which are represented by an alphabetic orthography (e.g., see discussions in Brady & Shankweiler, 1991; Leybaert, 1993; Paul & Quigley, 1994a; Shankweiler & Liberman, 1989; Templeton & Bear, 1992). One of the debates between the proponents of whole-language researchers and those associated with the phonics and other bottom-up skills is whether the knowledge of the alphabet system needs to be taught or allowed to develop during the process of reading (e.g., see discussions in Adams, 1990a, 1990b, 1994).

It is argued here that fluent word reading, representing a working knowledge of the alphabet system, is critically dependent on the use of a phonological-based code in short-term working memory (e.g., see Hanson, 1989, 1991; Leybaert, 1993; Paul & Quigley, 1994a; Tzeng, 1993). This line of research is the impetus for the passage and discussion at the beginning of the chapter (Hanson). As discussed in Chapter 6 on ASL/English bilingualism, it has implications for the teaching of English as a second language. Most important, the major emphasis is on whether the development of English literacy of students who are deaf is similar or different as compared with that of students with typical hearing ability.

In this section, the purpose is fourfold: to describe briefly (1) the nature of the coding strategies used by individuals who are deaf; (2) the reason why the use of a phonologically based code is important for reading; (3) the case for the qualitative similarity of literacy; and (4) the relation of the development of a phonologically based code to literacy instruction. There is a reasonable amount of research on the nature of the coding strategies used by individuals who are deaf. Summaries can be found elsewhere (e.g., Conrad, 1979; Paul & Jackson, 1993; Paul & Quigley, 1990, 1994a). Research on deafness revealed four types of coding used by individuals during either working memory (WM) tasks or during reading tasks. The types of codes are presented in Table 3-4.

Most students with hearing impairment used a nonphonologically based code (relative to a phonetic language such as English). Students who are deaf and who use predominantly a phonological (speech)-based code are better readers than other students who use predominantly a nonphonologically based code (e.g., see Hanson, 1989, 1991; Tzeng, 1993; cf., Gibbs, 1989). Why is the use of a phonologically based code so important? In my view, an eloquent response has been provided by Lillo-Martin et al.:

> In reading and listening, individual words of a sentence must be retained while the grammatical relations among words are determined. Evidence suggests that working

memory is most efficient for verbal material (including written material) when the processing involves phonological coding. For readers suffering from impaired phonological coding in working memory, processing individual words and putting these words together into phrases and sentences can be computationally overloading, impairing overall reading performance. (1991, p. 147)

It should be emphasized that the use of coding is related to the requirements of the task, for example, reading. Thus, the short-term working memory of individuals who are deaf is not deficient per se, but rather, might not be equipped to handle verbo-sequential information effectively. For students who are deaf, it is the inability to use peripheral hearing as an aid in developing the phonological and morphological systems of English. Surprisingly, the relationship between the use of a phonologically based code and literacy ability can also be stated in a similar manner for other individuals with disabilities, for example, learning disability or developmental disability (e.g., see research reviews in Brady & Shankweiler, 1991; Shankweiler & Liberman, 1989). In fact, there seems to be an interrelationship among the use of a phonologically based code, working memory, knowledge of the alphabet system, and literacy ability. This seems to be evidence for an overall qualitative similarity with respect to the development of literacy. Of course, the reasons *why* students who are deaf have difficulty with the use of a phonologically based code are quite different than those associated with individuals with learning disabilities or developmental disabilities. Nevertheless, one source of this difficulty is with the morphophonological system of English.

One of the most important questions for the teaching of literacy is: Can deaf students *learn* to use a phonologically based code in working memory? If the answer is NO, then there are legitimate arguments for a *psychology of deafness*. That is, it can be argued that

TABLE 3-4   Types of internal mediating codes

Internal Code	Brief Description
Sign (e.g., Odom, Blanton, & McIntyre, 1970)	Use of static signs from the English-based signed systems.
Dactylic (e.g., Locke & Locke, 1971)	Use of fingerspelling; 23 different handshapes representing the letters of the alphabet.
Visual (e.g., Blanton, Nunnally, & Odom, 1967)	Use of the configurations associated with the shapes of printed letters; also known as graphemes; analogous to the sight word approach.
Phonological (e.g., Conrad, 1979; Hanson, 1989)	Representations of subvocalizations or the auditory-articulatory movements.
Multiple (e.g., Lichtenstein, 1984, 1985)	Any combination of the codes described above.

English is an unrealistic goal for most students who are deaf (see detailed discussion of this issue in Chapter 6). On the other hand, if the answer is YES, then there is some evidence that working memory for verbo-sequential items can be improved. In addition, there is evidence that teaching students what the alphabet is about, giving them a working knowledge of vowels and consonants, has a marked effect on the acquisition and development of English literacy skills (e.g., Brady & Shankweiler, 1991; Shankweiler & Liberman, 1989).

Future researchers need to be concerned with methods to increase students' knowledge of phonology and morphology. The question of whether phonology can be by-passed is an open debate. The central problem remains, at least relative to most mainstream theories of literacy: It is important to improve students' access to the sound system of English, the system on which the alphabetic principle is based. As stated eloquently by Liberman, Shankweiler, and Liberman (1989):

> Proper application of the alphabetic principle rests on an awareness of the internal phonological (and morphophonological) structure of words that the alphabet represents. . . . Not surprisingly, then, awareness of phonological structures is normally lacking in preliterate children and adults; the degree to which it does exist is the best single predictor of success in learning to read; lack of awareness usually yields to appropriate instruction; and such instruction makes for better readers. That some children have particular difficulty in developing phonological awareness (and in learning to read) is apparently to be attributed to a general deficiency in the phonological component of their natural capacity for language. Thus, these children are also relatively poor in short-term memory for verbal information, in perceiving speech in noise, in producing complex speech patterns, and in finding the words that name objects. All children will benefit from instruction that is intelligently designed to show them what the alphabet is about. (p. 1)

A Final Word

This chapter attempted to show that the literacy development of students who are deaf is qualitatively similar to that of hearing students. This finding has pervasive implications for the use of instructional and curricular materials; that is, similar methods and materials should be used with students who are deaf. This focus on qualitative similarity is important also for other students with disabilities. In essence, there seems to be some fundamental knowledge necessary for the development of English text-based literacy.

One way to view this fundamental knowledge is to think of literacy as a social-cognitive interactive process in which there are interactions between the student and the text and the students and others in a classroom or other group settings. Such interactions depend on, at least, a working knowledge of both word identification and comprehension skills. In addition, although spoken, conversational proficiency in English is important, literacy is much more than just a knowledge of the spoken form of the print. Relative to students who are deaf, there seems to be a need to increase their access to the sound system of English. That this is difficult—and almost impossible for some students—has provided the major impetus for the development of American Sign Language/English bilingual programs. One of the major strategies of these bilingual programs is to teach English through the use of writing and reading activities. Some insights on this technique plus others on the nature of writing are addressed in the next chapter.

Further Readings

BRADLEY, L., & BRYANT, P. (1985). *Rhyme and reason in reading and spelling.* Ann Arbor, MI: University of Michigan Press.

CARR, T., & LEVY, B. (Eds.). (1990). *Reading and its development: Component skills approaches.* New York: Academic Press.

CHALL, J. (1983). *Stages of reading development.* New York: McGraw-Hill.

CLAY, M. (1979). *Reading: The patterning of complex behavior.* Portsmouth, NH: Heinemann.

JENSEN, J. (Ed.). (1984). *Composing and comprehending.* Urbana, IL: National Conference on Research in English.

Kozol, J. (1985). *Illiterate America.* New York: Doubleday.

Chapter *4*

The Development of Writing

> Chances are good that the very first person who invented speech did not do so because she or he was itching to hear someone else hold forth. Similarly, it is a good bet that the person who invented written language did not do so because she or he was yearning for a good book. There would seem to be something fundamentally human about the desire to communicate. Why not capitalize on this desire in beginning instruction on written language? Although this is not at all a new idea, it is worth examining anew in context. (Adams, 1990a, p. 375)

The passage above by Adams (1990a) is representative of the growing interest in and emerging perspective of writing, particularly the development of writing in young children. This is one of several perspectives of recent attempts to understand writing and its relationship to reading, language, and cognitive development (e.g., see discussions in Czerniewska, 1992; Irwin & Doyle, 1992; Mason, 1989). In fact, the existence of multiple views on writing seems to suggest that this endeavor is a more complex activity than previously thought.

Prior to the burgeoning interest in research on American Sign Language and the English-based signed systems, much of the research on the language development of children and adolescents who are deaf focused on written language productions (e.g., see reviews in Kretschmer & Kretschmer, 1978; Paul & Quigley, 1994a). It was hypothesized that a good, consistent understanding of their knowledge of English can be gleaned from the analyses of writing samples. Although some insights are possible, they must be interpreted with caution for several reasons. As argued by Chomsky (1957, 1965, 1988), language performance or production (in this case, speech or sign) does not provide a complete, accurate picture of language competence. This argument can be extended to the *production* of written language. There are many individuals who can neither read nor write well, but who still have proficiency in a language, particularly its conversational form.

In fact, there is some research on this issue with students who are deaf. It can be inferred from the work of Everhart and Marschark (1988) that the written language of these students is not reflective of their proficiency in the use of English-based signed systems or in the use of sign communication in general. In essence, these researchers remarked that "literalness evidenced in written English need not be indicative of the more general cognitive literalness assumed from such results by previous researchers" (p. 191).

The plan for the chapter is as follows. A brief discussion of the major views of writing is presented, using, as much as possible, the framework provided in Chapter 1: cognitive information-processing, naturalism, and social-constructionism. The latter two views seem to focus mostly on the process of writing; however, comments are often made about the products and processes of writing. After this, the chapter focuses on a representative sample of the research on written language with both children and adolescents who are deaf *and* those who are hearing. The information in this chapter is related to that presented on reading in Chapters 2 and 3. The intent is twofold: (1) to highlight why writing is an extremely difficult task for many, if not most, students with severe to profound hearing impairment and (2) to provide a conceptual framework for the instructional strategies discussed in Chapters 7 and 8.

Models of Writing

As discussed in Chapter 1, the depiction of models is dependent upon the metatheoretical views of the individuals performing this task. Whatever scheme is used, it is important to note that there is a marked influence of the knowledge level of the individual on the development of literacy skills. Hillocks (1986) differentiated four major types of knowledge. The first type is labeled declarative knowledge of substance, which refers to the information base for writing a piece of work. The second type is called procedural knowledge of substance, which refers to the tasks of recalling, ordering, and transforming the available information base. The third type is labeled declarative knowledge of form, which is the knowledge of grammar, genre, and style. Finally, the fourth type is procedural knowledge of form, which is the ability to search for and produce the appropriate form. These labels are somewhat similar to those used to describe metacognitive aspects of the reader (e.g., see Paris, Wasik, & Turner, 1991). Although the scheme discussed by Hillocks (1986) is considered feasible, there are other ways of viewing the knowledge of writers as discussed in a review by Montague (1990).

Perhaps a productive way to understand the scheme of Hillocks (1986) is to discuss literacy within the framework of current theoretical perspectives. Based on a synthesis of the research literature, it is possible to separate the component of writing from reading and discuss it relative to the three broad theoretical models. As mentioned in Chapter 1, cognitive information-processing theorists attempt to show that both reading and writing are interactive and consist of a number of subprocesses. These theorists are interested in exploring the effects of subprocesses on performing special tasks. Within this model, there is an attention component; thus, competence in reading and writing is defined as the amount of attention that needs to be given to the use of the subprocesses. The less amount of attention needed—say on short-term memory tasks—the more effort and attention can be given to the important task of comprehension. This makes writing a more efficient process for the student.

In discussing subprocesses, the act of writing is said to entail planning, composing (also translating), and revising (also reviewing) (e.g., see Flower & Hayes, 1980). For example, during the planning stage, students might use their prior knowledge to choose a topic, generate ideas, identify their audience, and devise a tentative organizational plan. The students begin writing during the composing or translating stage. This is often described as tentative writing because there might be several drafts. Revisions can occur during and after composition. Writers attempt to polish, alter, expand, and clarify their manuscripts. It should be highlighted that these are not necessarily discrete stages. Writers can revise their plans or plan their revisions (e.g., see discussion in Tierney & Pearson, 1983). Relative to subprocesses, there are other concepts that have been proposed, for example, idea and text production, identifying choices, making decisions, and carrying out the plans (e.g., see Scardamalia, Bereiter, & Goelman, 1982). The focus is on dividing a complex psychological process into smaller components for analysis and description.

Relative to the attention issue, or limited capacity processors, writers operate on several levels that include activities such as selecting topics, planning and organizing ideas, making decisions on what information to include, and engaging in self-monitoring during the stages of composing and revising their productions (e.g., see discussions in Hillocks, 1986; Montague, 1990). Within this purview, it is typically argued that writers must not expend too much effort and time on the lower-level aspects of writing such as mechanics (e.g., spelling, grammar, punctuation, etc.). These lower-level skills should become automatic processes so that writers can focus on the far more important higher-level skills such as organization, intent, and audience.

With a focus on the scheme of planning, composing, and revising (e.g., Flower & Hayes, 1980; Tierney & Pearson, 1983), there are two major forces that have changed the face of writing instruction and writing evaluation. First, there has been a shift in the teacher's role—moving from an expert concerned with the correction of errors on the products of writing to a catalyst, facilitator, and even a participant in the writing process with the students. The second force has been the effects of this process of evaluation (planning, composing, revising) on the development of theories of writing (e.g., McCormick, Busching, & Potter, 1992). In essence, the very act of reviewing or revising is a reaction to the evaluative aspects of writing by either the teacher or the students' peers. It has been argued that this evaluative component needs to be on-going and dynamic, taking place throughout the entire writing process, which results in a *finished* product.

Another perspective on this evaluative aspect relative to the concepts of planning, composing, and revising has been presented by McCormick et al. (1992), who interpreted the work of Flower and Hayes and colleagues:

The act of writing is assumed to be a goal-directed thinking process, guided by the writer's own growing network of goals. In order to create text, the writer engages in four kinds of mental processes: *planning, translating* mental images into words, *reviewing* what has been written, and *monitoring* the entire process. Knowledge of topic (specific domain knowledge), knowledge of audience (reader's background, beliefs, and values), and the availability of writing plans (a generalized sense of how to produce the text) are stored in the writer's long-term memory. The specific writing task creates additional kinds of knowledge: the writer's concept of the "rhetorical problem" at hand and the writer's concept of the "text produced so far." (McCormick et al., 1992, p. 313)

There is still much research to be done relative to the specific links between reading and writing (e.g., see discussion in Fitzgerald, 1992). The cognitive information-processing perspective has dominated the research on short-term memory and reading comprehension in deafness, as discussed in Chapter 3. Nevertheless, there are growing efforts to understand writing from other perspectives. A description of the reading-writing connection within the cognitive information-processing framework has been provided by Tierney and Pearson (1983):

... what drives reading and writing is this desire to make sense of what is happening—to make things cohere. A writer achieves that fit by deciding what information to include and what to withhold. The reader accomplishes that fit by filling in gaps ... or making uncued connections. All readers, like all writers, ought to strive for this fit between the whole and the parts and among the parts. (p. 572)

The naturalistic position has been influenced by the cognitive work of Piaget and the language work of Chomsky, especially with the focus on innate cognitive and linguistic structures. Some of the more salient aspects include the assumptions that the child constructs his or her own knowledge, and that this process proceeds through developmental stages. As discussed in Chapter 1, this position also seems to be an outgrowth of a cognitive information-processing approach known as top-down approaches. One prominent example is the psycholinguistic-transactional model of Goodman (e.g., 1985), more popularly known as the whole-language approach. Goodman also incorporates the transactional view of Rosenblatt (1989) in his model, which he claims is essentially a language learning model applied to literacy (see discussion in Chapter 1).

The naturalistic position is most heavily influenced by phenomenological philosophy (e.g., see discussion in McCormick, 1988). As was noted in Chapter 1, phenomenological theory has also influenced cognitive information-processing models known as interactive approaches. However, the most pervasive effects can be noted with naturalistic models. In essence, phenomenological theorists maintain that individuals need to interpret the natural world and give it personal meaning. Meaning resides in the self and all events and objects of the natural world are interpreted in a subjective manner. The tools for interpretation are speech and written language. It is argued that language is a natural part of the world.

This heavy emphasis on language is also related to the development of reading and writing, as mentioned previously, relative to Goodman's model. In fact, it is argued that reading and writing are based on the acquisition of oral language. Thus, from a psycholinguistic perspective (e.g., Goodman, 1985), oral and written language share similar basic characteristics. The major characteristic—and one that forms the basis of the whole-language approach—is that both oral and written language are and should be developed naturally. This has been interpreted to mean that language acquisition proceeds from whole to part and that there is no hierarchy of skills. As remarked by McCarthey and Raphael:

... words are learned before letters, stories are read before sentences, meaning is acquired within the context of reading and writing. Learning to read and write involves actively reading and writing, rather than learning to master specific skills or participating in formal instruction. (1992, p. 9)

It seems that naturalistic theories form the foundations of many ASL/English bilingual programs (see Chapter 6). The main problem with this model for bilingual programs is the interpretation of *oral* language. This is interpreted broadly by ASL/English bilingual proponents to include any form of conversational language (i.e., speech or sign). However, as argued in Chapter 6, that is not the interpretation of naturalistic theorists. In fact, naturalistic theorists emphasize the reciprocal relationship between oral and written language, and the *oral* aspect has referred to the spoken component of a language. As discussed also in Chapter 6, this oral-literacy (reading/writing) reciprocity is not the same as the sign-literacy (reading/writing) one.

The third major area is social constructionism. Several influences on this philosophy can be delineated, for example, the works of Vygotsky (e.g., 1962; see discussion in McCormick, 1988; and other phenomenologists) and literary critical theorists. The main tenet is that knowledge is socially constructed; that is, it is a social artifact that is maintained and supported by a community of scholars in agreement. In essence, knowledge is not based on the quantitative measure of an objective reality; rather, it is the result of social interactions. Thought, language, literacy, and learning (i.e., all higher-level cognitive processes) are all social and cultural in nature. Initially, there is an internalization of interactions that occurs between individuals. Subsequently, this internalization process occurs within the individual. The internalization process is dependent upon the guidance of adults or the collaboration of peers with advanced skills or knowledge. Thus, mature members of a particular culture can play an important role in assisting in the learning acquisition process of the less mature members.

The last point has important implications for teachers working on literacy development. Some children might not learn effectively via a naturalistic approach, that is, one in which they are totally responsible for their learning. An example of this situation has been discussed by McCarthey and Raphael (1992):

... children may scribble in their early attempts to write. Simply leaving them alone to explore print and "naturally" develop their writing ability may not be effective for all learners. Vygotskian perspectives suggest that students learn about the functions of print, and about the conventional forms that allow print to communicate, through interaction with a more knowledgeable adult or peer. Through the modeling and thinking aloud of the more expert person, students learn the role of writing within our culture, the relationships between writing and reading, different ways of thinking when planning to read and write, and so forth. (p. 17)

Consider, for example, the task of answering questions on different levels, known as Question-Answer Relationships, QARs (e.g., Raphael, 1984). Within this framework, the teacher can ask the question and model his or her response to the question. This modeling behavior might include strategies such as rereading a paragraph, considering the sources or

TABLE 4-1   Major principles of three broad paradigmatic views of writing

Principles of the Cognitive Information-Processing View

- Reading and writing are interactive and consist of a number of subprocesses.
- Attention is devoted to studying the effects of subprocesses on performing special tasks.
- Writers must not expend too much effort and time on the lower-level aspects of writing such as mechanics (e.g., spelling, grammar, punctuation, etc.). These lower-level skills should become automatic processes so that writers can focus on the far more important higher-levels skills such as organization, intent, and audience.

Principles of the Naturalistic View

- Phenomenological philosophy has heavily influenced this perspective.
- Individuals need to interpret the natural world and give it personal meaning.
- Learning to read and write involves actively reading and writing, rather than learning to master specific skills or participating in formal instruction.

Principles of the Social-Constructionist View

- Knowledge is socially constructed; it is the result of social interactions.
- Thought, language, literacy, and learning are all social and cultural in nature.
- Mature members of a particular culture can play an important role in assisting in the learning acquisition process of the less mature members.

information available from the text and the reader's mind in answering the question, and considering the completeness or accuracy of the answer. It should be underscored, however, that within a social-constructionist view, both the teacher and students contribute to the social construction of knowledge or, in this case, to the answers to the questions.

The major principles associated with these three broad paradigmatic views of the development of writing are delineated in Table 4-1.

Critique of the Three Broad Theoretical Views

The critique presented here is similar to the one provided in Chapter 1 on theories mostly associated with the reading comprehension framework. The difference is that this critique focuses on the macro metatheoretical positions (cognitive information processing, naturalistic, and social constructionist) rather than on the macro positions within a framework such as cognitive information processing (e.g., bottom-up, top-down, and interactive or parallel dual processing). Much of the ensuing information is based on the critiques of Antonacci and Hedley (1994), McCarthey and Raphael (1992), Mitchell (1982), and Samuels and Kamil (1984).

There are several concerns associated with the cognitive information-processing approach. It should be recalled that this approach focuses on the differences between mature learners of literacy and those who are novice or poor readers and writers. Although we have a better understanding of the differences and skills that the novice or poor learners need, there is a very limited understanding of the manner in which the novice or poor learners become more skilled, and, it should be added, whether poor learners can reach functional or high levels of literacy, that is, text-based literacy.

It seems that cognitive information-processing theorists have neglected to include the relationship between the processes of writing and the nature of the writing activities, specifically the goals and purposes. In addition, the writing processes vary relative to other factors such as the experiential and educational background of the writer and the context in which writing occurs. As noted by Calkins (1983, 1986), Graves (1983), and others:

> Denying the importance of such factors may lead to decontextualized learning of subskills or routines, much as we see in some workbook pages from basal reading series. (McCarthey & Raphael, 1992, p. 9)

Perhaps the biggest weakness of the cognitive information-processing models is the notion of linearity, often associated with bottom-up or top-down models and sometimes with interactive models (see discussions in Chapters 1 and 2). This focus is often interpreted as support for the teaching of subskills either prior to or after the process of reading and writing. In many cases, the teaching of subskills might be separate from the meaningful act of literacy. In this sense, the application of the cognitive information-processing models to literacy instruction has been said to be limited (McCarthey & Raphael, 1992; Rosenblatt, 1989). There is too much emphasis on the cognitive aspects and not enough attention has been paid to the social aspects, that is, the environment in which literacy interactions occur.

With its heavy focus on biology, a major problem with the naturalistic approach is its validity, that is, empirical support for the invariant stages (e.g., Piaget, 1980). In addition, it is an open question whether literacy development is related to the physical development of the individual. This debate relates to the Chomsky-Piaget dialogues concerning the notion of maturation versus that of construction (e.g., see Piatelli-Palmarini, 1980). Furthermore, it has led to a split into two major camps of language researchers. One group, primarily linguists by training, is specifically interested in linguistic theory (mostly deductive approaches). The second group, primarily psychologists or psycholinguists, are interested in the data and processes of children (i.e., child language researchers). Finally, the naturalistic approach depends on the acceptance of the notions of assimilation and accommodation; however, there is much debate on the operation of these biological notions (see discussion in Flavell, 1985).

Perhaps a major concern with the naturalistic approach is the seemingly minor role that teachers play in the cognitive and language development of children. The child is construed as an active constructor of meaning, and this meaning-making endeavor is considered to be primarily personal in nature. The contributions of the teacher in a social environment is acknowledged; however, the child is deemed mainly responsible for acquiring and deriving meaning. The breadth and depth of these meanings are related to the physical development of the child in this sociocultural environment. As noted by McCarthey and Raphael (1992):

> While this perspective may recognize that the teacher is critical in enriching or structuring the environment, it is difficult to infer exactly what should be done instructionally.

In sum, while this perspective suggests the kind of environment in which students may acquire the knowledge bases identified by information processing theorists, it fails to provide pedagogical information about how learners actually acquire new knowledge, relying heavily on the belief that such knowledge is simply acquired "naturally." (p. 15)

At first glance, social constructionism appears to be the real *balanced* view because it avoids the assumption that knowledge is totally objective or totally subjective. Social constructionists argue for a *consensus*, which consists of both objective and subjective information to be synthesized, discussed, and agreed upon. This theory also focuses on the importance of recognizing and respecting the diversity of cultures in school classrooms.

The major concern with the social-constructionist view is the ability to test the theory. This framework does not lend itself to either specific components or holistic approaches. Because of the complexity of the social interactions in the classrooms, neither quantitative nor qualitative measures might be sufficient. As discussed in Chapter 5, the main tools of testing social constructionism might be mainly in the critical domain rather than in the empirical (quantitative) or interpretative (qualitative) domains. Perhaps a productive way to understand the complex interactions of children, culture (home and classroom), and literacy is to adopt the format used by literary critical theorists (e.g., deconstructionism).

Table 4-2 presents a critique of some issues relevant to the broad metatheoretical views on the development of writing.

TABLE 4-2   Critique of the three broad views of writing

Cognitive Information-Processing

- Better understanding of skills that novice or poor learners need; however, very limited understanding of the manner in which the novice or poor learners become more skilled.
- Failure to include the relationship between the processes of writing and nature of the writing activities, especially goals and purposes.
- A major problem is the notion of linearity, especially in bottom-up and top-down models and sometimes with interactive models.
- Application to instruction seems to be limited.

Naturalism

- One major problem is validity, due to its focus on biology—for example, support for the stages of Piaget.
- Open question whether literacy development is related to the physical development of the individual.
- In this view, the teacher plays a seemingly minor role in the cognitive and language development of children.

Social Constructionism

- Considered to be a balanced view because it avoids the assumption that knowledge is totally objective or totally subjective.
- Focus is on reaching a consensus, which consists of both objective and subjective information to be synthesized, discussed, and agreed upon.
- Major concern is the ability to test the theory.

Research on Written Language and Hearing Students

In this section, there is a discussion of the representative sample of research studies that have been conducted within each perspective. The focus here will be on writing with the understanding that the bulk of the research has been on reading-writing connections. Previously, much research attention was devoted to writing, separate from the process of reading. This line of inquiry yielded information relative to the products of writing. Until quite recently, this has been the predominant view of the written language development of students who are deaf (e.g., see reviews in Paul & Quigley, 1990; 1994a).

The cognitive information-processing theorists have contributed to our understanding of the underlying structures of both reading and writing. Surprisingly, there is a limited amount of research on the underlying processes *common* to both reading and writing (e.g., Mason, 1989; McCarthey & Raphael, 1992). As mentioned previously, there is consensus, within this view, that the foundations of literacy (reading and writing) require, at least, a working knowledge of the morphophonological system of English. This is the system on which written language is based, that is, the alphabet system (e.g., see discussions in Liberman, Shankweiler, & Liberman, 1989; Templeton & Bear, 1992). This line of research has led to some understanding of the interrelationships among short-term memory, the use of a phonological coding strategy, and reading comprehension (see Chapter 3; see also Hanson, 1989, 1991; Paul & Jackson, 1993).

Another view of the cognitive information-processing contributions can be gleaned from research reviews and metatheoretical analyses (e.g., Hillocks, 1986; McCarthey & Raphael, 1992; for students who are deaf, see reviews in Paul & Jackson, 1993; Paul & Quigley, 1994a). Relative to reading/writing connections, it has been argued that good writers are invariably good readers and that good readers have the potential to become good writers. In essence, good readers do produce more syntactically mature passages with a rich vocabulary than poor readers. It has also been shown that enriched writing experiences tend to affect the reading comprehension levels of students.

There is much research on the effects of reading on writing (e.g., see research review in Adams, 1990a, 1990b). For example, the nature of what students read influences the quality and complexity of their written language productions. Perhaps the most interesting revelation is that good readers are able to produce complex syntheses based on a variety of sources. That is, the synthesis works of good readers are typically reflective of the influences of reading various text materials. It should be highlighted that *reading* in this sense refers to the ability to think critically and reflectively across a broad range of sources.

Finally, within cognitive information-processing models, there has been a comparison of novice versus poor readers with the assumption that such comparison will shed light on what is necessary for improving the literacy development of poor readers. Much of the focus has been on *text* features such as word identification, word meaning, and anaphora. It has been shown that knowledge of text features has a marked influence on reading comprehension and, in some cases, can lead to an improvement of writing. As discussed in Chapter 3 and later on in this chapter, much of the research on deafness and literacy has been influenced by this line of inquiry.

Within the naturalistic paradigm, there has been research interest in children's early writing and their understanding of the concepts of written language (e.g., print awareness, boundaries of words, etc.) This has resulted in a reconceptualization of the role of children's language proficiency in the development of literacy skills (e.g., Clay, 1979; Harste, Burke, & Woodward, 1982). For example, it has been shown that children attempt to make sense of reading and writing quite a long time prior to the beginning of formal instruction in these areas. Children have strategies that they use to understand text or construct meaning, and it seems that some of the strategies require risk taking.

Within the whole-language paradigm, it has been found that children as writers discover meaning as they engage in the writing process. There is a connection between the emerging text and the use of the thought processes. A number of researchers have shown that the development of writing is dependent upon or related to several factors, for example, the drawings of children and the social interactions between and among writers (e.g., Calkins, 1983, 1986; Graves, 1983). Thus, the classroom environment and the interactions within it are important for developing the language, literacy, and learning potential of children (see also, the discussion in Bloome, 1989). As a result, it appears that future investigations will focus on classroom interactions in order to deepen our understanding of the development of literacy.

Despite the many forces that have influenced the naturalistic paradigm, it is safe to conclude that the bulk of this research is driven by a qualitative methodology (e.g., see discussion of this methodology in Lincoln & Guba, 1985). In addition, the naturalistic paradigm seems to emphasize the major roles that language plays in the development of cognition, literacy, and other learning areas. The focus on the importance of language is one of the main reasons for the appeal of this paradigm to proponents of ASL/English bilingual programs (see Chapter 6).

A good summary of the major research findings of this paradigm has been provided by Harste, Burke, and Woodward (1982). Three points are made here: (1) Similar to oral (i.e.. spoken language), written language develops in a natural manner; (2) children in literate (i.e., reading and writing) societies become engaged very early in making sense of and using print; and (3) children's perceptions of print can be labeled as organized and systematic; that is, they seem to have a logical, hypothesis-testing approach similar to oral language acquisition.

There has been little research on the understanding of the reading-writing connections from a social-constructionist perspective. Rather, much of the research has centered on the role of dialogue or culture in the development and use of literacy practices. The issue of how literacy is valued is discussed in the next chapter on literary criticism. The exemplar used here for social constructionism is the work of Heath (1982), who investigated the effects of three types of socioeconomic environments on background information that children bring to school. It was found that mainstream children, or those associated with the typical middle socioeconomic class, already possess literacy behaviors important for beginning schooling. For example, the ability to respond to questions in which the person asking the question already knows the answer, to label and categorize objects and items, and to listen quietly to stories read by others. Children from the other types of environments did not have the same quantity and quality of school-type literacy experiences. As a result, these students were not as successful in school as the mainstream children.

The influence of the home environment on literacy has been a topic for many research investigations within other paradigms (e.g., Brown, 1973; Cazden, 1965; Milner, 1963). For example, Cazden's work showed that it was important to use full grammatical sentences when responding to the verbal expressions of children (for the various viewpoints on this issue, see Bates, 1976). In addition, if adults model adult grammatical sentences in response to the telegraphic speech of children, this has a positive effect on measures of grammatical development of children. Milner (1963) showed the effects of the home environment on the development of language and the quality and quantity of interactions between parents and children. As expected, children with high scores on measurements reside in homes in which they were highly engaged in conversations and positive interactions with parents. The influence of the home environment has also been an important issue in psychosocial research on deafness (e.g., see reviews in Lane, Hoffmeister, & Bahan, 1996; Paul & Jackson, 1993). There is also some current research on literacy development of children who are deaf and their parents within the reading/writing connection paradigm (e.g., see relevant discussions in McAnally, Rose, & Quigley, 1994; Schirmer, 1994). There is still a need to conduct research within the purview of social constructivism in which the focus is on the meaning-making of both the teacher and students in a sociocultural, interactive setting.

In sum, social-constructivist theorists and researchers can address critical questions about the quality and content of environment necessary for promoting literacy development. They can also explore the role of the teacher in the reading/writing connection paradigm. The importance of interactions, experiences, and other aspects of the environment, both home and school, has been highlighted by the work of Heath (1982), mentioned previously. Heath has stressed the necessity of understanding the culture of children and providing relevant experiences :

> . . . knowing more about how these alternatives are learned at early ages in different sociocultural conditions can help the school to provide opportunities for all students to avail themselves of these alternatives early in their school careers. (p. 73)

Major highlights of the research on written language and hearing students are presented in Table 4-3.

Stages of Written Language Development

On one hand, the use of the word *stages* is reflective of an empirical, particularly quantitative, world view of the development of writing. Indeed, much of the information in this area has been dominated by quantitative research methods relating mostly to a comparison of the products relative to chronological age, mental ability, or some other yardstick. An inspection of the products of writing does not necessarily preclude the manner (i.e., process) in which writing can or should be developed.

With the above remarks in mind, it is possible to present a summary of the investigations that have been conducted on writings of children with normal hearing specifically during the elementary years. Several researchers have found that, in general, children's writings increased in both quantity and complexity in a steady manner (e.g., Hunt, 1970; Loban, 1976; see also the review in Ruddell & Haggard, 1985). The early writings of children seem to resemble their spoken language. This has been the impetus for emerging

TABLE 4-3 **Major highlights of the research on written language and hearing students**

Cognitive Information-Processing

- Foundations of literacy (reading and writing) require, at least, a working knowledge of the morphophonological system of English, the system upon which the written language is based (alphabet system).
- This line of research has led to a better understanding of the interrelationships among short-term memory, the use of a phonological coding strategy, and reading comprehension.
- Good writers are invariably good readers, and good readers have the potential to become good writers.

Naturalism

- Research has focused on children's early writing and their understanding of the concepts of written language (e.g., print awareness, boundaries of words, etc.). This has resulted in a reconceptualization of the role of children's language proficiency in the development of literacy.
- Children as writers discover meaning as they engage in the writing process.
- The classroom environment and the interactions within it are important for developing the language, literacy, and learning potential of children.

Social Constructionism

- Little research data are available on the understanding of the reading/writing connections.
- Much of the research has focused on the role of dialogue or culture on the development and use of literacy practices.
- Potential exists for addressing critical questions about the quality and content of environment necessary for promoting literacy development. Can also explore the roles of the teacher.

views of literacy, particularly those based on the naturalistic approach with whole language as its prominent metaphor.

From age nine to fifteen, there is an increase in several language variables. For example, there is a progression from conjoined sentences to embedded sentences. An increase has been noted in the length of the written language productions and in the use of clauses, particularly the use of subordinate and adverbial clauses (except for time and cause). Interestingly, this growth in clauses also mirrors its growing use in the spoken language of children. Nevertheless, the developmental increase of each language variable mentioned above was greater in the written domain than in the spoken domain. In addition, children gained control over the use of syntactic structures, and thus, their writings contain the more complex structures.

Although the stages of written language development are not sharply defined, it is still possible to observe differences that occur between spoken and written language relative to issues such as spelling and syntactic complexity. Many theorists and scholars are in agreement on the importance of the relationship between oral and written language development even though they disagree about the nature of this connection. Perhaps it comes as no surprise that some researchers believe that the strength of this relationship can be seen by examining the written language productions of children with severe to profound hearing impairment (e.g., see discussion in Ruddell & Haggard, 1985). This is a traditional view, which is often held by many researchers interested in children who are deaf and those who are hearing (e.g., see review in Paul & Quigley, 1994a). The major tenets of this view have been discussed in a synthesis by Danielewicz (cited in Ruddell & Haggard, 1985):

> Danielewicz's extensive review... suggests that children progress through stages of writing development in which they 1) *unify* spoken and written language, making few distinctions between the two; 2) *distinguish* between spoken and written language by reducing coordinating conjunctions; 3) *strip* features of spoken language from written productions; and 4) *add* features typically associated with written language. (p. 68).

In the following section, this traditional view is examined, specifically as it has been applied to the research on deafness. In addition, other views of writing, along with additional research foci, are discussed, although this research with children who are deaf is still in the beginning stages. Nevertheless, the personal bias of the present writer is that a deeper understanding of the written language development of children with severe to profound hearing impairment requires a deeper understanding of the intricate and complex relation between oral (i.e., spoken) and written components of the *same* language. The present writer is also in agreement with many researchers that written language models need to include both cognitive and social components. Finally, the social component should be discussed relative to classroom interactions between the teachers and students and between students and students.

Research on Written Language and Students Who Are Deaf

Whether the focus of writing research has been product-oriented or process-oriented, it is clear that students who are deaf have extreme difficulty in learning to write well. The following remarks by Moores (1987) still hold true today: "The evidence suggests that the problems deaf children face in mastering written English are more formidable than those they face in developing reading skills" (p. 281). These remarks are accurate if it is accepted that writing entails more than just reading skills as is purported within a cognitive information-processing approach.

Perhaps a compelling way to show the writing problems of students who are deaf is to present a sample of their written language productions. These samples are drawn from the longitudinal research of Quigley and his collaborators (e.g., Quigley, Wilbur, Power, Montanelli, & Steinkamp, 1976) and from the present author's work. The authors of the samples are 18-year-old students with prelingual, profound hearing impairment. The story theme is going on a picnic.

Sample 1

The family have plan to go to picnic, they packed the foods for lunch. Two children were exciting and will have a fun at there. Father puts a big basket in his car and all of they left the house but the boy saw a dog stay outside and excited with wagged his tail. He tamed and hug it then he took it in the car. They left to the Picnic. Father drove there fabout 6 miles away then arrived. They took off from the car. A little girl ran to the swing. Father and his son played a baseball. The boy fall on the ground and got hurt. Mother yelled "Time for lunch" They ate lots and they tasted so good. (Quigley & Kretschmer, 1982, p. 84)

Sample 2

Once a day a family named Smith wanted to have a picnic out in hot day. The family wanted to have a picnic so badly so they had to make sandwiches. They had a dog who wanted to go so badly and Mr. Smith asked Mrs. Smith how did the dog know that they planned to have a picnic. Mrs. Smith looked at the dog and saw him looking at something, she looked at the table and saw a basket then she found out the answer and replied the answer to her hudsband and he called the place where they planned to have a picnic at and he told him that if the dog is allowed on the picnic? The man went outside and took a look at the sign and went back to telephone and replied that the sign said not. Mr. Smith thanked him for telling him and he was dissapoint because the dog can't go and he told him that he can't go, he understand him and there is nothing for him to do. Mr. Smith told his family to get ready so Mrs. Smith and her daughter helped her, make food and pack food in the basket and Mr. Smith and his son went up in the house to get baseball, glove and ball.

They all got in the car and Mr. Smith started the motor and his son told him to stop and he went out said good bye to the dog.

When they arrived at the picnic they started gobbling then they played baseball.

Sample 3

Mike and Jane got up the bed and ate breakfast. They helped Mother to made enough sandwiches. Mike helped his father to put things in the car. Mother put sandwiches into the basket. Jane gave sandwich to Spot to eat. Then, Jane, Mike, Mother and father got ready to go and they drove to store and bought some meat. Spot followed the car, Mike saw him in the sidewalk. His father told him that he let spot go with Mike. Spot was too exciteing to go with his family. They arrived the park. Jane, Mike and Spot played different game. Jane stopped playing and returned to help mother to put everythings. Her mother cooked hamburgers. Jane called Mike and her father to come for dinner. They ate hamburgers and drinks some tea. After dinner they packed them and get ready to go home. They put thing in the car His father started the car and went to back home His father and Mike cleaned the car and his mother washed the dishes. They had lots of fun.

Note: Samples 2 and 3 are from the data bank of Quigley et al., (1976) and Paul (1987).

Relative to the written language samples above, it should not be surprising that the research on written language productions of students who are deaf reveals low levels of achievement similar to those of their reading ability. At least two major themes can be inferred from the research synthesis, particularly a synthesis of the most recent research: (1) Most students who are deaf are operating with a rule-governed, albeit inadequate, system of English, and (2) similar to their reading difficulty, the students are struggling with both low-level (e.g., mechanical) and high-level (e.g., organizational) skills.

Before discussing the research on written language and deafness, it is important to present some problems with the analyses of written language samples. To elicit writing samples, investigators have employed two general methods: free response and controlled response (see also the discussion in Chapter 9 on assessment of literacy skills). In free-response studies, students are required to produce spontaneous samples of writing, perhaps following a discussion of a topic, a viewing of a film or videotape, or a completion of a field trip or some other experiential activity. Within a controlled-response framework, the investigator is attempting to elicit a certain response from the students. For example, the investigator might present pairs of sentences that differ in one language structure (e.g., a syntactic structure). The students are required to judge the grammaticality of the sentences.

Despite efforts to improve these measures, there are still a number of problems associated with the use of written language samples (e.g., see discussions in Kretschmer & Kretschmer, 1978; Paul & Quigley, 1994a). For example, Paul and Quigley (1994a) provided a summary of the problems:

1. Typically, some external stimulus is used to elicit a written sample—a picture, picture sequence, short film, request to write a story or letter, and so forth. The validity and reliability of these techniques often are unknown. If it is found that certain vocabulary items, morphological structures, syntactic structures, or other linguistic units of interest do not appear in the writing samples elicited, it is difficult to determine whether this is due to the deaf child's inability to produce such structures, or whether it is merely that the stimulus used did not elicit them.
2. Some linguistic units (e.g., infinitival complements—Mary wanted *to make a million dollars*) might appear in the written productions, but in insufficient numbers or variety to allow for study and analysis.
3. Some constructions (e.g., some types of relative clauses) appear in linguistic environments such that it is difficult to understand them and their role in a sentence.
4. As probably every teacher of the deaf knows, the written language productions of many deaf children are often as unintelligible as their spoken language. (p. 175)

The research on writing is presented with respect to three broad areas: traditional/structural, transformational generative grammar, and the process approach. This framework is reflective of the influences of theories on written language research. Both the traditional/structural and the transformational generative grammar views are representative of a product-oriented approach. However, transformational generative grammar (TGG) proponents are interested in describing the underlying rule system that is used by students who are deaf. The TGG approach is related to the framework of cognitive information processing. As the name implies, research within the process approach is representative of the more recent models of the writing process, especially reading and writing connections and the influence of social-constructivist theories. In addition to exploring the connections between reading and writing, process-oriented proponents employ analyses that go beyond the sentential level of the product-oriented proponents.

Traditional/Structural

These early studies explored the content of single sentences. Within a traditional/structural perspective, the emphasis was on prescription, or the *correct* way to use words in sentences. Using structural analyses, researchers were interested in describing the surface or text features of written language sentences. This was a heavy emphasis on the products within the framework of behaviorism (e.g., see discussion in Paul & Quigley, 1994a). There was little interest in the process of writing or in analyses beyond the sentence level. Consequently, teachers provided feedback to students with regard to what is called the mechanics, or lower-level skills, of writing as discussed previously.

Much of the research during this period was focused on comparing the written language productions of deaf students with those of their hearing counterparts. It should come as no surprise that the writings of students who are deaf were considered to be inferior, especially with reference to certain variables such as sentence length, sentence complexity, and the use of words. In addition, it was observed that the writings of students who are deaf varied greatly from standard English (e.g., Heider & Heider, 1940; Stuckless & Marks, 1966; Templin, 1950).

In general, students were exposed to visual stimuli such as pictures, picture sequences, or short films. Then, they were required to write their reactions to these stimuli. The written language samples were analyzed with respect to certain areas; of interest here are the results associated with factors such as productivity (amount), sentence complexity, and errors.

Relative to productivity (e.g., sentence length), the levels of written samples of high-school age students were judged to be equal or inferior to those of average 10-year-old hearing students (e.g., Heider & Heider, 1940; Myklebust, 1964; Simmons, 1963; Stuckless & Marks, 1966). There were no differences between students who were deaf and those who were hearing in the total number of words used in sentences or passages.

Relative to sentence complexity, the students' written productions were also described as rigid or stereotyped. It was observed that the students used several redundant or recurring phrases or sentences. Examples included *They had an idea, I see a . . .* , and *There is a . . . .* In addition, there was limited use of compound and complex sentences involving conjoined phrases or subordinate clauses. In essence, some researchers have characterized the written language samples of students who are deaf as stilted (e.g., Wilbur, 1977, 1987). It has also been argued that the stilted productions are the results of unsound teaching practices. The stilted productions here are analogous to the presence of deviant structures in the language of second-language learners, due to instruction that has been focused on unnatural language structures within the developmental process (e.g., see Chapter 6; see also McLaughlin, 1984, 1985, 1987).

Perhaps the most interesting findings were the types of errors reported. Students made errors of addition (adding unnecessary words), omissions (omitting necessary words), substitutions (using inappropriate words in place of other words), and word-order deviations (inappropriate word order). It should be noted that the researchers during this period only described or listed the types of errors. There were no discussions of why and how students produced these interesting errors. With a focus on description, rather than explanation, it was presumed that these students' writings deviated from standard English.

This idea is still expressed today; some teachers/educators believe that the writings of some students who are deaf reflect their use of American Sign Language (i.e., interference errors; see discussion in Paul & Quigley, 1990, 1994a). Nevertheless, as discussed in Chapter 6, the concept of interference is not a widely-accepted view among researchers/ theorists of second-language learning and second-language literacy development (e.g., see research reviews in Bernhardt, 1991; McLaughlin, 1984, 1985, 1987).

Transformational Generative Grammar

Influenced by the thinking of Chomsky (1957, 1965, 1988), linguists interested in deafness attempted to explain why students were producing certain types of errors. The reason for this focus is because of Chomsky's insistence on differences between performance (i.e., actual spoken utterances and written productions) and competence (i.e., the underlying in-tuitive knowledge of the language user). Chomsky argued that a better understanding of language development can be obtained by referring to the rule-governed system under which the user is operating. It should be highlighted that this is still a cognitive informa-tion-processing approach with an emphasis on innate mechanisms (namely, the Language Acquisition Device, or LAD). In addition, Chomsky has been influenced by what is called dualism or Cartesian/Newtonian philosophy (see discussions in Paul & Quigley, 1994a; Rosenblatt, 1989; see also Chapter 1 of this text).

Within this framework, researchers elicited written language samples (or responses) from students who were deaf using both free-response and controlled-response measures. Free-response measures require the students to respond in writing to a visual stimulus such as a picture or film. These can be considered open-ended measures. Controlled methods are close-ended measures because of the focus of specific types of responses on forced choice measures, for example, multiple-choice tests. Using controlled methods, researchers can construct test items that permit a perusal of specific linguistic units such as relative clauses or determiners (e.g., see Hunt, 1965; Marshall & Quigley, 1970; Quigley, Wilbur, Power, Montanelli, & Steinkamp, 1976).

For this chapter, the focus is on written language errors that can be described and ex-plained relative to rule categories within the purview of generative grammar such as mor-phological and transformational rules. The use of morphological rules might concern areas such as inflections (e.g., *-ing*, *-ed*) or derivations (e.g., *-ness*, *-ment*). Transformational rules refer to the underlying mechanisms that language-users apply in the production and comprehension of structures such as relative clauses (e.g., clauses starting with *that, who*) and verb processes (e.g., passive voice: The boy *was bitten* by the dog). Only a few high-lights are presented here; for an in-depth discussion of this line of research, the reader is re-ferred to other sources (e.g., see research reviews in Paul & Quigley, 1994a; Quigley, Wilbur, Power, Montanelli & Steinkamp, 1976; Taylor, 1969).

Relative to morphology, using free-response measures, it was observed that the scores of students who were deaf improved with the advancement of age. The students seemed to have the most difficulty with verb inflections. This can be seen in the following examples:

1. *She fly* instead of *she flies* (present tense omitted).
2. *The table broked* instead of *The table broke* (redundant use of past tense marker).

In general, the students either omitted, overgeneralized, or used the inflections inappropriately.

Another prevalent area of difficulty was with the use of plurals. It was not uncommon to find examples such as the following:

1. *sheeps* for *sheep* or *six boy* instead of *six boys.*
2. Problems with the use of possessives such as *'s* and *s'*.

Despite these errors, one of the strongest conclusions made was that the patterns of errors were similar to those found in the writings of much younger hearing children and in individuals who were learning English as a second language (e.g., see King, 1981; Paul & Quigley, 1994a).

For transformations via the use of free-response measures, the work of Taylor (1969) is representative of the types of results. Taylor focused on three types of transformational rules: conjunction, nominalization, and relative clauses (some examples of these structures were presented in Chapter 3). At first glance, it was observed that there were relatively few variances in these areas. However, Taylor argued that this finding was due more to students' rarely using these structures as opposed to the fact that they had little difficulty. More important, there was no significant (or noticeable) improvement with age; that is, the students did not show any real proficiency in the use of these complex structures. Some types of transformational errors are illustrated in Table 4-4.

One of the most salient conclusions of this early research on written language was that students who were deaf were producing correct (from their perspective) sentences from rules that were not based on those of standard English.

Relative to the use of controlled methods, a substantial body of data is available on the two broad areas of interest here: morphology and transformation. The reader is also referred to the work of O'Neill (1973) as representative of the research on phrase structure rules and the lexicon—two other important areas. In relation to morphology, Cooper (1967) reported that for students who are deaf, knowledge of inflectional morphemes was superior to their knowledge of derivational markers. These data support those documented by Taylor (1969) using free-response methods. Morphology is highlighted here because it is an area that has received some research attention relative to the use of the English-based signed systems (e.g., see the seminal works of Bornstein, Saulnier, & Hamilton, 1980; Crandall, 1978; Looney & Rose, 1979; Raffin, 1976).

Relative to transformational rules, two areas are highlighted: negation and the use of the passive voice (verb processes). Schmitt (1969) reported that most of his deaf subjects, between the ages of 8 to 17 years, had little difficulty with the negative marker *not* in English sentences. Nevertheless, the researcher hypothesized that a number of the younger students, particularly the 8-year-olds, were operating with what he called the *no negative rule*. This meant that students seemed to be ignoring the marker *not* and treating the negative sentences as if they were affirmative sentences. Consider the differences in meanings in the following examples with and without the *not*.

1. *The boy did not hit the ball* interpreted as *The boy hit the ball.*
2. *The girl did not write the letter* interpreted as *The girl write the letter.*

TABLE 4-4   Examples of transformational errors of deaf students (Taylor, 1969)

Conjunction

Omission
- A ant see a tree a bird.
- Ant walk found animals.

Misplacement
- The dove got out of the tree and took a leaf threw it down.
- The ant ran to its home and get the scissors and hit a man's leg.

Deletion
- The tool hurt the hunter and yelled.
- The hunter scared the dove and flew away.
- The ant went off and ride the dragonfly.

Nominalization

Gerunds and Infinitives
- The ant like to played with insects.
- The man began screamed.
- He cannot know how to swimming.
- The hunter missed to shoot the dove.
- The ant saw him what he was doing.

Relativization

Nonuse of pronoun
- The ant held the thing look like circle.

Copying Phenomenon
- There was a little hole underground which a smart ant lived in it.
  [Based on: There was a little hole underground. A smart ant lived in the hole.]

Schmitt (1969) also studied the use of passive transformational rules. The students were required to select one of four passive sentences that correctly illustrated the action of reversible passive sentences. An example of a reversible passive sentence is *The boy was hit by the ball*, for which the reverse is also acceptable, *The ball was hit by the boy*. The students were required to *fill-the-gap* in sentences to produce passive sentences to describe pictures correctly. Schmitt reported that few of his subjects younger than 14 years old could pass the tests. Even many of the older students, at 17 years of age, had difficulty understanding the meaning of passive sentences or producing them correctly.

Schmitt's findings were supported also in a research project by Power and Quigley (1973). These researchers concluded that the majority of students who are deaf were operating with a defective rule for the processing of passive sentences. They stated this rule as "passive reversal of subject-object order to process meaning of such sentences is signaled only by *by;* tense markers are free to vary" (Power & Quigley, 1973, p. 76). Thus, many of these students persist in interpreting all sentences in terms of the standard subject-verb-object order of the English simple sentence.

Based on these lines of research, Quigley and his collaborators have constructed a set of instructional materials for teachers to use in developing syntactic knowledge in children and youth who are deaf (see discussion in Paul & Quigley, 1994a). Despite the shortcomings of these materials, it should be underscored that the materials were based on the longitudinal research project of Quigley, who was heavily influenced by the thinking of Chomsky and Transformational Generative Grammar. Difficulty with TGG's cognitive-dualistic approach notwithstanding, it was never intended that these students could learn about syntax solely via the use of these materials. In my view, Chomsky would not have approved the use of any instructional materials because one of his major arguments is that language cannot be taught to children. The development of these and other language materials is/was an attempt by researchers to respond to the needs of teachers in the classrooms.

More importantly, it should be underscored that for children who are deaf difficulty with English syntax is complex and is influenced by several major factors, two of which are knowledge and processing capabilities. Both of these issues have been discussed in depth in Chapter 3. A related issue is the exposure to a reasonably complete and unambiguous representation of English via the use of a signed system (e.g., see discussion in Drasgow & Paul, 1995). Relative to the development of a conversational form of English, this last issue has not received the attention that it deserves (see Paul & Quigley, 1994a; see also the discussion in Chapter 6).

In sum, although we have learned much about the syntactic and other language difficulties of students who are deaf via the use of traditional/structural and TGG approaches, we have made few significant gains in either teaching or developing this knowledge as measured by traditional, standardized tests, including the recent use of the Test of Syntactic Abilities (Quigley, Steinkamp, Power & Jones, 1978; see the research results in Tzeng, 1993).

Major highlights of the research on writing and deafness discussed previously are illustrated in Table 4-5. Because of these findings and others, some researchers and scholars have argued for a shift in our investigations of the written language productions of students who are deaf. This is the topic of the next section.

TABLE 4-5   Highlights of early research on deafness and writing

Highlights

- For students who are deaf, knowledge of inflectional morphemes was superior to knowledge of derivational markers. [Cooper, 1967].
- A number of younger students, particularly the 8-year-olds, were operating with the *no negative rule*. [Schmitt, 1969].
- Many of the older students, at 17 years old, had difficulty understanding the meaning of passive sentences or producing them correctly. [Schmitt, 1969].
- Many students who were deaf persisted in interpreting all sentences in terms of the standard subject-verb-object order of the English simple sentence. [Power & Quigley, 1973].
- Because of the limited usefulness of some of the major findings for instruction, some researchers/scholars have argued for a shift in our investigations of the written language productions of students who are deaf.

The Process Approach

As discussed previously, the process approach has been influenced mainly by naturalistic and social-constructivist models. However, it is possible to see the influences of the cognitive information-processing models, particularly within cognitive-interactive views such as those expressed by Tierney and Pearson (e.g., 1983) and others (e.g., see reviews in Mason, 1989; McCarthey & Raphael, 1992). Research in deafness seems to have been motivated mainly by cognitive-interactive and naturalistic models. The common denominator is the focus on the intersentential level. In addition, many researchers and educators have described writing relative to a focus on planning, composing, and revising. This is based on the cognitive-interactive composing model of Tierney and Pearson (1983; see also the discussions in Flower & Hayes, 1980; McCarthey & Raphael, 1992; Paul & Quigley, 1994a).

The emphasis on the intersentential level is due to the assumption that these analyses permit a more in-depth understanding of the relationship between form (e.g., morphology, syntax) and meaning (i.e., semantics). Thus, it is presumed that studying the interactions between syntax and semantics on the intersentential level might shed more light on the literacy problems of students who are deaf. As argued by Mason (1989), Rosenblatt (1989), and McCarthey and Raphael (1992), this is still related to the notion of componential analyses (i.e., reductionism) within the purview of cognitive information-processing models.

Wilbur's (1977) reanalysis of the data of the Quigley, Wilbur, Power, Montanelli, and Steinkamp (1976) study is representative of this line of research. Wilbur found that these students produced more syntactic errors on the intersentential level than on the sentential level. This researcher hypothesized that the students were receiving instruction that placed too much emphasis on producing correct single sentences. As a result, the written language productions of students who are deaf were considered to be stilted or unimaginative. In essence, the writing of students who are deaf was devoid of metaphorical expressions and usage of words. Within a cognitive-interactive paradigm, Wilbur argued that students needed additional instruction in the development of meaningful paragraphs or passages in which organization and content are stressed.

The work of Gormley and Sarachan-Deily (e.g., Gormley & Sarachan-Deily, 1987; Sarachan-Deily, 1982, 1985) represents the early shift to the new paradigm on writing as a process; however, this research is still heavily oriented to the cognitive-interactive view because of its instructional implications and list of writing components. Gormley and Sarachan-Deily (1987) placed students who are deaf into two groups: good writers and poor writers. The assignment of students to their respective groups was based upon the ratings (typical general impressions) of their teachers and one of the investigators. The researchers conducted in-depth analyses of the writing of the two groups. They described their data relative to three areas: content, linguistic aspects, and surface mechanics. *Content* represented items such as introduction, supporting statements, summary, conclusion, and identifying an audience. In one sense, content referred to the higher-level, albeit traditional, components of writing. *Linguistic aspects* referred to word order, omission of parts of speech, and violation of semantic relations. Surface mechanics included items such as spelling, punctuation, capitalization, legibility, and minor grammatical errors such as articles and possessives. It is possible to label linguistic aspects and surface mechanics as the lower-level components of writing.

Gormley and Sarachan-Deily reported that both good and poor writers committed numerous errors in the lower-level components: linguistic aspects and surface mechanics. In fact, they found no significant differences between these two groups on surface mechanics and on some of the linguistic aspects. Relative to the content area, however, the groups differed significantly. The researchers documented that the compositions of good writers were more developed, cohesive, and appropriate than those of poor writers. It seems that good writers were more concerned that their writings were readable and understandable. In essence, this research seems to suggest that the real differences between good and poor writers are in the higher-level components of writing, which were argued to be the more critical areas of written language. Nevertheless, it should be noted that both groups produced a number of errors in the lower-level aspects of writing.

In sum, Gormley and Sarachan-Deily argued that writing should be considered a communication process, and this should be the major focus of all writing instruction. They also noted that it is important to encourage students with hearing impairment to read and revise their manuscripts. In relation to the composing model with the focus on planning, composing, and revising, the researchers suggested that improvements in the lower-level aspects of writing will occur if students become engaged in the rereading and revision processes of writing.

This focus on the aspect of revision was also of interest to another researcher (Livingston, 1989). This study is discussed at length here because it is reflective of the transition between the lingering focus on products to the emerging focus on the process of writing. Livingston (1989) was interested in examining whether the revisions had any positive effects on the final drafts produced by the students. The suggestions for revisions could come from the teacher or from the student writers themselves.

The subjects for this study were 22 high-school students between the ages of 16 and 21 years old. The students were required to write one story per month, and this continued for three months. After completing the first draft of the story, each student consulted with the teacher individually in *conferences*. In these meetings, the teacher's role was to provide suggestions and feedback with a focus mainly on clarification of the content of the manuscript. There should have been little or no suggestions for students relative to their *grammatical errors*. After the conferences, students composed a second draft of their manuscripts, which were then read by their classmates or peers.

Livingston (1989) examined two areas: (1) the differences between the first and second drafts and (2) the teacher-student interactions during the conferences. To analyze the differences between drafts, the researcher focused on syntactic changes and on areas such as deletion, substitution, and addition (for the protocol, see Bridwell, 1980; Sommers, 1980). Livingston found that the students, themselves, initiated most of the revisions; in fact, they did this more often than teachers. Most of the changes in the drafts involved additions and substitutions. Livingston was also able to compare these changes with those found in the research on writers with typical hearing. The hearing writers made fewer additions and more deletions than the writers who were deaf. Nevertheless, both groups were similar with their syntactic revisions.

Finally, Livingston noticed that teachers' suggestions were not reflective of the process-oriented view of writing. It seems that the emphasis was mostly on the sentence level rather than on the discourse level. That is, teachers concentrated on improving sentence construction (i.e., lower-level skills) and not on the organization and purpose of stories (i.e., higher-level skills). This was particularly interesting because some of the stories written by these students had no clear purpose. In addition, some teachers provided feedback on the first drafts without holding conferences (i.e., discussing feedback) with students. As is typical of such procedures, this resulted in the students' misunderstanding of the nature and intent of the written remarks. Some teachers attempted to correct the grammatical errors of the students. This led the students to simply incorporate the corrections into the next draft without any real, meaningful discussions or generalizations.

A more recent study also seemed to incorporate analyses on both a product and process level. Klecan-Aker and Blondeau (1990) analyzed the written compositions of eight students whose hearing impairment ranged from severe to profound. The students were between 10 and 18 years old (10.10 years to 18.1 years) and were receiving oral/aural program services in a public-school. The students were asked to write stories and were given the following instructions: "I want you to write a story. Remember as you write that stories have a beginning, middle, and end" (p. 277). The researchers imposed no time limits.

In analyzing the stories, the researchers employed several measures that focus on intrasentential and intersentential levels, for example, T units (a syntactic unit measuring syntactic complexity and maturity; Hunt, 1970), story grammar components (Stein & Glenn, 1979), cohesion, and developmental level of writing (Klecan-Aker, 1988). Relating the data on T units to those on hearing students (Klecan-Aker & Hedrick, 1985), the researchers reported that students with hearing impairment produced fewer clauses and words per T unit than did their counterparts with typical hearing. The students with hearing impairment did quite well with story grammar components such as setting, consequence, and ending. Focusing on conjunctions for the cohesion aspect, the investigators reported that students with hearing impairment produced more coordinating conjunctions (and, and so, and then) than subordinating conjunctions (because, that, when). These results are essentially similar to those reported in the earlier research on the products of writing. Finally, the researchers found no strong relationship between development level of the stories and the ages of the students with hearing impairment.

The results of this investigation should be interpreted with caution. Firstly, the sample size was small (n = 8). Secondly, the students in this study were those exposed and educated within an oral/aural philosophy. For a better understanding of research on different types of students who are deaf, the reader is referred to other sources (e.g., Moores, 1987; Paul & Quigley, 1990; 1994a).

Within the process paradigm, the current research on deafness is still focused on higher-order skills of writing (e.g., organization and intent), although there seems to be a proclivity toward naturalistic research employing a qualitative paradigm and focusing on reading/writing connections. This research is also heavily influenced by the work of Goodman (1985), particularly the whole-language approach. The emphasis on developing higher-levels skills can be seen in studies that examined the free writing of children who are deaf in kindergarten (e.g., Andrews & Gonzales, 1991), in the elementary and secondary grades (e.g., Kluwin & Kelly, 1991), and in postsecondary programs (e.g., Brown & Long, 1992). These investigations revealed improvements in the writing samples of these children, especially in the areas of content and grammatical structures such as syntactic complexity.

Another line of recent research, which parallels the development in reading/writing research on hearing children, is the focus on children's responses to literature (e.g., for hearing children, see Morrow, 1988; Yaden, Smolkin, & MacGillivray, 1993; for children who are deaf, see Andrews & Taylor, 1987; Lemley, 1993; Williams, 1994: Williams & McLean, 1996). This line of research is based on reader response theory, which has been influenced pervasively by literary critical theory and social constructionism (see Chapter 5). Reader response theorists argue that there is no one right interpretation of a particular text. In effect, children's responses are based on personal experiences, knowledge, and perspectives (e.g., see the work of Lemley, 1993).

This process involves the reading of the text or attending to it if it is read aloud and making a response via either the conversational or written form (i.e., speaking, signing, or writing). The response is also shared with others. This sharing of response is at the heart of social-constructionist theories. Children can see similarities and differences between their personal responses and those of others. This sharing leads to the social construction of meaning or knowledge within a particular context or setting.

A representative line of work in this area is that of Williams (1994; Williams & McLean, 1996). This line of investigation is discussed in some detail because it depicts the shift in examining the reading/writing connections of children who are deaf using qualitative research methodology. In addition, this paradigm shift also acknowledges no separation of the reading/writing process.

Williams examined three classrooms of preschool children for six months for a larger study (1994). The focus here is on the five children with profound hearing impairment in one classroom, ranging in age from 4.11 to 5.7 years. The children used simultaneous communication as their mode of communication; that is, they signed mostly but they also employed speech and other gestures. The researcher videotaped activities surrounding picturebook reading in the classroom and free-choice reading in the classroom library. The researcher also recorded field notes and conducted interviews with the classroom teacher. The videotaped data were transcribed and coded. Transcriptions included sign and spoken communication and even body movements—all of which were considered reader responses. Trustworthiness in data collection and analysis was established (e.g., see discussion in Lincoln & Guba, 1985).

In general, Williams (Williams & McLean, 1996) reported that the range of responses were similar to those reported by Hickman (1979) on children in kindergarten and first grade. In summarizing her results, Williams (Williams & McLean, 1996) noted that:

> The children in this study were clearly interested in children's picturebooks. They attended and responded to children's literature in meaningful ways. They transacted with books on an individual level, and they interacted around books with one another and with their teacher in socially-constructed ways. Their severe receptive and expressive language delay did not prevent them from enjoying, responding to, and learning from children's picturebooks. Response to literature as a pedagogical approach is a very powerful medium for both language and literacy development, and it should be considered as a viable instructional practice in classrooms for young deaf children. (p. 3)

Approaches to literacy based on the naturalistic and social constructionist models tend to empower children in the classrooms (e.g., see Schirmer, 1994; see also Chapter 5). Chil-

TABLE 4-6 **Highlights of research on writing as a process approach**

Highlights

- Students were receiving instruction that placed too much emphasis on producing correct single sentences. Students needed additional instruction in the development of meaningful paragraphs or passages in which organization and content are stressed. [Wilbur, 1977]
- The real differences between good and poor writers are in the higher-level components of writing. Improvements in the lower-level aspects of writing will occur if students become engaged in the rereading and revision processes of writing. [Gormley & Sarachan-Deily, 1987]
- Teachers' suggestions were not reflective of the process-oriented view of writing. Emphasis was mostly on the sentence level rather than on the discourse level. Some teachers provided feedback without holding conferences (i.e., discussing feedback) with students. [Livingston, 1989]
- Reader response theorists argue that there is no one right interpretation of a particular text. In effect, children's responses are based on personal experiences, knowledge, and perspectives. [Lemley, 1993; Williams, 1994, Williams & McLean, 1996]

dren are given choices with respect to their reading and writing activities. They are encouraged to take risks and become predominantly responsible for their progress. This has led one researcher to argue that naturalistic approaches can be placed within the cultural paradigm whereas cognitive information-processing can be placed within the clinical category (e.g., Lemley, 1993). However, in many classrooms for students who are deaf, the teacher is still the main agent of control, and classroom activities still evolve around the structure and agenda of the teacher, especially if the teacher has normal hearing (e.g., see discussion in Lane, Hoffmeister, & Bahan, 1996).

Despite the growing influence of process approaches to writing, children who are deaf still need to have assistance in their understanding of lower-level skills (e.g., Dolman, 1992; Kelly, 1995). Otherwise, this marked emphasis on process in writing might lead to the same result as the pervasive emphasis on top-down aspects in reading-comprehension theories. Whether the focus is on cognitive information-processing, naturalism, or social constructionism, the end goal should be virtually the same: good readers and writers. And, in the present writer's view, this means a facility in the use of bottom-up and top-down skills. Which group of theories most likely leads to the development of effective instructional practices is an open question. Nevertheless, all three major groups have contributed to our understanding of the process of literacy.

Highlights of research on writing as a process approach with children and adolescents who are deaf are illustrated in Table 4-6.

The Reading-Writing Connection: Future Directions

Despite the amount of research on both students who are deaf and those who are hearing, there is still a great need for further research on the interactive nature of oral and written language. With respect to children and adolescents who are deaf, we know very little about the contributions of the conversational form of a language to the corresponding written form. In addition, very little is known about the development of both lower-level and higher-level skills. It is not clear whether these students can learn these lower-level skills of reading/writing in functional and social settings only. It might be necessary for them to be exposed to direct teaching activities as indicated by some cognitive information-processing approaches.

To obtain a better understanding of the reciprocal relationship between oral and written language, it is necessary to conduct research within a social-cognitive paradigm. However, this will not provide a complete story. More research is needed also within the purview of social-constructionist theories. In my view, naturalistic and social-constructionist models are most conducive to classroom interaction research; however, as discussed previously, social-constructionist models are difficult to test empirically (e.g., McCarthey & Raphael, 1992).

Ruddell and Haggard (1985) have proposed research needs with respect to hearing students. More specifically, these areas are of immense importance for students who are deaf, given the general dearth of inquiries in these areas, and given the view that research on these students can benefit from the models used with hearing students (e.g., King & Quigley, 1985; Paul & Quigley, 1994a; cf., Lane, Hoffmeister, & Bahan, 1996). As suggested by Ruddell and Haggard (1985), there is a need for:

1. Research examining the relationship between children's preliterate experiences with text and reading acquisition.
2. Research examining the relationships among children's perception of reading instruction, text, and reading acquisition.
3. Longitudinal study of the process through which children develop lexical control during the elementary school years.
4. Longitudinal study of the relationship between lexical control and reading comprehension.
5. Qualitative research examining the relationship between children's metalinguistic awareness of oral and written language functions and reading acquisition.
6. Ethnographic research studying the relationship between the literacy support systems in home and community environment and reading and writing acquisition.

A Final Word

The intent of this chapter was to discuss theories and research on writing within the purview of three broad models: cognitive information-processing, naturalism, and social constructivism. Much of the research on both children and adolescents who are deaf and those who are hearing has been conducted within the cognitive framework; however, there is a growing trend to use naturalistic and social-constructionist paradigms. It was argued that these two latter models should be utilized in order to understand the instruction of literacy within classrooms. The cognitive approach, albeit important, has not been very effective in improving the literacy skills of children. This approach, however, has provided implications for practice, particularly in the direct or precision teaching of skills, both lower-level and upper-level.

In all fairness, it can be argued that none of the models discussed has led to much improvement in the reading/writing achievement levels of children and adolescents who are deaf. As indicated in this chapter and the one on reading, the problem for all models is to engender instructional activities that would enable these students to develop both lower-level and higher-level skills. There seems to be a reciprocal relation between these two sets of skills. The chapters on instructional practice (Chapters 7 and 8) are based on the basic tenets of these three models.

The present chapter also provided a perspective on relating the theories, research, and practice within these models to the overall macro paradigms of reading comprehension and literary criticism. More important, there was a discussion of the relationships to clinical and cultural perspectives of deafness. Some researchers have argued that reading-comprehension models, specifically cognitive information processing, can be considered clinical because of their heavy focus on remedying the literacy deficiencies of these students (e.g., see discussions in Lemley, 1993; Paul & Quigley, 1994a). On the other hand, both naturalistic and social-constructionist models are considered to be culturally oriented with a focus on understanding students' response to literacy and empowering the students in this process.

This empowerment issue should be viewed with caution. In most classrooms for students who are deaf, much of the agenda and many activities are still established and controlled by teachers, particularly hearing teachers (for an interesting perspective, see Lane, Hoffmeister, & Bahan, 1996). Nevertheless, this issue of empowerment is important for a number of reasons. It is examined along with others such as accessibility and enlightenment in the next chapter on literary critical perspectives.

Further Readings

BAKHTIN, M. (1935). *The dialogic imagination.* Austin, TX: University of Austin Press.

BLEICH, D. (1978). *Subjective criticism.* Baltimore, MD: Johns Hopkins Press.

FREDERIKSEN, C., & DOMINIC, J. (Eds.). (1981). *Writing: Process, development and communication.* Hillsdale, NJ: Erlbaum.

HUCK, C. (1987). *Children's literature in the elementary school* (4th ed.). New York: Holt, Rinehart & Winston.

ROSENBLATT, L. (1978). *The reader, the text, and the poem.* Carbondale, IL: Southern Illinois University Press.

ROUTMAN, R. (1988). *Transitions, from literature to literacy.* Portsmouth, NH: Heinemann.

Chapter 5

Literary Critical Perspectives

Why should teachers be interested in critical theory? . . . I believe it addresses itself to questions which are of vital concern to all teachers: why do some children persistently fail in school? Why are some pupils so unmotivated and so difficult in the classroom? Why do we teach what we do? Why are schools organized as they are? These are urgent and familiar questions. Critical theory attempts to explain the origins of everyday practices and problems, but it goes further. It claims to offer replies to those awkward questions which ask what should be done. What should be the relationship between teacher and pupil, teacher and teacher? What should be taught? How should schools or classrooms be organized? Critical theory is not simply explanatory, but is committed to enabling change towards better relationships, towards a more just and rational society. (Gibson, 1986, p. 2)

In Chapter 1, three modes of metatheoretical research perspectives were briefly mentioned: empirical, interpretative, and critical. As indicated by the passage above, this chapter focuses on the third mode, the critical. For most scholars and educators in the field of deafness, this might either be an unfamiliar mode or one that is often misconstrued as polemic arguments (for an earlier discussion of polemic arguments re: reading and deafness, see King & Quigley, 1985). Nevertheless, the critical perspective has been used to justify and support the establishment of American Sign Language/English bilingual programs for students who are deaf (e.g., for reviews see Lane, Hoffmeister, & Bahan, 1996; Paul & Quigley, 1994a, 1994b; see also Chapter 6). Thus, to obtain insights into the rationale for ASL/English bilingual programs or the call for more Deaf persons in leadership or decision-making positions, it is important to understand the basic tenets of the critical perspective to which theorists, researchers, and educators ascribed.

The critical perspective is not a scientific argument; however, it is a logical, and perhaps an ethical, one. As discussed later, critical theorists are concerned with certain issues such as empowerment, enlightenment, and emancipation. In addition, there is an attempt to illustrate situations that are oppressive to selected members of the population. One goal of these attempts is to improve the educational and social welfare of underrepresented or *powerless* groups.

Because of the enduring difficulty that students with severe to profound hearing impairment have with the acquisition of literacy skills, it might be that English (either spoken, signed, or written) is an unrealistic goal for these students. As indicated in the works of Paul (e.g., Paul, 1994a, 1994b, 1995a, 1995b; Paul & Quigley, 1994a), this should not be interpreted *as surrendering to nature* or *giving up*, but rather, that the focus should be on alternative methods to develop literate thought in these individuals. Literate thought refers to the ability to think critically and reflectively. Ignoring this concern might result in English literacy skills representing an oppressive situation for individuals who are deaf, as discussed later. Paul and Quigley (1994a) proposed two questions from a critical theoretical framework (mentioned in Chapter 1):

1. Is it possible to develop literate thought without possessing high-level skills in text-based literacy, that is, the ability to read and write printed materials?
2. Is literate thought sufficient for participation in a scientific, technological society, such as the United States? (p. 299)

Additional questions that should be addressed are: What is literate thought? How does it relate to literacy? What are the goals of literate thought and literacy? Are these goals affected by the values of educators? Are they affected by the goals of the larger society?

These questions provide the springboard for the bulk of the discussion in this chapter. It should be noted that it is possible to operationalize the questions and to use the scientific method to address them. However, an in-depth response to the questions proceeds beyond science and into the world of philosophy or metatheory (e.g., see discussions in Ritzer, 1991, 1992). Any discussion on values is related to the domain of ethics, essentially a philosophical domain, which is considered to be the science of the study of morals. This discussion is critical relative to the issue of oppression, which is an often-used word in describing the education of students who are deaf, especially with respect to the use of signed systems, language, and literacy (e.g., Drasgow & Paul, 1995; Johnson, Liddell, & Erting, 1989; Lane, 1984, 1988; Lane, Hoffmeister, & Bahan, 1996; Paul & Jackson, 1993).

The major purpose of this chapter is to delineate some salient highlights relative to critical theory and apply them to the framework of literacy. Despite the brevity of this chapter, the reader should gain an understanding of the literary critical framework, including its place within the three broad literacy perspectives discussed in Chapters 1, 2, and 4, namely, cognitive information-processing, naturalism, and social constructionism. In addition, it is necessary to describe the influences and interrelations of other concepts such as phenomenology (see Chapter 1) and deconstruction. Subsequently, the literary critical framework is applied to the situation of deafness, particularly in relation to the teaching of English literacy skills and the establishment of ASL/English bilingual programs.

This chapter addresses and attempts to answer the questions posed above. More importantly, it provides another perspective for viewing the literacy difficulties of students with severe to profound impairment. It should be highlighted that this perspective is primarily *ethical* in nature, although it is based on the interpretation of the available *scientific* data. This perspective might also be construed as a broad description of literary critical theory or, from another perspective, a critical discussion of the research data available on the development of literacy skills in students who are deaf.

In any case, there is no claim that the interpretation proffered here is the best or correct one. In fact, such a claim undermines a basic principle of critical theory; that is, any position is relative to the specific conditions or the power base of the individual or group stating the position. The application of critical arguments in education is not new; it can be seen in the ongoing debates on the merits of inclusion (e.g., Paul & Ward, 1996; Stainback & Stainback, 1992). The chapter also offers implications for further research in the development of literate thought in students with severe to profound hearing impairment.

Critical Theory: A Brief Introduction

To obtain a sense of the purview of critical theory, specifically with its focus on empowerment, emancipation, and enlightenment, consider the following passage:

> A person may possess the capacity to function in one group, in one community, perhaps in more than one, but not necessarily in others; a functional literate may be rendered dysfunctional as community or societal demands for attainment in reading and writing change—as of course they will. To be schooled once, as most of us know, is not to be functionally educated forever, not in times of rapid social and technological change. We mandarins of print culture who have earned our high literacy through serious engagements with books and struggles with the pen could possibly be rendered illiterate by the electronification of the word, unless we keep up or hold on to power.
>
> Literacy changes in nature more or less in pace with technological changes . . . Industrializing societies demand more readers able to comprehend and make use of information and more writers able to provide it. Information societies will demand many more readers, though what *reading* means may change; they may, perhaps, demand more, or perhaps, fewer, writers, depending on whether the means for producing information are decentralized or centralized. The nature of literacy is as subject to *political change*—to alterations of power—as it is to technological change. [emphasis on *political change* added] (Robinson, 1990, pp. 15-16)

There is little question that some scholars in the field of deafness would agree that this passage has pervasive implications for the situation with children who are deaf, specifically if one adheres to a cultural (DEAF-WORLD) view of deafness (e.g., see discussion in Johnson, Liddell, & Erting, 1989; Lane, 1984, 1988; Lane, Hoffmeister, & Bahan, 1996). That is, it is possible that current educational practices are not conducive to producing literate people who are deaf because of the all-encompassing emphasis and value placed on the printed word. Obviously, literacy may be defined differently by members of the DEAF-WORLD; however, one should keep in mind that the definition of literacy can be subject to political change as indicated above.

The reason for including the above passage is to illustrate the point that critical theorists are concerned with ideas, assumptions, beliefs, and values that are often either taken for granted or considered the *mainstream* point of view. The focus is not on explaining the problems spawned by this approach, but rather on resolving or managing them. In essence, this critical analysis of problems is said to enable individuals to become empowered and to gain control of their lives. In one sense, critical theorists are very concerned with social, political, and economic inequities that result from oppressive practices and ideas (e.g., see discussions in Foucault, 1973; Gibson, 1986; Habermas, 1984). In this chapter, some educational practices related to the development of literacy, that is, reading and writing, are examined critically.

Beginnings and General Nature of Critical Theory

It is important to address the question: What is critical theory? Several perspectives have been offered on the nature, methods, and implications of critical theory (e.g., Gibson, 1986; Ray, 1984). Although the foundation of critical theory can be gleaned from the writings of Karl Marx (e.g., see discussion in Gibson, 1986), it has evolved much beyond this original building block. It might be more accurate to state that the origins of critical theory can be found in the writings of individuals associated with the Frankfurt School. That is, these scholars constituted a group associated with the Institute of Social Research, which was founded in 1923 at the University of Frankfurt in Germany (Gibson, 1986). Important influential figures, who often disagreed vehemently, were Adorno, Horkheimer, and Marcuse. A later, significant influence on critical theory has been the work of Habermas, who was not a member of the Frankfort School but, nevertheless, is an often-quoted writer.

There is no one critical theory; this term is often used (metatheoretically) to refer to a host of theories that have been influenced by the critical framework. Critical theorists seem extensively involved with *theory* itself. They expend a substantial amount of time and energy on assumptions, methodology, and implications. Nevertheless, they are convinced that there is no separation of theory and practice, especially when discussing theories about the human condition or human nature. This should call into mind Lewin's dictum that "There is nothing so practical as a good theory" (Marrow, 1969, n.p.). However, the difference is that Lewin was interested in applying scientific theory and methodology to social issues whereas critical theorists do not accept this type of application.

One of the problems asserted by critical theorists is that practitioners are not always aware of the underlying theoretical or metatheoretical assumptions of their practices. This can lead to a gross misunderstanding of the use or implication of the practices. In addition, there might be a breakdown of communication because of assumptions that are derived from different world views. More important, as is discussed later, these misunderstandings and miscommunications can result in inequalities and inaccessibility for certain segments of the population, typically the underserved or underrepresented groups or groups without much socio-economic and political clout.

Critical Theory and Science

An understanding of critical theory requires a comparison of its assumptions to those traditionally associated with science or the scientific method. To make this comparison, there needs to be an understanding of the scientific method. Unfortunately, or perhaps, fortunately, there is much debate on what constitutes the scientific method (e.g., Argyris, Putnam, & Smith, 1985; Borg & Gall, 1983; Lincoln & Guba, 1985; Travers, 1978). There seems to be a perception that the scientific method is positivistic (i.e., reductionistic) and objective (i.e., separation of knower and the knowledge). As discussed in Chapter 1, this places the method mostly in the empirical domain. Besides the experimental approach, this domain also encompasses the use of quantitative investigations (i.e., experimental, quasi-experimental, and descriptive).

Some scholars take issue with this interpretation (e.g., Argyris et al., 1985; Lincoln & Guba, 1985). They feel that the interpretative domain is also a part of the scientific inquiry. The interpretative domain is considered to be mostly subjective; however, it is based on logical analyses of data within a specified context or situation. There is no separation of the knower and the knowledge. For discussion purposes, social constructionism combines elements of both the empirical and interpretative domain. In other words, social constructionism is, at least, both objective and subjective and related to critical theorizing.

In any case, critical theory is a reaction against the *positivistic* and *objective* assumptions of the scientific method. Proponents argue that this approach to human nature is fruitless or, worse, a distortion of reality. There is no value-free knowledge because there is no separation of the knower and knowledge relative to social and educational issues. It is impossible to express this knowledge in language that is *neutral* and *objective*. Objectivity is an agreed upon condition subject to an individual's social and educational status. Thus, subjectivity and relativity are acceptable and unavoidable, specifically in relation to human issues. The following passage serves as an exemplar of this position (Gibson, 1986):

> Critical theory argues that in human affairs all 'facts' are socially constructed, humanly determined and interpreted, and hence subject to change through human means. In education, for example, such notions as 'achievement', 'failure', 'progress', 'ability', (and 'education' itself) are neither objective, nor natural, nor disinterested terms. Rather they are categories, constructed by, and serving the interests of, certain groups. When claims are made about 'unchanging human nature', or about 'eternal truths', or 'natural behaviour', or the 'organic community', critical theory's claim is that certain sectional views and beliefs are being passed off, wrongly, as universally valid. (p. 4)

Enlightenment, Emancipation, and Instrumental Rationality

Two other concepts that should be discussed together relative to critical theory are enlightenment and emancipation. With enlightenment, critical theorists focus on uncovering the interests of certain individuals or groups. Although this can refer to needs, it is possible to discuss advantages and disadvantages of certain conditions. For example, Lane (1988; see also Lane, Hoffmeister, & Bahan, 1996) refers to the paternalistic views of hearing educators of students who are deaf, alluding to their need for control (mostly social and political). He compares these views with those held by the European colonizers in Africa, who were motivated by self-economic values. Banking on this theme, it can be argued that it is in the best interest of current White South Africans to deny voting privileges to all Black South Africans. Analogously, Lane is implying that certain practices and beliefs of hearing educators are serving the interests of these educators and may not be in the best interest of the students who are deaf.

Relative to the education of students who are deaf, it can be inquired: What are the *interests* of individuals who promote the use of English-based signing? What about the interests of those who favor the use of American Sign Language as a first language for all children with hearing impairment? Finally, for the purposes of this text, what are the interests of educators and scholars who promote a narrow view of literacy, that is, as the ability to read and write text-based English? Does this narrow view cause difficulty for some individuals who are deaf?

The above questions revolve around the issues of accessibility and oppression. As an example, it might be that the use of English literacy alone prevents these individuals from accessing knowledge and skills that would allow them to enter specific social, economic, and political realms of mainstream society. Of course, it is also the case that certain members of mainstream society (those in power positions) might support the assumption that literacy skills are important for maintaining the standards of society. These arguments should not be taken lightly, especially in light of the growing understanding of literate thought (Olson, 1989) and in view of the historical accounts of oppression relative to the use of sign language with individuals who are deaf (e.g., Lane, 1984; Lane, Hoffmeister, & Bahan, 1996).

With enlightenment comes the notion of emancipation. Exposing the *true interests* of certain individuals or specific rules, laws, or policies should lead to emancipation. With this knowledge, individuals should become empowered and should gain control of their lives. It can be argued that a lack of exposure keeps individuals *in the dark* and might even contribute to behaviors that can best be described as an external locus of control (see Weiner, 1974; see also the discussion relative to deafness in Paul & Jackson, 1993). That is, certain members of society might feel helpless or feel that their situation depends either upon the power of others or upon luck. These individuals might stop trying to achieve or refuse to become involved because they have no internal locus of control, that is, no faith in their internal ability or skill.

The last concept to be discussed relative to this brief introduction of critical theory is instrumental rationality. Instrumental rationality is a major concept for critical theorists, especially for individuals in the field of sociology, who have engaged in a considerable amount of metatheorizing (e.g., Ritzer, 1991, 1992). Instrumental rationality is considered to be the dominant approach of most institutions, for example, education, science, and government. There is an emphasis on methods and products, rather than on processes and purposes (e.g., see related discussions in Foucault, 1973; Gibson, 1986; Habermas, 1984). Proponents of this view are interested mostly in *how* to do it questions rather than questions that focus on *should* we, *why* should we, or *what* are the implications for certain subgroups of the population. As noted by Gibson (1986):

TABLE 5-1   Summary of major principles relative to critical theory

Critical Theory

- There is no separation of theory and practice, especially for theories about the human condition or human nature.
- Practitioners are not always aware of the underlying theoretical or metatheoretical assumptions of their practices.
- A reaction against the postivistic, objective assumptions of the scientific method.
- There is no value-free knowledge; no separation of the knower and knowledge relative to social and educational issues.
- Subjectivity and relativity are acceptable and unavoidable, specifically in relation to human issues.
- Enlightenment is the result of the focus on uncovering the interests of certain individuals or groups. In other words, whose interests are being served?
- Enlightenment leads to emancipation. With the knowledge of true interests, individuals should become empowered and should gain control over their lives.
- Instrumental rationality is a major concept and the source of counterattacks by critical theorists. Instrumental rationality is the emphasis on methods and products, rather than on processes and purposes. Proponents of instrumental rationality are interested primarily in *how* to do it, rather than the queries of critical theorists such as *Should* we do this? *Why* should we do this? or *What* are the implications for certain subgroups of the population?

It is the obsession with calculation and measurement: the drive to classify, to label, to assess and number, all that is human. As such, it is the desire to control and to dominate, to exercise surveillance and power over others and over nature. Because of its preference for the intellectual over the emotional, it represents the devaluation and marginalisation of feeling. It is a kind of intellectual activity which actually results in the decline of reason itself, and it therefore stultifies, distorts and malforms individual and social growth. (p. 7)

Is it possible to observe these effects in the literacy instruction of students who are deaf? This leads to a discussion of the application of critical theory to literacy in the ensuing sections.

Table 5-1 presents a summary of the major principles relative to critical theory.

Critical Theory and Literacy

Critical theory has been applied to numerous areas, for example, education, culture, schools, literature, and literacy. With the focus on the concept of literacy, it is necessary to also discuss some aspects of the debate on the nature and importance of literature. It is assumed that a literate person is one who is conversant about the *great* works of literary figures (e.g., see discussion in Gibson, 1986). Thus, in some educator's eyes, it is important to read (and write), mostly because of the information and understanding that comes from the reading of *great literature*. In this sense, there is some overlap in critical theory between literature and literacy. The concept of literature is discussed later.

To establish a context for the discussion of questions posed earlier in this chapter (e.g., those by Paul & Quigley, 1994a), it is important to address a few—what some critical educators and scholars would call basic— questions, What is literacy? Why is literacy important? These questions can lead to several others: What is illiteracy? Is illiteracy a problem for individuals in this society? Why? Most people want to think of these questions in a rapid-fire simple manner—either you can read or you cannot. Either you can write or you can express yourself in speech (sign) only. If you cannot read and write, you cannot get a diploma, degree, or a decent-paying job (e.g., see discussion in Robinson, 1990). But, as Flavell (1985) has argued, the deep, complex concepts in life are difficult to define and describe, and perhaps that is why they are deep and complex.

One perception of literacy is to define it as functional literacy. This is evident in one description of which many educators of children who are deaf might be aware:

> The primary goal of education for typical (non-multiply handicapped) prelingually deaf children should be literacy—the ability to read and write at a mature level the general language of society, which in the United States is English. (Quigley & Kretschmer, 1982, p. xi)

With little doubt, this definition (or some other version of it) has been very influential in the instruction of reading and writing skills to students with hearing impairment (e.g., Moores, 1987; Paul & Quigley, 1990). In fact, much of this book is concerned with this description. It is related to a widely accepted definition of functional literacy (Hunter & Harman, 1979):

> A person is literate when he has acquired the essential knowledge and skills which enable him to engage in all those activities in which literacy is required for effective functioning in his group and community and whose attainments in reading, writing, and arithmetic make it possible for him to continue to use these skills toward his own and the community's development. (p. 14)

If these definitions are accepted, then it should be clear that the focus is on teaching reading and writing, or text-based literacy skills. In other words, in order to be *literate*, students who are deaf need to read printed-English materials, texts, and so on, and be able to express themselves in written English. It can be inferred that illiteracy is the inability to read and write text-based English. Ending on this note, however, would undermine the complexity of terms such as reading, writing, literate, illiterate, and even functional literacy.

Consider these questions: What does it mean to read? Would someone be labeled literate if she or he could read only the back of a cereal box? How about just the newspaper? What about *Moby Dick*? What about the works of Shakespeare? One possible interpretation (a traditional one) is to argue that there are levels of literacy (e.g., see discussions in Olson, 1989; Robinson, 1990). Given the fact that a high level of literacy is extremely difficult, a plausible goal for most students with severe-to-profound hearing impairment is functional literacy, and reading the newspaper might be considered as one manifestation of this goal.

There are several problems with this interpretation. *Reading* the newspaper does not necessarily correspond to one level of reading. What is being referred to is a level of understanding or comprehension. As indicated by the major theories of literacy discussed in this text, this level of understanding is not determined solely by the contents of the text. Furthermore, it is doubtful that functional literacy should really be the desirable goal for any student, let alone students with hearing impairment. For example, being able to *read* a newspaper written on the sixth-grade level can be taken literally to mean being able to reason or think on a sixth-grade level. One response is that many individuals are capable of thinking and reasoning at levels that are higher than their *reading* and *writing* ability. Consequently, one beneficial endeavor is to rewrite (actually, modify or scale down) high-level materials and information to a functionally literate level, say a sixth-grade level, so that these individuals can have access to the contents of these materials.

This is not a new line of thinking. High-interest, low-vocabulary books and other printed materials do exist. In addition, a number of classics (with apologies to critical theorists!) have been rewritten to a lower grade level than that of the original version. Thus, students and individuals can read the *classics* (or other so-called complex or great materials) with little or no assistance. Setting aside the argument that scaled-down classics (or complex materials) are not classics (or complex materials), it can be wondered why—if this is such a feasible, beneficial idea—there is not a widespread movement to make all reading materials accessible to individuals at the so-called average reading level, whatever that is.

Perhaps another crucial perspective on this issue—and one germane to critical theorists—is the description and implications of illiteracy. There are, at least, two descriptions. One, illiteracy can mean, in the traditional sense, the inability to read and write at a functional level, which has been described. Two, this term can also refer to an *unawareness* or *lack of knowledge* of the great works in several genres, for example, literature, history, and science. The awareness or, rather, understanding of great, complex works is often used to describe learned or literate individuals. It can be argued that learned or literate qualities are necessary for a high-school diploma and a college degree and for access to an important level of socioeconomic and political status (e.g., Adams, 1990a; Olson, 1989; Robinson, 1990).

Within this perspective, functional literacy might not be much better than survival literacy (e.g., reading street signs, medicine labels, etc.). Why bother with functional literacy if one cannot obtain a reasonable job in a changing, highly-literate technological world? If illiteracy is associated with poverty and powerlessness, then functional literacy might be equated with little power and the working poor. As is discussed later, this obsession with functional literacy is present in the education of students who are deaf. The question to be addressed is: Is this an oppressive situation?

Within a traditional view, many educators believe that a functional level of literacy is better than survival literacy and might even be a stepping stone for higher levels of literacy, including literature. There are several implications. One, a high level of thought is not possible without being able to read (and write) text-based materials (i.e., print). This is similar to one of the two questions presented previously from Paul and Quigley (1994a). To paraphrase: Can individuals engage in literate thought without having the ability to read and write text-based materials? Two, there is a reciprocal relation between literature and high thought because of the *greatness* of literature. That is, literature is great because it contains high-level thoughts that are appreciated by high-level thinkers. In essence, it is critical (no pun intended) to pass on, teach, and transmit these enduring, high-quality thoughts to all members of the present culture. In fact, preserving these thoughts or ideas is the hallmark of a cultured, advanced civilization. It is also averred that text-based literacy itself is necessary for advancing society, especially to the stage of technological prowess. These two broad implications are examined critically in the ensuing sections.

Literature and High Thought

Why is literature, especially great literature, important for high thought? For that matter, why is it important to discuss and learn about any great work, whether in history, philosophy, or science? Literature is the example used here; the arguments can be extended to other areas. As noted by Gibson (1986):

> There is a 'common-sense view' of literature which goes something like this. There exists an undeniable canon of great works that constitute 'Literature' (with Shakespeare the most obvious and unquestionable element). These works are the products of men (and occasionally women) of undeniable genius. These authors somehow offer almost magical transcendence, as they overcome the local limitations of their time (and ours) to provide universal, timeless truths about the human condition. Those truths can be grasped by a straightforward reading of literature by men and women in all ages. Literature is not simply enjoyable; it feeds the imagination, it enhances the quality of our lives, it links us to our culture, it deepens our understanding, refines our feelings, aids empathy. It is a personal resource for the healthy development of mind and spirit that enables us to cope with conflict, see more clearly and express our feelings more authentically. Indeed, somehow it makes us better persons. (pp. 90-91)

What is the response of critical theorists to the above passage? The following is based on the interpretation offered by Gibson (1986). Additional perspectives can be found elsewhere (e.g., Foucault, 1973; Godzich, 1994; Habermas, 1984; Robinson, 1990). Critical theorists argue that there is no such entity as *literature*. Any body of work is constructed by various individuals at varying periods to serve the specific interests of these persons and others who agree with their views. There are no universal, timeless, enduring truths; however, a particular point of view or ideology might be sustained by certain groups who happen to have a great deal of power and control. Texts do not contain *objective* truths; they are interpretations and these interpretations are influenced by specific ideologies or philosophies of powerful individuals and groups. There is also a discussion by many critical theorists on why texts are not necessarily written by authors; however, that debate is beyond the scope of this text.

What about having knowledge of these great works? From a critical theoretical point of view, *knowledge* of these texts or their interpretations does not equate to high thoughts. Rather, this knowledge merely reflects a commitment to the resulting ideology from another period of time. In one sense, this is useless knowledge because it is essentially situation or context bound and not really applicable to current times. In another sense, *this type of knowledge is not really possible.* All knowledge and interpretations are socially constructed; an understanding of any text requires the construction of meaning in a particular context, for example, a classroom setting or a book store.

Let's apply the above discussion to a fairly typical classroom situation, a situation that distorts reality or actually represents the best interests of the teacher, according to critical theorists. The students in this hypothetical class have just finished reading *Gulliver's Travels,* a project assigned to the whole class. The teacher is poised to ask questions about their understanding of this book. In this sense, the teacher is considered the *expert,* who has the inside track to the meaning and understanding of this book. The children are expected to demonstrate their understanding of the book via the answers to the teacher's questions. The teacher is in control, determining *which questions* are important to ask and *what* is important for the students to remember. Finally, the teacher attempts to relate the high-level interpretations of this book to children (e.g., the author is really talking about the social and political oppression in England during his time, etc.).

In essence, high thought refers to a process of complex thinking and reflecting, not to the memorization or understanding of great thoughts. This leads us to the question of whether high thought is possible without the ability to read text-based materials. This is examined in the next section.

Some of the major points regarding literacy, literature, and critical theory are presented in Table 5-2.

TABLE 5-2   Major points regarding literacy, literature, and critical theory

Literacy and Critical Theory

• Literacy is defined broadly in critical theory. Text-based literacy refers to reading and writing skills. A literate person is one who can engage in literate thought, i.e., thinking creatively and reflectively.
• Many individuals are capable of thinking and reasoning at levels that are higher than their reading and writing levels. Thus, text-based literacy does not seem to be a prerequisite for development of skills in literate thought.
• Examination of the following questions are important: Is text-based literacy necessary for a technologically based society? Is text-based literacy an oppressive situation for some members of the population? Whose interests are being served by the predominant focus on text-based literacy?

Literature and Critical Theory

• There is no such entity as literature or great literature.
• There are no universal, timeless, enduring truths; however, particular views or ideologies are often held and espoused by individuals or groups in power positions.
• Texts do not contain objective truths; rather, these texts are interpreted by powerful individuals or groups.
• Knowledge of 'great literature' does not equate to high thought, but rather reflects a commitment to these ideas or views from another period of time.
• All knowledge and interpretations are socially constructed.

Literate Thought

Again, literate thought refers to the ability to think or reason critically and reflectively. Philosophers and other scholars have expended a great deal of energy on the relationship between thought and language (e.g., see discussions in Byrnes & Gelman, 1991; Cromer, 1988a, 1988b; Snyder, 1984). This has been an ongoing debate since the time of the Greek philosophers:

> The Platonic school of thought held that principles such as one finds in language are immutable and unaffected by man's mortal mental structures. By contrast, Aristotelians felt that such principles were affected and defined by the constraints or limitations of the organism that must use them. Obviously, these same positions are represented today, articulated in our contemporary idiom. (Snyder, 1984, p. 108).

One line of the current debates focuses on the contributions of cognitive science to the understanding of this relationship. Variations of this debate focus on the relationships between language and literacy and the relationships among thought, language, and literacy.

With respect to these variations, there has been growing evidence of the significance of the reciprocal relationship between the conversational (i.e., speech) and written forms of the same language, particularly a phonetic language such as English (e.g., Templeton & Bear, 1992; Nickerson, 1986; Shankweiler & Liberman, 1989). This is one of the main tenets common across all cognitive information-processing theories of literacy, despite differences in the manner in which this relationship should be established and developed. Some scholars argue that knowledge and use of text-based literacy skills exert a pervasive influence on the manner in which words are organized in an individual's mental lexicon (i.e., in the mind). For example, it has been documented that English reading skills contribute to an understanding (and appreciation) of the phonological and morphological properties of spoken English. This understanding leads to the development of advanced reading skills because of the increased and growing awareness of the alphabet system, the system upon which literacy is based (e.g., Shankweiler & Liberman, 1989). It should be highlighted, however, that much of our understanding of an individual's mental lexicon has come from psycholinguistic research that examines the spoken errors and uses of words (e.g., for an accessible, readable account, see Aitchison, 1994).

There have been also several extensive reviews on the reciprocal interactions of reading and writing. In fact, this line of research probably has contributed to the differentiation among the three broad theories (actually, metatheories) of literacy: cognitive information-processing, naturalism, and social constructionism (e.g., see discussion in McCarthey & Raphael, 1992; see also Chapter 1). Despite these differences, it is generally agreed that reading and writing influence each other (e.g., Adams, 1990a; Tierney & Pearson, 1983; see also the various perspectives in Irwin & Doyle, 1992). As indicated by Adams (1990a):

> In support of this foray, research indicates that children's achievements in reading and writing are generally quite strongly and positively related. Further, across evaluations of beginning reading programs, emphasis on writing activities is repeatedly shown to result in special gains in reading achievement. . . . the supportive relations between reading and writing surely run in both directions . . . (p. 375)

The foregoing discussion seems to suggest that there is a relationship between literate thought and literacy, that is, the ability to read and write text-based materials. Are text-based skills a necessity for developing abstract, comprehensive, precise thinking abilities? Perhaps the dictum of Francis Bacon is applicable here, "Reading maketh a full man, conference a ready man, and writing an exact man" (Beck, 1980, p. 181).

Several reviews can be found in the literature regarding the examination of the relationship between literate thought and text-based materials (e.g., Olson, 1989; Wagner, 1986). There is a growing consensus that the ability to read and write, albeit important, is not essential or necessary for the development of the ability to engage in critical and reflective thought. Although literacy skills interact with thinking skills—and it seems difficult to separate the two groups—it has been argued that literacy skills are manifestations of individuals who can engage in logic or reasoning activities. That is, text-based literacy is one avenue that people can use to demonstrate their ability to address complex topics and interactions involving areas such as law, philosophy, and science. From another perspective, it is possible for individuals to develop complex, deep understandings in these areas despite their inability to access the information in print-related materials.

It is not difficult to find examples of this situation. In the present writer's view, the most obvious example is the philosopher Socrates, who purportedly left no written records of his thought (Plato performed this task) and who did not engage in much reading activity. No one would claim that Socrates was not *literate,* at least not in the sense of being learned or well informed.

There is additional documented support for the ability to engage in literate thought without accessing printed materials. For example, historical researchers have reported numerous accounts of individuals who participated in the discussions of texts or printed documents that were read or orally presented to them (e.g., see discussion in Olson, 1989). These events were quite common during earlier periods (and even later) after the invention of the printing press. Literacy was not a common skill, and in many cases, there were few copies of texts or materials available. Basically, the *reader* or *speaker* was a person whose major role was to read or present the information to a group of individuals. The reader or speaker did not actively engage in discussing the information. It was the responsibility of members of the group to participate in the debate of the merits of the information, particularly when some documents required a vote or action to be taken.

It might be wondered whether information presented in an *oral* or *conversational* (including signing) mode is really as complex as the information that is captured in print. On one hand, there is some research that reveals that written information is decontextualized, less redundant, and more complex, especially with respect to the use of complex sentence structures (e.g., see discussions in Adams, 1990a; Shankweiler & Liberman, 1989). Despite the importance of the reciprocity between speech and print, two possible implications of this research have been proffered: (1) written language is not simply speech written down, and (2) the ability to read and write requires another set of skills that proceed beyond those needed for spoken language comprehension.

It should be highlighted that much of the research on the complexity issue has focused on the structure of the language of print versus that used in spoken language and the skills needed to comprehend this information. However, complexity has another, equally as important, aspect, namely, the *content* of the information. It has been shown that the content of information presented or delivered in the conversational mode (speaking or signing) can be as complex and difficult as information presented in the written mode (e.g., see discussions in Olson, 1989; Wagner, 1986).

It is not difficult to find examples. Consider the following excerpt from a presentation presented by the present author without explicit notes (Paul, 1994c), which was recorded verbatim by real-time captioning.

> Descriptions of the reading achievement of deaf students have been based on the results of their performance on standardized tests, both of general achievement and reading. Despite improvements in the construction of the tests and the implementation of early intervention, there are two general themes that can be gleaned from the findings. One, the overwhelming majority of 18- to 19-year-old deaf students do not read above a fourth-grade level. Two, this plateau has been in existence since the beginning of the formal testing movement in the early 1900s. I want to emphasize that these two themes are not simply the results of either poor instruction, poor signing skills, or, even, poor students. Literacy is an unbelievably complex activity, and we need to investigate whether this endeavor is a realistic goal for the overwhelming majority of students with severe to profound hearing impairment. (November, 1994)

Other examples include the use of *talking books* for people who like to listen to classics or other books, rather than to read them, or the use of complex recorded materials for individuals with varying levels of visual impairment. It is not uncommon for an individual with severe visual impairment to *listen* to newspapers or other printed materials on audiotapes.

It might be easy to convince educators and scholars about the complexity of the information in the conversational mode; however, they might remain unconvinced about the development of literate thought in this mode only. Part of the reason for this uncertainty has to do with the widespread uses of literacy in professions such as medicine, law, science and industry, and, of course, education. In addition, there is a permanence to this information; it can be referred to periodically because it is captured on paper (or computer screen). Furthermore, scholarly discussions and debates seem to evolve about information presented in text-based materials.

With the availability and ease of modern technology, it is possible to capture the complex contents of learned information presented in the conversational mode (speaking or signing). With the advent of computers and interactive video, this medium can be just as efficient and effective as print (e.g., see discussion in Montague, 1990). Indeed, this type of medium might be preferred by many individuals to make use of printed materials an obsolete and ineffective endeavor. Some scholars have argued that a fixed medium such as print is not sufficient for meeting the complex challenging needs often associated with the calls for educational reform (e.g., see relevant discussion in Ellsworth, Hedley & Baratta, 1994). It is argued that only the use of electronic media can meet these challenges that include the following concepts:

1. Inclusion (an education program that includes children with special needs and varying abilities in typical classroom settings, (for example, see discussions in Friend & Bursuck, 1996; Paul & Ward, 1996).

2. Individualization (an educational approach that attempts to meet the individual needs of all students, regardless of level of ability).

3. Engagement (a process that encourages students to become engaged in active, creative construction rather than passive reception of information—one of the major tenets of social constructionism).

The crux of the foregoing discussion is that it should be possible for individuals to develop high levels of critical and reflective thinking skills without having adequate skills in text-based literacy. In essence, these individuals can be exposed to the same amount and diversity of learned, complex information that is preserved on video and audio tapes or diskettes (e.g., compact diskettes). These recorded materials can perform the same functions as books and more. Learned debates, discussions, and instruction can be organized around these materials. Individuals need to be able to access these materials, to take them home for review, and to become engaged in meaningful discussions.

Assuming that literate thought is possible with an electronic medium, at least two major questions might be raised. One, is it cost efficient to duplicate everything that is already available in print; that is, to present all information in several forms—print, video and audio recordings, Braille, and sign? If there are bilingual education programs, does that mean all information has to be duplicated by translation into the home language of the students? Two, is literate thought, without text-based literacy skills, sufficient for participation in a scientific, technological society such as the United States (from Paul & Quigley, 1994a)?

Addressing these questions in depth is beyond the scope of this text; however, some remarks need to be made. There is always somewhat of a cost factor involved whenever someone suggests a change in what can be called traditional, standardized representations of information, that is, the use of newspapers, magazines, books, and other types of recorded materials. At present, perhaps text-based literacy is a power issue; it might be mostly valued and used by individuals in power positions (e.g., see previous discussion in this chapter).

In my view, there is nothing magical about the type of preservation of information; sometimes I prefer to hold a book; other times, I prefer to read my computer screen; and still other times, I prefer to watch real-time captioning on television (and preserve that information on a videotape). However, my choices are a matter of taste, not necessity. That is, I can probably obtain nearly everything I need via the use of journals and books.

However, for individuals with text-based literacy problems, choice is basically an accessibility issue. In addition, it might even be an oppression issue, especially if it is clear that the same individuals could have reached high literate thought levels via the use of conversational information and other text-based information captured on audio and video media. From one perspective, this is a good example of what some educators mean when it is remarked that we need to pay closer attention to the *learning styles* of students (e.g., see discussion in Ellsworth et al., 1994). Some students prefer to listen/watch and speak/sign whereas others prefer to read and write and so on. Why should text-based literacy be the most valued mode of accessing or receiving information when research has shown that conversational forms of information can be just as complex and intricate?

As for literate thought being sufficient for living in a scientific, technological society—that depends upon the values of the larger mainstream society. At present, it might be

TABLE 5-3   Some major points regarding literate thought and critical theory

Literate Thought and Critical Theory

- There is a reciprocal relationship between text-based literacy and literate thought; nevertheless, literate thought can occur without text-based literacy.
- Information presented orally or in the conversational form of a language (i.e., speech or sign) can be just as complex as the information that is captured in print. However, there is a tendency for information in print to contain more complex grammatical structures such as longer sentences, complex syntactic structures, and so on. To deal with this level of complexity and with the notion of print, the individual will need to learn skills that are different from what is needed for interactions via the conversational form of the language.
- With the availability and ease of modern technology, it should be possible to capture the complex contents of learned information presented in the conversational mode. Media such as computers and tape recorders can be just as effective and efficient as print.

difficult to participate in such a society without text-based literacy skills because of the general lack of accessibility and because of educational programs that are not oriented to utilizing predominantly electronic media. In essence, there is still a need to investigate "whether the possession of high-level text-based literacy skills is the hallmark or an epiphenomenon of an advanced civilization—one that possesses scientific and technological prowess . . ." (Paul & Quigley, 1994a, p. 301).

Table 5-3 presents some major points of the discussion of literate thought and literacy.

Clinical and Cultural Perspectives

The intent of this section is to relate these two macro paradigms, clinical and cultural, to the two broad perspectives on literacy and deafness: reading comprehension and literary critical. In conducting this kind of analysis, there is always a risk of oversimplification. In addition, some educators might think that paradigm choice is not an issue that crosses the minds of teachers. Perhaps not. However, if it is an issue, then it presents a dilemma for educators because of the persistent low literacy achievement levels of students who are deaf. Several questions need to be addressed by educators: Is literacy a realistic goal for most students with severe to profound impairment? If it is, is it worth the effort in time and resources? Furthermore, as mentioned previously, is literacy an oppressive issue for many students with severe to profound impairment?

To reiterate briefly, it has been discussed (Chapter 1) that reading-comprehension theorists, researchers, and educators are most interested in investigating the decoding and comprehension skills of students. These individuals are attempting to understand how and why some children develop these skills and why others have extreme difficulty. The major goal of the reading-comprehension perspective is to improve the text-based literacy ability of students.

There are some major assumptions common across these reading-comprehension theories (including those with naturalistic principles). All theorists seem to agree, in general, that a working knowledge of the language of print (i.e., conversational English) is critical during the literacy stages (see reviews in Paul, 1993a, 1994b; Paul & Quigley, 1994a; Samuels & Kamil, 1984). This working knowledge includes the components of a language that have been delineated: phonology, morphology, syntax, and semantics. Knowledge of the culture (e.g., school, environment) and of the topics of the texts is also important. With a focus on improving and teaching literacy, it is safe to conclude that reading-comprehension theories can be placed within the clinical paradigm. Some theories, particularly those that focus on identifying deficiencies, seem to be more clinical than others (e.g., see discussions in Lemley, 1993; Paul, 1995a, 1995b; Paul & Quigley, 1994a). In any case, there is the assumption that literacy skills are the cornerstones of academic success and success after compulsory education.

As discussed in this chapter, literary critical theorists are not concerned with the improvement of literacy. They desire to know how literacy is valued and utilized by certain groups of individuals within particular contexts. Within this framework, literacy skills (i.e., reading and writing) are subsumed under a broad definition of literacy (or being literate). In some societies being literate might include the ability to read and write as one expression of literate thought. This broad notion of literacy also includes the values and beliefs of affected societies toward the functions of reading and writing. This broad perspective also renders it difficult to construct a theoretical model due to the varying views that emerge across the different cultures. In essence, critical theorists aver that there are no universal theoretical models.

Because of the emphasis on the interactions and usage of individuals with literacy, several scholars in deafness have placed this framework within the cultural paradigm (e.g., Lemley, 1993; Padden & Ramsey, 1993; Paul, 1994a, 1994b). Literary critical theorists, researchers, and educators consider the act of literacy as a social phenomenon. They also argue that the emphasis should be on developing literate thought, rather than on specific literacy skills. The mode of literate thought (e.g., reading, writing, computer, and mathematics) might be relevant for specific purposes depending on the needs and values of the members of a specific subgroup. However, the development of literate thought, itself, is highly dependent upon the development of a first language, particularly the conversational form of that language. Given what is known about language development, the earlier the acquisition, the more wide-reaching the results.

Literate Thought and Deafness

Literate thought has become an issue with students who are deaf because of the results of research on how well these students can acquire English (e.g., see Allen, 1986; King & Quigley, 1985; see also Chapter 3 of this text). This *how well* concept really contains two aspects, the conversational form and the literacy form (i.e., reading and writing). However, much of the available information concerns the results of secondary language measures. There is some evidence relating to the use of English-based signed systems.

Detailed summaries of the research on oral/manual communication systems can be found elsewhere (e.g., Moores, 1987; Paul & Quigley, 1994a; Wilbur, 1987). There is evidence that some students can acquire English at respectable levels; however, most of them have extreme difficulty with reaching functional literacy levels. One implication of this research is that there is no superiority associated with either oral English or total-communication approaches for the overwhelming majority of students with severe to profound hearing impairment. Another implication is that ASL should be developed initially and used to teach English as a second language for all deaf students (e.g., Johnson, Liddell, & Erting, 1989). This latter implication is related to the assumption that all children who are deaf should be considered as members of a cultural group in which ASL is the language of choice (e.g., see discussion in Lane, Hoffmeister, & Bahan, 1996). It is argued further that ASL is a bona fide language and is the easiest language form for most students in the United States to learn.

In defense of the second implication regarding the use and acquisition of ASL, at least three points should be made. One, practitioners have difficulty adhering to the principles of some of the signed systems (as discussed briefly in Chapter 3). This leads to an inconsistent and unsystematic use of the systems (e.g., see review in Drasgow & Paul, 1995). Two, these systems do not fully represent the English language. Assuming that students have limited or no residual hearing, it would be difficult for the students to internalize principles of phonology and the suprasegmental aspects of speech via the use of the signed systems, even when they are accompanied by the use of speech. Three, it is important to acquire a first language at as early an age as possible.

In essence, if educators wear a clinical hat predominantly, the end result for many students might be that they will not acquire the conversational form of English by the time they start formal schooling. Indeed, they might not acquire this form of English after 12 years of school. Thus, students who are deaf are expected to read and write a language without ever having a working knowledge of it in the conversational form. No current theory of literacy supports this process despite the fact that this is the focus of several ASL/English bilingual programs (see Chapter 6).

Even knowledge of American Sign Language might not be sufficient for learning English as a second language. According to critical theorists, this is a good argument for the case of oppression. For example, consider that acquisition of text-based literacy skills is an unrealistic goal for some, perhaps most, students who are deaf because of difficulty in accessing this form. This lack of access might lead to an impoverished development of cognition, particularly critical thinking and reasoning skills. This could occur because of the inordinate amount of time and resources expended on conveying information and using the literate form.

Thus, this can be considered an unfair treatment of this subgroup of the population. It can be argued that the sole use of literacy prevents many of these individuals from reaching a high level of literate thought, which is possible via other communication and information modes. The problem is that these individuals might not be able to demonstrate a high level of thinking via the printed mode. Therefore, if text-based literacy is a major requirement for entrance into the prestigious socio-economic level of society, critical theorists argue that this represents an oppressive situation.

The issue for students who are deaf might be: What is the language that can be acquired at as early an age as possible in order to enable the students to achieve literate thought? When educators wear a clinical hat, the predominant focus is on developing English, the majority language of mainstream society. When educators wear a cultural hat, the predominant focus might be on developing literate thought in any language (or mode) that is accessible to the students.

Should not literate thought be the higher goal, rather than the acquisition of a particular language such as English, almost at any cost? Who really decides which hat should be worn? Must there be a choice between literate thought and text-based literacy? Can the selection of a hat initially and subsequently depend on the evolving needs of children who are deaf and their parents? Is it possible to oscillate between the two hats, and occasionally create a third one, whatever that might be?

The difficulty with or impossibility of *either–or* situations has been recognized quite some time ago by a famous philosopher of education, John Dewey (1938):

> Mankind likes to think in terms of extreme opposites. It is given to formulating its beliefs in terms of *Either-Ors*, between which it recognizes no intermediate possibilities. When forced to recognize that the extremes cannot be acted upon, it is still inclined to hold that they are all right in theory but that when it comes to practical matters circumstances compel us to compromise. Educational philosophy is no exception. (p. 17)

The quote by Dewey seems to suggest that *either–or* dichotomies can become a no-win situation. Furthermore, with this type of dichotomy, the emphasis is on resolving conflicts. Not all conflicts can be resolved permanently, especially conflicts within education and the social sciences. Managing conflicts might be the more productive approach, and this requires flexibility and tolerance with respect to various, competing philosophies.

Instructional Practices

In discussing instructional practices, this section returns to some critical issues, for example, empowerment, accessibility, and instrumental rationality. Discussions of literacy instructional practices are based on those used with students who are deaf (e.g., McAnally, Rose, & Quigley, 1994; Schirmer, 1994) and those used with hearing students (e.g., McCarthey & Raphael, 1992). The goal here is to relate the discussion to the critical issues mentioned above.

It is safe to categorize much of the research and practice of literacy instruction with students who are deaf into three broad areas, natural, structural, and some combination (e.g., King & Quigley, 1985; McAnally et al., 1994; Schirmer, 1994). These areas are most often associated with the array of language instructional methods used with children and adolescents who are deaf (e.g., McAnally et al., 1994); however, they are applicable to literacy instruction. The structural approach is often associated with concepts such as direct instruction and precision teaching (e.g., for reading, see Carnine, Silbert, & Kameenui, 1990). Some basic principles include explicit teaching of rules and strategies, selection and sequencing of examples, and the notion of covertization (i.e., internalizing rules and principles; see also Chapters 7 and 8). The natural approach is intent on exposure to a literacy environment that enables children to acquire literacy in a natural, non-teaching manner. There is no implicit or explicit teaching of rules or generalizations.

Relative to our purposes here, the aspects for discussion are (1) the notion of best method and (2) the aspect of teacher control. These two aspects are interrelated; in addition, they can be related to the three broad categories of reading/writing models: cognitive information-processing, naturalism, and social constructionism.

The present writer has discussed the notion of best method elsewhere (e.g., see discussions in Paul & Quigley, 1994a; Quigley & Paul, 1994). The emphasis here is on how this notion might cause problems for students who are deaf, especially those who have difficulty developing reading and writing skills. As might be expected, the notion of best method assumes that there is a separation of the method and the use of the method during classroom interactions. This idea is most often associated with cognitive information-processing models (e.g., see McCarthey & Raphael, 1992; see also Chapter 1 of this text). It is also assumed that the search for the best or most efficient method is a desirable, enduring goal. Thus, the low literacy levels of students who are deaf are presumed, in part, to be due to the dearth or lack of good, effective methods of instruction.

There is a belief that the pursuit of better methods of instruction leads to or has led to the improvement of literacy achievement. The point, of course, is to remedy the deficiencies of text-based literacy in children and adolescents who are deaf. In essence, the teaching of text-based literacy skills is often considered to be a school-long, worthwhile, endless activity; that is, it needs to be pursued from preschool to graduation.

The belief that literacy is a school-long, actually life-long, activity is also shared by educators who work with students with typical or normal hearing (e.g., see discussions in Adams, 1990a; Anderson et al., 1985). The problem here is that many poor readers and writers, including students who are deaf and others in special education programs, do not reach high levels of literacy or even functional literacy levels in text-based literacy after 12 to 13 years of school. This relentless pursuit, fueled by the high value placed on literacy by the larger society, is influenced also by the notion of instrumental rationality, discussed previously. This makes it difficult for parents and educators to accept the reality that many students who are deaf might not be able to develop these text-based skills. The seemingly inordinate amount of attention placed on achieving text-based literacy also precludes the search or the development of acceptable, alternative ways to present and address complex information.

In essence, there seems to be no recognition of the issue of accessibility because of the focus on and value of only text-based literacy approaches and materials. In addition, little or no consideration is given to the fact that prolonging this situation might cause serious cognitive and language delays, especially in students who are deaf. Finally, because of this driving force of finding the ultimate effective method or methods, many educators might not even be aware of the growing consensus that the notion of good or bad methods is itself misguided (e.g., Prabhu, 1990; see also the discussion in Paul & Quigley, 1994a; Quigley & Paul, 1994). This is especially true from the perspective of either the naturalistic or social-constructionist model.

The pursuit of a best method also does not address adequately one of the questions posed previously by critical theorists, <u>Whose interests are being served?</u> It has been argued that text-based literacy skills might be serving the needs or interests of the larger mainstream society. This heavy *clinical* bias makes it difficult to consider the individual needs of minority cultures or of certain subgroups. Perhaps the most devastating effect is the assumption that certain members of minority or other subgroups are *deficient* because of their inability to read and write English. This deficiency is often extended to include the ability to think and reason adequately. In short, this assumption ignores the real possibility of a *difference* relative to the use of text-based literacy skills; a difference that requires alternative modes of receiving and expressing information (for another interesting perspective, see Lane, 1984, 1988; Lane, Hoffmeister, & Bahan, 1996).

The last issue to be discussed is teacher control, especially as it relates to empowerment and the three broad models of literacy. The behaviors of teachers in the classroom can be related to the style of teaching. For example, within some cognitive models, the teacher has a very active, directive role in the classroom instruction of literacy. Examples that can be found in Chapters 7 and 8 concern the direct teaching of lower-level and higher-level skills of reading and writing. The classroom is structured and activities proceed according to the agenda and style of the teacher. As discussed in Chapters 1 and 4, this model is a traditional one based on the notion that there is a separation of knowledge and the knower, of the content and the teacher, and of the method and delivery of instruction. Some characteristics of this view have been listed by Calfee (1994, p. 22):

Instruction
Teacher directed, student recitations
Individual work based on uniform processes and outcomes
Student is the recipient of information; teacher is the source
Uniform pacing for entire class or ability groups; micro-management of objectives
Organization
Hierarchical structure, principal as manager
Individual work by isolated teachers
Separate grade levels; pull-out programs and specialists to handle problem causes (sic)

These characteristics can be found in a majority of classrooms for both general and special education students (e.g., Calfee, 1994; Cooper, Heron, & Heward, 1987). Teachers have a tremendous amount of power over students, and it seems that students have little voice in their education. Some scholars have argued that this situation is the case for students who are deaf, particularly because most of the educators have normal hearing. In this view, there is considered to be a hearing agenda, which does not consider or meet the needs of students who are deaf (e.g., Lane, Hoffmeister, & Bahan, 1996).

In a naturalistic classroom, the student is said to be completely responsible for his or her meaning-making or learning. The teacher is present to *facilitate* or *guide* this process. This situation fits the basic tenets of naturalism, namely, that knowledge is ultimately constructed and interpreted by the individual. Thus, knowledge is subjective; there is no separation of knowledge and the knower, the method and delivery, and so on. In essence, there is no such thing as a method and the notion of best method is a fallacy.

The situation is somewhat similar in a social-constructionist classroom, except that the teacher plays a larger role than in the naturalistic environment. That is, the teacher and the students participate together to construct knowledge or meaning. There is still no absolute or one meaning available; any meaning is a socially agreed upon phenomenon based on the experiences, knowledge, and sharing of information from all participants.

There are some common characteristics for both naturalistic and social-constructionist classrooms. As indicated by Calfee (1994, p. 22):

Instruction

Teacher as facilitator of student learning and production

Cooperative learning, group framing and solving authentic problems

Student as constructor of meaning; teacher as guide to resources *(for social-constructionism, both are constructing meaning and act as guides to resources)* [added by present author]

Pacing accommodated to student needs and interests; framed by long-term goals

Organization

Mutual decisions, principal as head teacher

Professional community of inquiry

Upgraded adaptations, schoolwide integrated services

In essence, literary critical scholars and educators tend to favor classrooms that are more naturalistic and social-constructionistic. It is argued that these types of classrooms are most likely to result in the rendering of services that lead to empowerment, enlightenment, and accessibility (as discussed in this Chapter). Some literary critical scholars of deafness argue that these conditions are most likely to occur when individuals who are deaf are involved in power positions such as teachers, administrators, and policy makers (e.g., see related discussions in Lane, 1988; Lane, Hoffmeister, & Bahan, 1996).

A Final Word

The intent of this brief chapter was to introduce the reader to some of the basic tenets regarding critical theories and to show how these theories have influenced our thinking on concepts such as literature, literacy, and literate thought. It is hoped that the reader has gained some understanding of the nature of critical theory, including its important issues such as empowerment, enlightenment, and instrumental rationality. Although critical theory is not based on the scientific method, it still employs the use of logical and systematic inquiry through the use of methods such as paradigm analysis and deconstruction (e.g., analysis of the language used in texts).

The notion of critical theory is important for understanding the current movement for establishing ASL/English bilingual education programs. This movement has been fueled mostly by sociopolitical goals despite the implicit assumption that it is possible to use ASL to teach English as a second language. Applying critical theory to literacy models should have provided some insights into how these models and practices are related to the overall macro models of clinical and cultural perspectives of deafness. Because of their focus on empowerment and instrumental rationality, literary critical scholars are most likely to favor models and practices within either the naturalistic or social-constructionist paradigm.

Perhaps the biggest contribution made by literary critical theorists, relative to deafness, is the focus on literate thought, that is, the ability to think critically and reflectively. It was argued that literate thought is dependent upon the development of a language at as early an age as possible. Furthermore, it was argued that literate thought is possible without accompanying text-based literacy skills. This is not a widely accepted conclusion, especially by individuals who wear predominantly the clinical, mainstream hat. The notion that text-based literacy might be an oppressive issue for many individuals with severe to profound impairment needs to be explored further. The resolution of the oppressive situation seems to be the intent of ASL/English bilingual education programs, the topic of the next chapter.

Further Readings

BARTON, D. (1994). *Literacy: An introduction to the ecology of written language.* Cambridge, MA: Blackwell.

DERRIDA, J. (1978). *Writing and difference.* London: Routledge and Kegan Paul.

FLANNERY, K. T. (1995). *The emperor's new clothes: Literature, literacy, and the ideology of style.* Pittsburgh, PA: University of Pittsburgh Press.

GRAHAM, R. J. (1991). *Reading and writing the self: Autobiography in education and the curriculum.* New York: Teachers College, Columbia University.

HABERMAS, J. (1974). *Theory and practice.* London: Heinemann.

JOHN-STEINER, V., PANOFSKY, C., & SMITH, L. (1994). *Sociocultural approaches to language and literacy.* New York: Cambridge University Press.

Chapter 6

Second-Language Literacy

The evidence from studies of second-language learning in preschool children indicates, as we have seen, that young children in a natural setting approach the task of learning a second language in much the same way they approach the task of learning their first language. In fact, they seem to progress through many of the same developmental stages as do monolingual speakers of the target language. Although the first language influences are noticeable, a number of studies indicate that children from different language backgrounds learning English as a second language make many of the same mistakes and go through essentially the same stages in acquiring various linguistic structures as do children learning English as a first language. Many authors believe that preschool children are guided in second-language learning, as in first language learning, by strategies that derive from innate mechanisms that cause them to formulate certain types of hypotheses about the language system being learned. (McLaughlin, 1985, p. 22)

The previous passage addresses briefly three major issues that have been part of the debate on developing English, that is, English literacy skills, as a second language in students who are deaf (e.g., see discussions in Paul & Quigley, 1994a, 1994b; Strong, 1988a; for a discussion on hearing second-language students, see Bernhardt, 1991; Cook, 1991; McLaughlin, 1984, 1985, 1987). The first issue concerns the setting in which the second-language learning occurs: contrived (i.e., classroom) or natural (i.e., outside the classroom). Is setting really important? Is setting itself an all-encompassing issue? More specifically, this issue is concerned with the language instructional methods used, for example, natural versus structural methods. In this chapter, the merits of the methods are briefly discussed. Although there are some fundamental aspects, there is an emerging view that this issue is too global or is an oversimplification of the complex teacher-students interactions that occur in classroom activities.

The second major issue can be labeled the qualitatively-similar-or-different hypothesis. Relative to students who are deaf, the question has been: Is development in L1 similar to development in L2? In Chapter 3, it was argued that English-as-a-first-language literacy development of students who are deaf is basically similar to that of typical hearing students learning to read and write in their native English language (e.g., see reviews in Hanson, 1989, 1991; Paul & Quigley, 1994a, 1994b). This seems to imply that much of what is known about teaching English-as-a-first-language literacy is applicable to teaching English-as-a-second-language literacy. There is evidence to suggest that theories of first-language literacy in English are relevant for understanding second-language literacy in English (e.g., for students who are deaf, see Paul, 1993a, 1993b; for hearing students, see Grabe, 1988, 1991). This evidence has come mostly from theories associated with the cognitive information-processing framework. At present, there has not been substantial evidence or research from theories associated with naturalism or social constructionism. Goodman's psycholinguistic-transactional model (i.e., one naturalistic model) has been used to explain second-language literacy with limited results (e.g., see reviews in Grabe, 1988, 1991).

Nevertheless, this second issue is not widely accepted, as can be seen in the various bilingual and bicultural models proposed for students who are deaf, particularly ASL/English models (e.g., see discussions in Lane, Hoffmeister, & Bahan, 1996; Luetke-Stahlman & Luckner, 1991; Paul & Quigley, 1994a, 1994b; Strong, 1988a). Without oversimplifying, it is possible to state that many ASL/English proponents believe that English literacy skills can be learned via explanations and interactions in American Sign Language only. Relative to literacy, some basic tenets of these bilingual/bicultural models are:

1. Students develop communicative and grammatical competence in American Sign Language initially.
2. The language of instruction and communicative interactions is ASL.
3. English is presented via print only, that is, by using reading and writing activities.
4. ASL is used to explain the grammar of English. Students use their knowledge and skills in their first language (ASL) to learn literacy skills only in the second language (English).

It is important to highlight here that neither spoken nor signed English is an integral part of these models. The reasons for omitting this area are discussed in detail in this chapter. In essence, the assumption is that it is possible to learn to read and write in English without ever manipulating the conversational form of this language. In Chapter 3, it was argued that this is not the case for learning to read and write in English as a first language. Is this situation different for students who are deaf learning English-as-a-second-language literacy skills?

The answer to this last question has been influenced by the debate on and interpretation of the third issue from the introductory passage. The third issue concerns the use of strategies that are derived from innate mechanisms. The intent is to show that second-language learning, similar to first-language learning, is guided by language-learning strategies. That is, individuals are developing and evaluating hypotheses about how their specific language works, namely, to come to an understanding of the underlying rule-governed system. Thus, strategies that an individual uses in acquiring their first language are applicable to the learning of the second language.

Relative to the third issue, it is possible to describe briefly the rationale for the majority of the ASL/English models. If students who are deaf learn ASL as a first language, they can use their first-language strategies to learn English *literacy* skills. Within this perspective, it should be highlighted that students who are deaf are applying the strategies in learning the conversational form of the first language (ASL) to learning the written form of the second language (English). To support this assertion, most proponents are appealing to the works of Goodman (e.g., 1985; specifically, the whole-language approach), Vygotsky (1962) and, most specifically, the linguistic independence hypothesis of Cummins (1977, 1978, 1979, 1984, 1989). The validity of this line of thinking is discussed in this chapter because the outcome has pervasive implications for the establishment of bilingual or English-as-a-second-language programs for students who are deaf.

Because most students who are deaf (i.e., with severe to profound hearing impairment) do not read and write above a fourth-grade level upon graduation from high school, there has been a growing movement for the establishment of bilingual and/or English-as-a-second-language programs (Luetke-Stahlman, 1983; Paul & Quigley, 1994b; Reagan, 1985; Strong, 1988a, 1988b). There is much controversy over the most beneficial model to adopt. Should students who are deaf be exposed to American Sign Language and English concurrently? Should ASL be taught as a first language in a typical interactive manner and then be used to teach English as a second language? Related issues concern the selection of participants (students and teachers) for the program, the roles of English speech and/or sign in developing English literacy, and the evaluation of the effectiveness of the program.

Several proponents of ASL/English bilingualism agree that ASL should be the first language for most, if not all, students who are deaf. Support for this assumption is based on four major points, gleaned from the literature on the acquisition of American Sign Language by some children and adolescents who are deaf (Paul & Quigley, 1994b, p. 222):

1. *ASL can be acquired naturally because it presents an adequate visual-motor feedback system similar to the auditory-articulatory loop of spoken language users (e.g., Cicourel & Boese, 1972a, 1972b).*
2. *ASL is the preferred language of use by deaf adults in most communicative situations (Reagan, 1985, 1990; Wilbur, 1987).*
3. *Children acquire ASL in a manner similar to that of hearing children learning a spoken language (Newport & Meier, 1985; Petitto & Marentette, 1991).*
4. *ASL (and other sign languages) are suited to the cognitive processing capacity of deaf individuals' brains (e.g., Bellugi, 1991; Poizner, Klima, & Bellugi, 1987).*

Relative to the three major issues presented in the passage at the beginning of this chapter, the plan for discussing second-language literacy for students who are deaf is as follows. First, a discussion of bilingualism and second-language learning with hearing students is provided. It is important to understand some basic principles of the theories and models that impact *second-language literacy*. Thus, the focus is on the nature of second-language literacy. This focus also necessitates a discussion of the research on both majority-language and minority-language hearing students. In addition, the research on deafness, albeit scanty, is synthesized and related to the current second-language learning and second-language literacy models. The chapter closes with future directions for research and instruction in this field and addresses some sociopolitical issues of this movement.

Bilingualism and Second-Language Learning: Description

It is appropriate to begin with a brief description of bilingualism and second-language learning. It should come as no surprise that a widely accepted definition of bilingualism or second-language learning does not exist (Bernhardt, 1991; Cook, 1991; McLaughlin, 1982, 1984, 1985, 1987). The notion of bilingualism has been examined from various perspectives, and it is generally agreed that psycholinguistic, sociolinguistic, cognitive, and educational variables should be considered in any description. What contributes to the difficulty of defining bilingualism or second-language learning are the debates on constructs such as the definition of language, the language goals of such programs, and language competence or proficiency (Cook, 1991; McLaughlin, 1987; Reich, 1986).

For the purposes of this chapter, bilingualism refers to proficiency in two languages. For example, an individual might have proficiency in two spoken languages such as English and French, two sign languages such as American Sign Language and French Sign Language, or a spoken language and a sign language such as French and Chinese Sign Language. Bilingualism is not an all-or-nothing phenomenon; it involves degrees of proficiency in various modes of the two languages such as speaking and signing, reading and writing. In addition, a distinction should be made between communicative proficiency and academic proficiency (e.g., Cummins, 1984). Communicative proficiency refers to the ability to use the language for ordinary, everyday purposes whereas academic proficiency refers to the ability to engage in the language of classroom discourse and school/academic texts.

Relative to deafness, the issue of bilingualism is further complicated by the relationship of American Sign Language to the English-based signed systems. There is no question that ASL is a bona fide language with its own grammar, which is different from that of standard English (e.g., Klima & Bellugi, 1979; Liddell, 1980; Wilbur, 1987). It should be emphasized that ASL is a visual-gestural language, executed without the use of speech, and that English is an auditory-articulatory language. Thus, the forms of the two languages are different.

It cannot be overemphasized that ASL is also different from the English-based signed systems. The various signed systems (e.g., Signed English, Signing Exact English, Seeing Essential English) are forms of English-based signing. That is, they were developed to represent in a manual manner the morphosyntactic structure of written, standard English (e.g., see illustrations and discussions in Paul & Quigley, 1994a; Wilbur, 1987). Two major differences among the systems are (1) the definition of a root word and (2) the selection of the signs and sign markers (i.e., prefixes, affixes, suffixes) for a particular word. There is contentious debate on which system(s) is/are truly representative of the grammatical structure of English and which can be considered a bona fide language. It is clear that the systems are not sign dialects of spoken English (for further discussions, see Drasgow & Paul, 1995; Paul & Quigley, 1994a and Wilbur, 1987).

A brief description of some major differences between ASL and the various English-based systems is as follows (Paul & Quigley, 1990):

> In using these systems, there is an attempt to create artificially a one-to-one correspondence between a word in English and a sign in ASL for the purpose of teaching English grammar to deaf students.
>
> Although the lexicon (i.e., vocabulary items) of ASL forms the basis of many signs in the English-based signed systems, it should be emphasized that there are several important modifications based on the structure of English. First, the signs are frozen. That is, they are executed only in their citation glosses (as presented, for example, in dictionaries of signs), and thus do not retain their original syntactic and semantic properties as evident in the context of ASL. Second, contrived sign markers are used to reflect inflectional and derivational morphology, and these are presented sequentially rather than simultaneously. Finally, certain kinds of linguistic and paralinguistic information conveyed by spatial and nonmanual dimensions in ASL are seldom used in signed systems. (pp. 136–137)

With the above description in mind and with the acceptance of the language status of the systems (and this is contentious), examples of ASL/English include any of the following: ASL/signed English, ASL/signing exact English, ASL/seeing essential English, ASL/Rochester method, and ASL/Linguistics of visible English (for a complete description and illustration of the systems, see Paul & Quigley, 1994a and Wilbur, 1987). For reasons beyond the scope of this text, ASL/pidgin sign English (or English-like signing or simultaneous communication or sign English, etc.) is not a bona fide example of bilingualism. In addition, spoken English (as in oralism) and one of the English-based signed systems does not constitute an example of bilingualism because this still involves the use of one language, English, in two different coding forms.

A useful conceptual framework for understanding bilingualism and second-language learning is the chronological principle developed by McLaughlin (1982, 1984). McLaughlin attempted to distinguish between bilingualism and second-language learning by labeling a period of acquisition as either simultaneous or successive. If an individual has been exposed to and or has learned (i.e., to a degree of proficiency) two languages prior to the age of two years, this is considered simultaneous acquisition or bilingualism. If an individual has been exposed to and has learned a second language after the age of three years, this is labeled successive acquisition or second-language learning. Learning a second language in a successive situation has been documented to be more difficult than learning two languages in a simultaneous situation (e.g., McLaughlin, 1984, 1985, 1987; Wong-Fillmore, 1989). Obviously, these issues are important for ASL/English bilingualism; however, an equally critical issue is how these two languages are acquired.

Theories of Second-Language Learning and Second-Language Literacy

In a previous work, the present writer has described two broad groups of theories on bilingualism and second-language learning (Paul & Quigley, 1994a). One group of theories is concerned with the ongoing effects of bilingualism on cognitive and educational achievement. Another group focuses on the development of the two languages (L1 and L2), including the development of literacy. In this text, the focus is on models of second-language learning and second-language literacy. As mentioned previously, much of the attention has been paid to Cummins' model (e.g., 1977, 1978, 1984). Although this model has its merits, it is argued that a better understanding of second-language literacy can be gleaned from the models and research that are based on first-language literacy, most of which have been influenced by a cognitive information-processing framework (e.g., Bernhardt, 1991; Grabe, 1988, 1991; Paul, 1993a, 1993b; Paul, Bernhardt & Gramly, 1992).

Second-Language Learning

The few models selected here deal with the broad notion of second-language learning, although some implications can be made for the development of second-language literacy. It needs to be emphasized that the selection of the models for discussion is subjective; however, it is based on common selections described in several theoretical and research reviews available (e.g., Beardsmore, 1986; Cook, 1991; McLaughlin, 1984, 1985, 1987). The influence of language-development theories on first-language acquisition can be seen. In addition, the models selected have influenced the types of bilingual/bicultural programs that have been established.

The Balance Theory

As is discussed later, some immersion (actually, submersion) programs have been influenced by the main tenets of the balance theory, proposed by Macnamara (1966). This theory is also known as genetic inferiority or verbal deprivation. Macnamara argued that individuals have a limited amount of language learning ability. The presence of two languages introduces the notion of competition; that is, individuals must divide their attention between the languages involved. Macnamara argued also that few individuals are able to learn two languages as well as native bilingual speakers. These speakers are those who are exposed to two languages simultaneously prior to the age of two years (e.g., see previous discussion of this issue). Macnamara highlighted the large body of data that shows that bilingual persons have difficulty learning the dominant or majority language of society. This difficulty manifests itself in lowered performances in all academic areas. It should be kept in mind that there is also a large body of data that contradicts these assertions of Macnamara (e.g., see research reviews in Lambert, 1972; Lambert & Tucker, 1972); however, the balance theory still has a number of proponents (see discussion on immersion programs).

Cummins' Models

The work of Cummins (1977, 1978, 1984, 1988) has been very influential in the field of deafness relative to ASL/English programs and also in other areas of second-language learning (e.g., see discussion in Lane, Hoffmeister, & Bahan, 1996). There are two models to be discussed here: the threshold model and the developmental interdependence model. Cummins' threshold model is actually an attempt to address the contradictions in the research literature on the effects of bilingualism on language and academic achievement (e.g., see conflicting views in Lambert, 1972; and Macnamara, 1966). Cummins suggested that the combined effects of the two languages in bilingualism produce desirable levels of cognitive and academic achievement. It should not matter whether the minority or the majority language is the initial acquired language. However, in order for benefits to be achieved, Cummins proposed that an individual needs to attain a certain threshold level in *both* languages. In fact, it is possible to trace the lowered performances of some individuals to the lack of proficiency in one of the two languages. Consequently, after acquiring a first language, an individual will not experience positive effects of bilingualism until reaching a threshold level in the second language.

Cummins' other popular model is termed the developmental interdependence model. To simplify, the main tenet of this model is that the development of skills in a second language is dependent upon the skills that have already been established in the first language. The alluring effect of this model for many ASL/English proponents is the corollary—if the first language is not developed adequately, then the introduction of the second language interferes with the further development of the first language. As a result, the inadequately developed first language impedes the development of the second language. This model attempts to address the situation of individuals who are struggling with two languages simultaneously. In essence, Cummins' intent is to show that it is extremely important to foster the continued development of the language of the home or the first language. Nevertheless, as is discussed later, it will be argued that ASL/English proponents have misinterpreted the main tenets of Cummins' model (see also, the discussion in Mayer & Wells, 1996).

Interlanguage

The interlanguage model is one of several second-language models that have been influenced by the work of Chomsky (1957, 1965). Selinker (1972) proposed this term to describe the interim grammars constructed by second-language learners as they move toward proficiency of the second language (see a recent discussion of interlanguage in Davies, Criper, & Howatt, 1984). In essence, Selinker endeavored to show that the spoken productions of these individuals could not be predominantly attributed to either interference or to the transfer of skills from the first language. Selinker (1972) also maintained that the interlanguage is a separate linguistic system that is distinct from the grammar of either the first or second language (i.e., the target language that the individual is attempting to learn). This system is the result of strategies that individuals used to acquire the target or second language.

Perhaps the most interesting argument Selinker puts forth is the assertion that the interlanguage contains *fossilized* (or frozen) features from the target language. For example, some second-language learners seem to persist in the use of certain words or phrases. The reasons for this persistence are still not clear; it might be due to problems with grammatical proficiency even though the individuals have attained communicative proficiency. In any case, Selinker's model should provide an interesting line of research for ASL-using students who are deaf and who are attempting to learn English as a second language.

It is argued later that the development of English as a second language by these individuals is essentially similar to the development of English by native speakers and users.

Nevertheless, it is possible to use Selinker's model to investigate some of the distinctive errors that are not developmental in nature, at least with respect to the first language. Selinker has concluded that fossilized features occur only in the development of the second language; they do not occur in the first language.

Second-Language Literacy

Similar to those of second-language learning, the models of second-language literacy have been influenced markedly by those of first-language literacy discussed in detail in Chapters 1 and 2. The influence can be seen mostly in the use of cognitive information processing and naturalistic (or social) models (e.g., Bernhardt, 1991; Grabe, 1988, 1991). In addition to Cummins' models discussed previously, there are two other approaches that address the development of second-language literacy, particularly reading: the vernacular advantage model and the direct approach to reading.

This section begins with a discussion of the latter two models. These two models address only the teaching of reading and provide some background for the L1 and L2 immersion models that are discussed later in the chapter. Indeed, these models and their variations form the bases for the types of reading programs in bilingual classes described in several texts (e.g., Bernhardt, 1991; Cummins, 1984; McLaughlin, 1985). Some of the more common programs include the following: simultaneous reading instruction, second-language-only reading, and first-language literacy programs (e.g., see discussion in McLaughlin, 1985). Some basic tenets of these reading programs are presented in Table 6-1.

TABLE 6-1   Basic tenets of some common bilingual reading programs

Descriptions of Reading Programs

First-Language Literacy Programs

Initially, the second-language learners develop skills in their home or first language. Subsequently, this serves as the basis for the later acquisition of skills in the second or target language. Also part of the minority-language immersion approach or the native language approach.

Second-Language-Only Reading

There is no reading instruction in the home or first language. Minority-language children are taught to read only in the second or target language. There is emphasis on developing oral, vocabulary, and syntax skills in the target language. Related to the direct approach to reading and transitional programs. Almost no use of the first or home language in this approach.

Simultaneous Reading Instruction

Attempts to utilize both languages during the school day. For example, one language might be used in the morning, and the second one in the afternoon. There are also two sets or parallel sets of instructional and reading materials available. Some programs employ the two languages together and use a grammar-translation method (based on the contrastive approach).

Source: Adapted from McLaughlin (1985).

Vernacular Advantage Model

The vernacular advantage model is concerned with the use of the mother tongue, or the first language of children from minority-language homes (i.e., children whose home or first language is not the language of the majority culture of society). This model asserts that the first language should be used to teach minority-language children (e.g., see discussions in Cummins, 1984, 1988; Rosier & Farella, 1976). It is suspected that children already have communicative proficiency for everyday use in the first, or home, language. The next step is to develop academic proficiency in this language (e.g., see Cummins, 1984).

One of the most important areas of academic proficiency is literacy. Thus, it is argued that reading and writing skills should be introduced and developed initially in the first language of the child. Similar to first-language learners, most children should be able to acquire proficiency in this first minority language within a reasonable amount of time. Subsequently, a working knowledge allows them to access academic materials presented in their home language.

After achieving a proficient reading level in L1, the students can be introduced to literacy in the second language, the language of the majority culture. The student will have been introduced to the oral form of the second language early in order to develop communicative proficiency. The crux here is that they will learn to read and write in their home language initially before learning to read and write in the second language. The advantage of this situation is that students can apply what they know about first-language literacy to the learning of second-language literacy (transfer skills) (e.g., Cummins, 1988; Gamez, 1979).

Direct Approach to Reading

Influenced by early bilingual models (e.g., the balance theory of Macnamara, 1966), some educators propose that only one language be used in the instruction of all students. That is, the main focus of education should be to enable second-language learners to develop both communicative and academic proficiency in the second language, the majority language of society (e.g., see discussions in McLaughlin, 1985; Paul & Quigley, 1994b). This approach assumes that there is or would be competition between two languages if they are employed simultaneously. Due to the limited amount of time and personal resources (i.e., intellectual, emotional), it would be best to emphasize one language only in the school setting.

In essence, within this framework, the most efficient approach for developing reading is the direct approach. That is, reading should be introduced in the second-language only. There is no real need to develop academic proficiency, particularly literacy skills, in the first or home language. As is discussed later, this approach is similar to submersion models found in some English-as-a-second-language programs. What is often misunderstood is that the evidence for this position comes from research on students whose first or home language is either the majority language of society or is equally as prestigious as the majority language (e.g., see discussions in Cummins, 1984, 1988; Genesee, 1987).

In sum, these two models take different positions regarding the issue of transfer skills from L1 to L2. Nevertheless, this is an area of intense debate, one that has brought to the forefront the influence of first-language reading models on second-language literacy development (e.g., Bernhardt, 1991; Grabe, 1988, 1991). This is the subject of the ensuing section.

Influence of First-Language Reading Models

The trends in first-language reading can also be observed in second-language reading. One can see the progression from text-based to reader-based to the current interactive social-cognitive models with influences from both cognitive (e.g., interactive) and social (e.g., naturalistic) models (Bernhardt, 1991; Grabe, 1988, 1991; Paul & Quigley, 1994a). However, many of the programs have been influenced initially by Goodman's model. The shift from top-down models (reader-based), particularly the psycholinguistic-transactional model of Goodman (1985; see discussions in Chapters 1 and 2), to interactive models has been slow because of the purported benefits of this top-down model. For example, Goodman's model has provided the impetus for extensive research on factors that affect the reading process in English-as-a-second-language, for example, conceptual knowledge, inference, and background knowledge.

Nevertheless, a number of criticisms have been made against Goodman's model and other top-down models. As discussed in Chapter 2, there are several problems that were not addressed adequately. Top-down (with a naturalistic or social bent) models in second-language literacy did not account for the degree of use of lower-level processing strategies. In addition, there was no detailed discussion of the relationship between lower-level strategies and higher-level (comprehension) strategies (e.g., Grabe, 1988; see also the discussion in Chapter 2).

Although *cognitive* interactive models are becoming in vogue, it is still necessary for these models (and subsequent ones) to address sufficiently major standard constraints associated with typical second-language learners, some of which are presented as follows (Grabe, 1988):

1. *They may or may not read in their first language; there is, in fact, surprisingly little current information on how, why, and what students read in other cultures.*
2. *If second language students do have literacy training, we still do not know how they approach reading in their first language as a social phenomenon; that is, do they view reading as a major academic, professional, and entertainment activity, or do they read much less, for far fewer purposes?*
3. *Second language readers are often assumed to transfer readily their first language reading abilities to the second language context; however, there is no adequate empirical evidence for assuming such a strong position.*
4. *Second language students coming from different orthographic traditions do appear to be affected by differing orthographic conventions, depending on their stage of reading skills acquisition.*
5. *Second language readers do not begin reading English with the same English language knowledge available to English-speaking children. (pp. 57–58)*

Point 5 above presents a clear distinction between first- and second-language readers of the same language (e.g., English). This point is applicable to many students who are deaf as well as to poor second-language readers. That is, many second-language readers and readers who are deaf do not have a working knowledge of the language of print, including text aspects such as vocabulary, morphophonology, syntax, and orthography (for second-language readers, see Bernhardt, 1991; for students who are deaf, see Kelly, 1995, King & Quigley, 1985, and Paul & Quigley, 1994a). Similar to poor first-language learners, second-language readers have both bottom-up and top-down difficulties. For example, the readers might overrely on text-based processing such as the use of a sight-word approach or over-rely on reader-based processes such as extensive guessing or use of context cues.

The importance of both bottom-up and top-down processing for both first- and second-language readers and writers has also been discussed by McLaughlin (1985), a well-known second-language theorist and metatheorist (e.g., see McLaughlin, 1987). This researcher remarked that:

> All children, when they begin school, have limited ability to use metalinguistic knowledge and conventional terms for describing language, are limited in their cognitive abilities, and are unfamiliar with the culture of the classroom and schooling. In addition, many children with limited proficiency in English in American schools do not have in their repertory certain of the sounds that occur in English, lack knowledge of English vocabulary, and have limited knowledge of the syntax of the English language. (p. 129–130)

It seems that this shift to an interactive theoretical framework (see discussion in Chapters 1 and 2 of this text) should have occurred sooner. In addition, the research on the importance of transfer skills, particularly bottom-up and top-down strategies, seems to have been established by early investigators. For example, a representative study on bilingual children (Spanish and English), conducted by Mace-Matluck and Dominguez (1981), revealed several points. Firstly, it was found that progress in reading can be rapid if children develop the ability to use two strategies effectively, that is, letter-sound correspondence and context cues (i.e., deliberate contextual learning). Secondly, bilingual children appear to use similar strategies for reading in the two languages. Initially, the children rely heavily on one or two strategies, then they add others at a later point in time. Finally, the researchers noted that certain foundation skills such as visual discrimination and phonological awareness are not language-specific. When these skills are acquired, they can be applied to both the first language and to English.

In sum, the interactive social-cognitive model of reading (e.g., see the model proposed by Bernhardt, 1991) can be used to explain much of the second-language reading process. In other words, second-language reading can also be viewed as an interactive process between the text and the reader. Similar to good first-language readers, good second-language readers are said to engage in the use of both bottom-up and top-down skills to construct a model of what the text means. Equally as important, the second-language reader needs to have access to the phonological code of the second language, which facilitates reading comprehension, particularly the comprehension of phrases and other longer discourse. Such access is also reflective of rapid, automatic word identification skills. These findings have important implications for the teaching of English literacy to students who are deaf, either as a first language or as a second language. Furthermore, in my view, these findings will still be applicable despite the growing contributions of naturalistic and social-constructionist models.

The Development of L1 and L2: Similar or Different?

To provide additional empirical evidence for social-cognitive interactive theories and some justification for the specific bilingual programs proffered in this chapter, it is necessary to address in some detail the question of development in L1 and L2. The focus is on answering the following inquiry: Is the development of English as a first language (i.e., L1) similar to the development of English as a second language (i.e., L2)? That is, do hearing or deaf second-language learners of English proceed through stages, make errors, or use strategies that are similar to those of native first-language learners of English?

Research on Hearing Students

Research on the development of English as a second language has been undertaken with respect to three broad groups: preschool, school-age children, and adults (e.g., see reviews in Cziko, 1992; McLaughlin, 1984, 1985). In general, this research has supported the notion of qualitative similarity between L1 and L2. This means that interference errors (errors caused by the structure of the first language) account for very little of the acquisition process of the second language (e.g., King, 1981; McLaughlin, 1984, 1985; Paul & Quigley, 1994a). The results of a sample of empirical investigations on hearing children and adults are synthesized in the ensuing paragraphs.

There is ample evidence from cross-sectional and longitudinal studies that the English L2 acquisition of children is similar to the English L1 acquisition of native users. For example, Natalicio and Natalicio (1971) examined native Spanish-speaking children in grades 1, 2, 3, and 10. The researchers focused on the acquisition of English plurals (e.g., boy, boys, woman, women), using a morphology test similar to that used by Berko (1958). The Berko Test has also been used with students with hearing impairment (e.g., see Cooper, 1967; Raffin, 1976). A brief description of the Berko Test can be found in Table 6-2.

TABLE 6-2   Brief description of the Berko Test

The Berko Test (Berko, 1958)

- Designed to evaluate children's knowledge of the morphological structure of English.
- Test contains 27 picture cards with accompanying sentences. Morphological structures assessed include plurals (girl to *girls*), singular and plural possessives (boy*'s* or boys*'*), past tense (want*ed*, *ran*), present progressive *(am running),* and derivational morphemes (*re* write).
- Example of a test item: There is a picture of an animal with bird-like features. Underneath this picture is another one with two of these creatures. The investigator remarks: "This is a wug. Now there is another one. There are two of them. There are two _____.
- Compound words are also part of the test. The test taker is required to describe, explain, etc. each word. Example: "A birthday is called a birthday because _____.

The subjects included 144 boys, half of whom knew Spanish as a first language, whereas the other half knew English as a first language. The researchers reported that both groups of students acquired the /s/ and /z/ plural allomorphs prior to the /iz/ allomorph. The native Spanish speakers produced more errors than the native English speakers. Nevertheless, the evidence for qualitative similarity indicated that there was little interference from the first language, Spanish.

One of the most extensive investigations in this area has been conducted by Dulay and Burt (1973, 1974a, 1974b). In their 1973 study, Dulay and Burt performed two analyses on the acquisition of morphological and syntactic structures. For the first analysis, they examined the errors in the speech samples of 145 Spanish-speaking children, ages 5 years to 8 years, who were learning English as a second language. The researchers focused on syntactic structures that were different in Spanish and English and attempted to classify errors in one of three categories: (1) developmental (i.e., similar to English L1 acquisition, (2) interference (i.e., reflecting Spanish structure), and (3) unique (i.e., deviant; could not be classified in the other two areas).

Dulay and Burt reported that most of the syntactic errors in English L2 were similar to those produced by English L1 learners (Category 1 above). As a result, Dulay and Burt proffered their creative construction hypothesis, which states that L2 learners are as creative as L1 learners. Finally, the researchers argued that the similarity of errors between L2 and L1 reflects the use of universal language processing strategies described in the research on first-language acquisition (e.g., see analogous arguments in Chomsky, 1975). As an example, it was noted that both L1 and L2 learners relied on word order of the target language to express semantic (i.e., meaning) relations. These results are similar to a later study (e.g., Dulay & Burt, 1974a).

For the second analysis, Dulay and Burt (1973) focused on the morphological aspects, particularly the order and degree of eight common morphemes as documented by Brown (1973). On the basis of the analyses of the speech samples of 151 Spanish-speaking children, ages 5 to 8 years, the researchers documented that the order and degree of the acquisition of the English morphemes were not similar to native English L1 acquisition. There seems to be some speculation that, at the morphemic level, L2 might not be similar to L1. This dissimilarity in the research on children has been addressed by McLaughlin (1984, 1985), as discussed later.

Nevertheless, as indicated by a number of subsequent studies, there seems to be little question that L1 is similar to L2 on the syntactic level (e.g., see reviews in McLaughlin, 1984, 1985; Paul & Quigley, 1994a, 1994b). For example, Gillis and Weber (1976) examined the acquisition of certain syntactic structures (e.g., negation, interrogatives, and imperatives) by two Japanese boys, ages 6 years, 11 months and 7 years, 6 months. The researchers analyzed the free, spontaneous speech samples of the subjects for five months. They concluded that the developmental stages of the two boys were qualitatively similar to those observed for first-languages learners as documented by Klima and Bellugi (1966). In addition, Gillis and Weber remarked that there was little evidence of interference errors due to the native language of the boys.

A number of scholars have reiterated these findings in extensive integrated reviews (e.g., Chun, 1980; Felix, 1981; Hatch, 1978; McLaughlin, 1984, 1985). Regardless of the linguistic background of the first language and amount of exposure to the second language, these reviewers have documented similar developmental stages for both English morphological and syntactic constructions for the second-language learners. The evidence is strongest for the acquisition of syntactic structures, whereas there are some differences relative to the acquisition of morphological structures.

At least two major reasons have been proposed for weak findings associated with morphology and, in some cases, syntax. There might be artifacts associated with the test used. For example, equivocal results have been obtained with Berko's Test (1958), described previously. Natalicio and Natalicio (1971) found evidence for L1 = L2 relative to morphology, whereas Dulay and Burt (1973) reported evidence to the contrary using the Bilingual Syntax Measure. Perhaps there needs to be an in-depth discussion of the construct and content validity of these tests (see Chapter 9 on assessment).

A second reason for the discrepant findings has been proffered by McLaughlin (1984, 1985). McLaughlin suggested that school-age children have less contacts with native speakers than adults. The greater incidence of interference errors and dissimilar developmental aspects might be due to the application of unsubstantiated instructional practices and methods. Teachers might be presenting grammatical lessons that do not follow the developmental sequence found in second-language learning. In essence, McLaughlin (1985) averred that the "more aberrant the input in the classroom is from input in natural communicative settings, the greater the likelihood of transfer from the first language" (p. 19). As discussed in the section entitled Analysis of Errors, another major factor might be the type of error analysis that is applied to the results.

The equivocal results associated with morphemes have been reported also in the research on adolescents and adults. Regardless of linguistic background, second-language learners performed similarly, that is, when compared to each other (e.g., comparing French L2 learners of English with German L2 learners of English). However, the evidence is not strong for L2 = L1 acquisition (e.g., comparing French L2 learners of English with English L1 learners).

In one study, Bailey, Madden, and Krashen (1974) explored the ability of English-as-a-second-language (ESL) adults to acquire eight English morphemes (based on Brown, 1973). The 73 adult subjects were between 17 and 55 years old and had varying linguistic backgrounds and levels of ESL proficiency. The researchers grouped the subjects into two categories: Spanish and non-Spanish speaking. It should be noted that the non-Spanish group contained speakers of 11 different languages: Greek, Persian, Italian, Turkish, Japanese, Chinese, Thai, Afghan, Hebrew, Arabic, and Vietnamese. Results revealed that the order of morphemic acquisition was similar for the two groups, regardless of proficiency level. In addition, Bailey et al. reported that the results were similar to those documented by young L2 learners in the work of Dulay and Burt (1973, 1974a, 1974b), discussed previously. However, Bailey et al., similar to that reported by Dulay and Burt, remarked that the developmental sequence was not similar to that documented for L1 learners in other studies (e.g., Brown, 1973; deVilliers & deVilliers, 1973). This suggests a qualitative difference between L1 and L2 learners, although there seems to be a qualitative similarity among L2 learners.

These findings have been supported by other studies on adolescents and adults (e.g., Krashen, 1981, 1982). A common hypothesis proffered is that there is interference of the native language, and this causes the discrepant findings between L2 and L1 learners. The order of acquisition in the second language (e.g., English) for the second-language learners seems to be dependent on the nature of the native language of the L2 learners. Thus, it is argued that the few studies that showed that L1 is similar to L2 for adults (i.e., a natural developmental order) have been confounded by artifacts associated with the test used (e.g., Hakuta & Cancino, 1977; Porter, 1977; Rosansky, 1976).

Despite the contradictory findings associated with morphology, the picture is clearer with respect to syntactical structures. In general, similar developmental stages have been noted for L1 and L2 learners relative to certain syntactic constructions such as negation and interrogation (i.e., use of questions). Some researchers have argued that it is different due to the nature of the first language (e.g., see discussion in Fillmore, 1979). However, there is substantial evidence to support the L1 = L2 hypothesis (e.g., Bongaerts, 1983; Cooper, Olshtain, Tucker, & Waterbury, 1979; McLaughlin, 1985).

Bongaerts' (1983) study is representative of this pattern. This researcher focused on three complex syntactic structures: (1) easy to see, eager to see (see analogous example by Chomsky, 1975), (2) promise, tell, and (3) ask, tell (Chomsky, 1969). The researcher examined the ability of Dutch adolescents between the ages of 14 and 18 years old. The findings were also related to those reported by d'Anglejan and Tucker (1975; French Canadian subjects) and by Cooper et al. (1979; Egyptian and Israeli subjects). All three groups experienced difficulty with the structures in which the meanings were not apparent. This is similar to the results for first-language learners and other language-impaired populations (e.g., Chomsky, 1969).

Finally, Bongaerts reported that the Dutch subjects had little difficulty with the *easy to see* construction. The researcher conjectured that this was because the construction was readily available within the first-language environment of the Dutch speakers. Nevertheless, Bongaerts argued that L2 is developmentally similar to L1 and that L2 learners do not apply their knowledge of the first or native language during the acquisition of the second language. Although L2 learners do apply the knowledge of their native language in the beginning, it seems that eventually they rely mostly on their knowledge of the second language during the acquisition process (e.g., see discussions in Bernhardt, 1991; McLaughlin, 1984, 1985).

Despite the few unequivocal findings on morphology, there is strong evidence for the developmental similarities associated with L1 and L2 learners, regardless of the first-language background of the L2 learners. The majority of errors are not due to the first-language structures. In fact, interference errors might be common in the early stages of acquisition and become less common as the second-language learners become more proficient in the second language. As noted by McLaughlin (1984):

> There seems to be little evidence from studies comparing language learning in children and second-language learning in adults that the two groups go through radically different processes. What evidence there is points to the conclusion that the processes

involved are basically the same. Older learners have the advantage of greater knowledge of semantic systems and strategies of conversations. (p. 66)

Nevertheless, it is important to provide some discussion on the analyses of errors as support for McLaughlin's assertions. The reason is simple: There is still a belief among teachers (according to research and heresay) that the poor written language productions of students who are deaf reflect their use of American Sign Language in trying to write English (e.g., see discussions in King, 1981; Paul & Quigley, 1994a). In other words, teachers and other educators believe that interference errors account for much of the English written language problems of students who are deaf.

Thus, it is not uncommon to find many ASL/English bilingual programs spending an enormous amount of time comparing and contrasting the two languages and *very little time on requiring students to manipulate the conversational form (speech and/or signs) of the second-language, English* (see reviews in Paul & Quigley, 1994a, 1994b). Comparing and contrasting the two languages (e.g., showing how each handles plurality, etc.) might be a good strategy; however, there is little research that this should be the *predominant* strategy. This problem can be better understood in light of the information in the next section on error analyses.

Analyses of Errors

In the second-language literature, at least three approaches to the analysis of errors have been identified: contrastive, interlanguage, and noncontrastive (Altenberg & Vago, 1983; Schachter & Celce-Murica, 1977; Sridhar, 1980). The contrastive approach focuses on the interactions of L1 and L2. That is, based on structural linguistics and behaviorism, this approach asserts that second-language learners are inclined to use L1 structures in their attempts to produce conversational L2 forms (i.e., speech or signs). This process results in *interference* errors. In other words, certain structures of L1 are incompatible with the interpretative or equivalent structures in L2.

The interlanguage approach asserts that there are specific fossilized structures that appear only in L2 productions. This phenomenon might occur because the learner has not attained grammatical proficiency. These errors are not made by native speakers of the target language.

The noncontrastive approach is considered to be a developmental model, based on the cognitive-linguistic model of Chomsky (e.g., 1957, 1965, 1975, 1988). That is, the errors made by the second-language learner are developmental in nature, similar to those made by young first-language learners of the same language. Thus, the errors are not deviant, as suggested by the contrastive or interlanguage approaches, but are part of the qualitatively similar developmental process that all learners proceed through in acquiring the target language or L2.

Although each approach has contributed to our understanding of second-language acquisition, there is still some controversy, particularly related to the instructional implications. At least five major reasons have been suggested for the controversial findings (Grabe, 1988, 1991; Lott, 1983; Richards, 1974a, 1974b, 1974c):

1. The complexity of the errors.
2. The limited knowledge of the processes involved in second-language learning.
3. Variability in factors such as type of teaching, age, attitude, and motivation of the student.
4. Influences of the first language on the target language.
5. The predictive power of the type of analysis of errors (i.e., contrastive, interlingual, or noncontrastive).

With respect to number 5 above, the focus in this section is on two types of analyses: contrastive and noncontrastive.

Richards (1974c) suggested that the discrepant findings related to the hypothesis of whether L2 is developmentally similar to L1 are due to the type of analysis employed. This researcher noted that contrastive errors analysis has the most predictive power at the level of phonology (and its influence on morphology) and the least predictive power at the level of syntax (and its relation to morphology). This can be seen in the studies reviewed previously in this chapter (e.g., Dulay & Burt, 1973, 1974a, 1974b) and in the research syntheses of other scholars (e.g., see discussions in McLaughlin, 1984, 1985, 1987; Schachter & Celce-Murcia, 1977; Sridhar, 1980).

Richards' hypothesis regarding type of analysis was supported by the work of Mukattash (1980) and others (see discussion in McLaughlin, 1984, 1985, 1987). In a representative study, Mukattash (1980) demonstrated the predictive power of noncontrastive error analyses at the syntactic level. This researcher studied the ability of first-year university Arabic-speaking students in understanding the Yes–No English constructions (see Table 6-3 for examples). The researcher instructed the adult second-language learners to change de-

TABLE 6-3   Examples of Yes–No questions

Questions with be—present and past

Is Mary going to the theatre?
Was John on the phone a minute ago?
Were you in the shoe store yesterday?

Questions with do—present and past

Does she like cream with her coffee?
Do you read novels often?
Did Rodney eat all of the ice cream?

Other types

Will you visit the zoo tomorrow?
Has she done her homework yet?
Have you seen this movie?
Shall I bake bread tonight?
Can you go to the athletic club with me?
May I go to the bathroom, please?

TABLE 6-4   Examples of errors from Mukattash's study

Errors Involving the Form of the Verb (e.g., tense and aspect)

Does he knew the answer?
Does he knows the answer?
Is Maha eating an apple when they came?

Substitution of do *for* be *and vice versa*

Is the girl know many languages?
Do(es)/did the house almost built?

Redundant Use of do *or* be

Is the house is almost built?
Do(es)/did the house is almost built?

Source: Adapted from Mukattash (1980).

clarative sentences (e.g., The man wanted a book) into Yes–No constructions. In the analysis of errors, it was found that most of the errors of the subjects involved the form of the verb (e.g., tense and aspect). Other common errors included the both-way substitution of the *do* form for the *be* form (i.e., *do* for *be* and *be* for *do*). In addition, there were examples of redundant uses of both the *do* and *be* forms. These last examples are reflective of the developmental strategy of overgeneralization or overextension (e.g., see discussion in deVilliers & deVilliers, 1978). This seems to support the overwhelming conclusion in most studies using noncontrastive analyses that very few of the errors during second-language acquisition are due to the interference of the first language. Examples of the errors from Mukattash's study are shown in Table 6-4.

Research on Students Who Are Deaf

It has been argued elsewhere (e.g., Paul & Quigley, 1994a, 1994b) that there is very little theoretical and empirical research on bilingualism, ESL, and deafness. What is available is in the form of anecdotal reports, descriptions of programs, and either polemic or metatheoretical arguments. The discussion here is limited to the development of English as a second language, particularly second-language literacy. Within this framework, information is presented in three major areas: (1) the effects of ASL on the subsequent development of English, (2) the comparison of English-as-a-second-language acquisition to English-as-a-first-language acquisition, and (3) the establishment of ASL/English bilingual education programs.

Effects of ASL on the Subsequent Development of English
Little is known about the long-term effects of having learned ASL in infancy and early childhood on the subsequent development of English literacy skills (e.g., see discussions in Paul & Quigley, 1994a, 1994b). This is true despite the fact that there is some speculation

that children who are deaf and whose parents were also deaf invariably become good readers and writers (e.g., see discussions in Lane, Hoffmeister, & Bahan, 1996; Moores, 1987; Wilbur, 1987). With respect to the limited research, the findings need to be interpreted with caution, for several reasons. One, most of the investigations were conducted prior to the period in which adequate descriptions of ASL grammar were available. Thus, the description or labeling of the signing behaviors of either the parents or the children must be suspect.

Two, the range of bilingual proficiency, if any, in either parents or children was not extensively studied and clarified. It is possible that the students who performed well on these assessments already possessed a range of proficiency in ASL and English. This can be inferred from the findings of later investigations (e.g., Hatfield, Caccamise, & Siple, 1978; Stewart, 1985). For example, Stewart (1985) explored the signing behaviors of high-school Canadian students. Teachers were asked to rate the signing behaviors of the students with respect to ASL or signed English (i.e., English-like signing, simultaneous communication, not Bornstein's system as described in Bornstein, Saulnier, & Hamilton, 1983). The students viewed two videotaped stories and were required to retell them. All students were judged to be bilingual (ASL and English); however, most of the students preferred to retell the stories in American Sign Language. The point here is that the observable signing behaviors of students do not indicate their overall proficiency, that is, overall with respect to number of languages—one or two.

A third reason—and perhaps the most important one—is that the implications of the results are not always clear, especially those that seem to undermine the complexity of English literacy skills. For example, suppose a study shows beneficial effects (typically, correlation) of knowledge of ASL and good English literacy skills. The simple, often-quoted implication is that knowledge of ASL leads to the acquisition of English literacy skills. Or, a related and commonly used implication is that students can use their knowledge of ASL to learn about the English language, particularly reading and writing. However, there is no clearly stated hypothesis why this should be true. Even more interesting is the implication that it is possible to learn English (or any other second language) without ever manipulating the conversational form (i.e., speech and/or signs). These issues are explored again in the discussion of the establishment of ASL/English bilingual programs in a later section of this chapter.

To assess the effects of ASL on subsequent English development, many early researchers focused on a design that compared deaf children of deaf parents (dcdp) with deaf children of hearing parents (dchp). Several of these studies were retrospective investigations (e.g., Brasel & Quigley, 1977; Meadow, 1968) The responses of the respondents (typically, parents) must be interpreted with caution, especially because they were responding to events that occurred 10 to 15 years previously. Focusing on academic behaviors in residential and day school settings, a number of these early studies documented that dcdp significantly outperformed dchp in several areas: educational achievement, intelligence, psychosocial development, literacy skills, and speech reading skills (e.g., Meadow, 1968; Quigley & Frisina, 1961; Stuckless & Birch, 1966). Even having only one parent who was deaf was reported to correlate with superior achievement scores when compared to deaf children with two hearing parents (e.g., Balow & Brill, 1975).

On the basis of these findings, two major variables were proffered to explain the differences: sign communication (presumably, ASL) and parental acceptance. The focus on these two variables undermines the complexity of developing English language skills in children and adolescents who are deaf and the complexity of psychosocial development (e.g., see discussions in Paul & Jackson, 1993; Spencer & Gutfreund, 1990). From another perspective, these variables should not be considered causal or all-encompassing. Furthermore, it should not be presumed that the variables are only present in parents who are deaf and who sign (presumably, ASL) to their children who are deaf.

Despite their shortcomings, a number of subsequent studies have shed light on these important factors: communication mode and parental acceptance. Although parental acceptance correlates with academic achievement, it can be present in homes in which the parents are either hearing or deaf (e.g., Corson, 1973; Messerly & Aram, 1980). Corson (1973) even reported that children of speech-using deaf parents performed better than those of sign-using deaf parents.

Relative to communication mode, there are two studies, which, in this writer's view, should cause educators to raise caution flags in the presence of overgeneralizations regarding emotional-laden issues. The work of Brasel and Quigley (1977) has provided some insights into the communication issue. These researchers examined four groups of students with hearing impairment. One group had deaf parents who used English-based signing (labeled Manual English or ME). A second group had deaf parents who presumably used ASL, which the researchers labeled as Average Manual (AM). This was probably an inaccurate description because they were comparing the two manual groups with respect to English language use. Needless to say, this label has been severely criticized (e.g., see discussions in Paul & Quigley, 1994a; Wilbur, 1987). The other two groups were labeled with respect to the use of oralism and hearing parents. The third group had hearing parents who fostered and used comprehensive oral methods (labeled Intensive Oral or IO). Apparently, this label was used to refer to the type of services and amount of parental involvement typically found in comprehensive oral programs such as Clarke School for the Deaf in Northampton, Massachusetts, and the Central Institute for the Deaf in St. Louis, Missouri. The fourth group had hearing parents who simply left the oral education of their children to the general school system (labeled Average Oral or AO). That is, the parents in this fourth group were not intensively involved with the education of their children.

This design allowed Brasel and Quigley to focus on the major variables discussed previously: parental acceptance and communication mode. It was presumed that high levels of parental acceptance were present in the ME and IO groups. The results revealed that the ME group of students performed significantly better than all other groups on almost all of the language and educational variables (including reading). The AM group and the IO group performed about equally. Finally, the scores of the AO group of students were significantly lower than those of all other groups. Brasel and Quigley concluded that early manual communication produced greater educational benefits than early oral communication for this research sample of students. Even more interesting is the finding that students who were exposed to ME outperformed those exposed to AM (presumably, ASL). This finding suggests that the extent and kind of manual communication are also important. These findings should be interpreted in light of my previous comments regarding causal and all-encompassing factors. In addition, Brasel and Quigley did not assess the bilingual proficiency, if any, of the ME group.

Nevertheless, despite the limitations of the Brasel and Quigley study, the extent and type of manual communication—actually, type of any communication—are factors worthy of further study. Most school systems do not adhere to a particular signed system; in fact, much of the signing behavior of teachers can be classified as simultaneous communication or English-like signing (speaking and signing simultaneously and following no specific rule system) (e.g., see discussions in Moores, 1987; Paul & Quigley, 1990; see also Chapter 3 of this text). Is this a critical issue? For example, it is not clear how English should be represented manually. The ME group in the Brasel and Quigley study had reading scores that were commensurate with other students with hearing impairment who were exposed to other signed systems (e.g., Signing Exact English or SEE II as in Babb, 1979; SEE I as in Washburn, 1983). In addition, should ASL be used to teach English as a second language? Why or why not?

Despite the scarcity of research, additional insights into these issues have been provided by the work of Luetke-Stahlman (1988a, 1988b). In essence, this researcher clarified further the issue of communication mode, relative to completeness of representation of English. For example, Luetke-Stahlman (1988a) investigated the performances of students on a battery of literacy tasks and a speech intelligibility measure. The battery of tasks included portions of several assessments, for example, *Woodcock-Johnson Psychoeducational Battery*, *The Johns Sight Word List for Third Graders*, and the *Northwestern Syntax Screening Test*. [Readers can access an in-depth discussion of the scientific merits of some of these tests and their applicability to students with hearing impairment in Bradley-Johnson and Evans (1991)].

Subjects for the study were students with hearing impairment between the ages of 5 to 12 years old. These students were exposed to a communication approach that was placed in one of two groups. Luetke-Stahlman labeled the approaches in one group as either languages or complete representations of a language, namely English. This group included oral English, cued speech, American Sign Language, seeing essential English (SEE I), and signing exact English (SEE II) (for a description of the approaches, see Paul & Quigley, 1994a; Wilbur, 1987). The second group included approaches that were not considered to be a complete representation of English, such as Signed English (SE) (e.g., Bornstein, Saulnier, & Hamilton, 1983) and pidgin signed English (PSE) (i.e., English-like signing). The researcher controlled for several important extraneous variables statistically, for example, age, aided hearing acuity, and unaided hearing acuity (for a description of these terms, see Davis, 1978; Meyerhoff, 1986).

Luetke-Stahlman found that students exposed to either languages (ASL or oral English) or complete representations of English (cued speech, SEE I, SEE II) performed significantly better than students exposed to SE and PSE on six of the seven measures used in the study. From one perspective, the findings indicate that *representation* of a language (such as English) is critical. Typically, representation refers to how a signed system represents an English word. Or, it can refer to how much of the English word is represented, either phonologically, as in oral English or cued speech, or morphologically, as in the signed systems. Within this framework, it is possible to place the systems on a continuum from

Least Representative					*Most Representative*		
I	I		I	I	I	I	I
EBE	SE		SEE II	SEE I	RM	CS	•

Note: EBE = English-based signing (English-like signing, simultaneous communication; has been known as pidgin sign English).
  SE = signed English
  SEE II = signing exact English
  SEE I = seeing essential English
  RM = Rochester method
  CS = cued speech
  • = all other oral methods involving the use of speech

For detailed discussions, see Paul & Quigley (1994a) and Wilbur (1987).

Figure 6-1   Representation of English via the Communication Systems.

least representative to most representative as shown in Figure 6-1 (e.g., see discussions in Paul & Quigley, 1990, 1994a; Wilbur, 1987).

From another perspective, Luetke-Stahlman has provided data on the benefits of knowing American Sign Language as a first language. This finding begs the question, Why should students who know ASL perform well on English tests, especially when they are in programs that do not emphasize bilingualism/biculturalism? It is clear that studies on classroom interactions and the use of signing are needed. What do classroom interactions tell us about the signing proficiency and use of both teachers and students? How does this relate to the teaching of English as a first or second language? More important, there is a need to understand the English language acquisition process of students who are deaf, especially students who know ASL as a first language. There is some quantitative evidence on this issue relative to the broad question of whether English-as-a-second-language acquisition of students who are deaf is similar to native English-language acquisition (i.e., L1). In addition, some researchers have attempted to demonstrate that English is a second language for most or all students who are deaf (presumably, students with severe to profound hearing impairment). These issues are the focus of the next section.

The Relationship of ESL Acquisition to First-Language Acquisition

What does it mean to say that English is a second language for most students who are deaf? One early line of research attempted to show that the performance of these students learning English is similar to that of hearing students learning English as a second language (e.g., Charrow, 1975; Charrow & Fletcher, 1974). It seems that this research thrust did not consider the possibility that English L2 acquisition might also be similar to English L1 acquisition. In addition, these early investigations were influenced by the notion of pidginization and the presence of nonstandard English usage.

The work of Charrow (e.g., Charrow, 1975; Charrow & Fletcher, 1974) is reflective of many of these early research endeavors. For example, Charrow and Fletcher compared the performances of three groups of students on a test of English as a second language: (1)

hearing students learning English as a second language, (2) deaf students of hearing parents, and (3) deaf students with deaf parents. The researchers were interested in testing three major hypotheses. One, they predicted that deaf students with deaf parents would outperform the deaf students with hearing parents. Two, they stated that there should be a strong similarity between the performances of hearing ESL learners and those of deaf students of deaf parents. Finally, the researchers focused on the performances of two tests, the Test of English as a Foreign Language (TOEFL) and the Stanford Achievement Test (SAT). They speculated that performances of deaf students of deaf parents on these two tests should resemble each other less than should the performances by deaf students of hearing parents on the same tests.

Charrow and Fletcher found evidence for the first hypothesis. Deaf students of deaf parents significantly outperformed deaf students of hearing parents on most of the subtests and on the total score on the TOEFL. The researchers did not proffer any reasons for this finding; however, as discussed previously in this chapter, there is no causal relationship between academic achievement and having deaf parents.

Much of the focus was on addressing the second and third hypotheses. The results, however, were mixed. For some subtests of both the TOEFL and the SAT, the performances of deaf students of deaf parents resembled those of the hearing second-language learners more than did the performances of deaf students of hearing parents. For example, there was a strong similarity on two of the TOEFL subtests, namely, English Structure and Writing Ability. But this similarity was not observed for the other subtests. Vocabulary and Reading Comprehension, which are also names of subtests (or sections) of the SAT.

The investigators concluded that the question of whether students who are deaf are acquiring English in the same manner as hearing second-language learners might be too broad to study. On the basis of the results of their study, Charrow and Fletcher argued that only some aspects of English acquired by students who are deaf are similar to those acquired by hearing second-language learners.

Charrow (1975) endeavored to identify and establish normative data for the nonstandard features of English language usage by persons who are deaf. The researcher labeled these features as examples of *Deaf English*. It was implied that persons who are deaf might be using a dialect of English, which is different from standard English. This implication was based on the occurrence of typical, consistent patterns of variant structures in the use of English. Furthermore, Charrow argued that there was an alternation of variant structures and standard English structures, and this was reflective of the process of pidginization (that is, the combination of grammatical aspects from two languages by a speaker/user who is proficient in only one of the languages). In sum, Charrow remarked that the range of grammatical forms, involving both standard English and Deaf English, appears to parallel the range of forms found in the speech of pidgin speakers.

In investigating the phenomenon of Deaf English, Charrow (1975) examined the performances of hearing students and deaf students of both hearing and deaf parents. The subjects were exposed to 100 sentences. Fifty of the sentences conformed to the rules of standard English and the remaining sentences were written by deaf teenagers and labeled Deaf English. The subjects were required to write the sentences from memory, one sentence at a time. Charrow reported that both groups of deaf students remembered more of the Deaf English sentences than did the hearing students. More interesting, there were no significant differences between the performances of the two deaf groups with respect to recall of both Deaf English and standard English sentences.

Charrow proposed an interesting, but unusual, conclusion. The researcher stated that students who are deaf do acquire most, if not all, of the rules of standard English syntax; however, the students were applying these rules in an inconsistent manner. In addition, it was argued that many of the variant structures (e.g., omission of articles such as *a, an*, and *the* and omission of past tense markers such as *-d, -ed*) found in the written language of the students were not the result of interference from the first language. These errors reflected the redundant, nonessential features of English that are difficult to acquire and easy to overlook. In sum, it seems that there is not much evidence that deaf students are learning English as a second language in the same manner as hearing second-language learners.

Previously, it was argued that the development of English by hearing second-language learners was similar to that of hearing, native first-language users. Since the works of Charrow and others, there have been a number of investigations on the English language acquisition of students who are deaf. As discussed in Chapter 3, much of the work in this area has been undertaken by Quigley and his collaborators (e.g., see research synthesis in Paul & Quigley, 1994a) with respect to students who are deaf learning English as a first language, particularly the acquisition of English syntactic structures. Quigley and his colleagues found that the English language acquisition of students who are deaf is quantitatively reduced, albeit qualitatively similar, when compared to that of first-language learners of English. Additional evidence has been provided in the area of vocabulary development (e.g., Paul, 1984; Paul, 1987, Paul & Gustafson, 1991; see also research syntheses in Paul, 1996; Paul & O'Rourke, 1988) and in reading achievement and development (e.g., see Hanson, 1989, 1991; Hayes & Arnold, 1992).

The focus here is on L2 acquisition, and there have been several more recent studies that have presented similar conclusions. Representative of this line of research is the work of King (1981), who explored the performances of students who are deaf on one component of language, syntax, and one mode of language, reading. King examined the performances of students who were either learning English as a first language or as a second language. Not only did King provide information on the similarity issue, but also, the researcher was able to offer additional insights into the existence of variant structures found in previous studies (e.g., Charrow, 1975; see review in Paul & Quigley, 1994a).

Eighty subjects participated in this study; 40 of them were subjects with hearing impairment between the ages of 8 and 13 years old, and 40 were hearing subjects between the ages of 8 and 11 years old. Twenty subjects from each group (i.e., deaf and hearing) were learning English as a first language, whereas the remaining subjects were acquiring English as a second language. The students learning English as a first language were exposed to English in the home and had not received any instruction in foreign-language learning. The students learning English as a second language were Puerto Rican Americans of Spanish descent. The researcher matched both groups of subjects relative to the following variables: language, type of school attended, amount of exposure to English, and type of instruction received. Specifically, the L2 subjects attended schools in which English was the primary language used. These subjects also received English instruction in content areas (e.g., science, social studies, etc.).

Similar to the findings of Quigley and his colleagues, King found that both deaf and heaing subjects (i.e., L1 and L2 learners) acquire English syntactic structures in a similar developmental manner. That is, the order of difficulty of the syntactic structures was similar for both groups. More interesting, King reported that both groups made similar errors. That is, the errors of the L2 learners were similar both to errors reported for other L2 learners (i.e., German, French, etc.) and to errors produced by younger, first-language learners of English. A sample of errors in this study and others are shown in Table 6-5. Thus, King provided evidence that the deviant structures are part of the acquisition process and suggested that many of them would either disappear or become rare as the subjects gained more profi-

TABLE 6-5   Errors made by deaf and second-language

Negation

No Daddy see baby.
Daddy no see baby.

Conjunction

John chased the girl and he scared. (her)
The boy hit the girl and (the girl) ran home.

Questions

What I did this morning?
The kitten is black?
Who TV watched?

Verbs

The boy was kissed the girl.
The boy saw the girl and the girl kiss the boy.
The boy is kiss the girl.
The sky is cover with clouds.
Tom has pushing the wagon.

Relativization

The dog chased the girl had on a red dress.
The boy saw the girl who the girl ran home.
The boy saw the girl who she ran home.
The boy helped the girl who her mother was sick.

Complementation

For to play baseball is fun.
Joe went to fishing.
Chad wanted go.
Bill like to played baseball.
The boy likes for fishing.

Source: Adapted from King (1981) and Quigley, Steinkamp, Power, & Jones (1978).

ciency in English. This interpretation is in line with the qualitative-similarity hypothesis. Finally, these findings provide additional evidence against interference as the major source of errors in second-language acquisition.

King also noted that there were no academic advantages associated with bilingualism. That is, knowing Spanish as a first language did not have any quantitative effects on the English syntactical development of the hearing students. For students who were deaf, the results for this issue were not clear. There are at least two points to keep in mind regarding this finding. Firstly, King stated that nearly all students with hearing impairment (L1 and L2) entered school with little or no proficiency in English and continued to have difficulty learning English. This finding can be explained within the purview of Cummins' threshold hypothesis, discussed previously. Secondly, none of the students with hearing impairment was enrolled in a bilingual educational program. In any case, the researcher hypothesized that there might be two reasons for the mixed results relative to these students. One of the groups of students who were deaf (L1 or L2) might have been an atypical group, that is, not representative of the respective population of students who are deaf. In addition, it might be that deafness overrides any positive or negative effects of being exposed to two *spoken* languages.

King's remarks on the effects of deafness have found some support from the findings of another study. Luetke-Stahlman and Weiner (1982) examined the performances of three Spanish females. They were primarily interested in the students' acquisition of the Spanish language and culture as it relates to exposure to five language/system conditions: (1) oral English, (2) English and signs, (3) oral Spanish, (4) Spanish and English, and (5) signs only. One subject was 4 years, 4 months old and had a bilateral, profound hearing impairment. The second subject was 3 years, 5 months old with a bilateral moderate-to-severe hearing impairment. The third subject was 4 years, 11 months old and also had a moderate-to-severe hearing impairment. In each of the five language/system conditions, all subjects were exposed to vocabulary items such as nouns, verbs, and adjectives. The subjects' performances on items in each of the language/system conditions were analyzed.

On the basis of the results relative to the five language/system conditions, the researchers concluded that the selection of a language or system to use in teaching Spanish children who are deaf should not depend solely on either the heritage of the students or the characteristics of their hearing impairment. Neither of these factors seems to be dominant in isolation. Consequently, the researchers suggested that language/system choice requires the consideration of several factors such as the language and/or communication system of the main caregiver, the amount of exposure to sign language and/or systems, the degree of usable aided hearing ability, and the language and/or system that has been evaluated to be most effective for the particular student.

Previously in this chapter, it has been argued that models of reading in English as a first language are applicable to understanding reading in English as a second language. Specifically, it was suggested that interactive theories of reading offer the best explanation for the reading process in English both as a first or second language. This also seems to imply that the developmental process in L2 English reading is similar to that in L1 English reading. In addition, it has been suggested that, similar to English language development, the reading development of students who are deaf is quantitatively reduced and qualitatively similar when compared to that of native hearing readers of English. Some evidence to support this later notion can be seen in studies that focus on comparing the performances of readers those who are deaf and those who are hearing on a reading achievement test and on comparing other measures (e.g., Hayes & Arnold, 1992).

Perhaps the strongest evidence to support the notion that the English reading development of both L1 and L2 readers who are deaf is qualitatively similar to that of hearing L1 readers has been gleaned from the research on the relationship between short-term memory (STM) and reading comprehension, a prominent line of research within the cognitive information processing framework (see also the discussion in Chapter 3 of this text). There is increasing evidence that students who are deaf who use a phonologically based code in STM are better readers than those who use predominantly a nonphonologically based code (e.g., Conrad, 1979; Hanson, 1989, 1991; Tzeng, 1993). The use of a phonologically based code reflects an individual's sensitivity to the morphophonological structure of words.

Why is the use of this code so important? To reiterate the remarks of Lillo-Martin, Hanson, and Smith (1991):

> In reading and listening, individual words of a sentence must be retained while the grammatical relations among words are determined. Evidence suggests that working memory is most efficient for verbal material (including written material) when the processing involves phonological coding. (p. 147)

Within the framework of interactive theories of reading, the use of a phonological code facilitates the development of rapid, automatic word identification skills. This leads to a working knowledge of the alphabet system of English, upon which the written language system is based. If readers have rapid word identification skills, they can devote most of their energy to top-down, comprehension processing—the real goal of reading. It is interesting to note that even good ASL-using readers who are deaf rely on the phonological code of English during reading activities (Hanson, 1989):

> The finding of phonological processing by deaf readers, particularly deaf readers skilled in ASL, makes a strong case for the importance of phonological sensitivity in the acquisition of skilled reading whether the reader is hearing or deaf. For deaf readers, the acquisition and use of phonological information is extremely difficult. They would be expected to use alternatives such as visual (orthographic) or sign strategy, if such were effective. Yet, the evidence indicates that the successful deaf readers do not rely on these alternatives. (p. 86)

Hanson (1989) concluded that, essentially, reading is the same for students who are deaf and for those who are hearing, including ASL-using students who are deaf and who are learning English as a second language (see previous discussion of Hanson's work in Chapter 3).

The Establishment of ASL/English Bilingual Education Programs

This section provides some basic underpinnings of current ASL/English bilingual or instructional programs. The influence of contrastive error analyses can be seen in the discussions of early and more recent investigations. In addition, a number of programs have cited the works of Cummins (e.g., see discussions in 1984, 1988) and Vygotsky (e.g., 1962) as support for ASL/English bilingual programs. Support has also been garnered from the transactional-psycholinguistic model of Goodman (e.g., 1985), specifically in the form of a whole-language philosophy (see discussion in Dolman, 1992).

From one perspective, it is surprising that a whole body of first- and second-language reading programs influenced by cognitive interactive theories has been virtually ignored by several ASL/English bilingual proponents (e.g., see discussion in Paul & Quigley, 1994a, 1994b). As is discussed later, it is hypothesized that this is due mainly to two major factors. Most proponents do not accept the notions (1) that reading for students who are deaf is qualitatively similar to that of hearing students and (2) that the importance of a phonological code applies to readers who are deaf. In addition, it is argued in this section that the works of both Cummins and Vygotsky might not be adequate enough to explain or address the literacy problems of L1 or L2 readers who are deaf (e.g., see also the discussion in Mayer & Wells, 1996).

Influenced by contrastive analyses and grammar-translation approaches, some of the early researchers attempted to encourage students who are deaf to compare and contrast their utterances in ASL and English. With this method, students are led to observe that what is acceptable in American Sign Language might not be acceptable in English (and vice versa). In some studies, the students are only exposed to English in the written mode. That is, all English language interactions are written on the blackboard (chalkboard) or overhead projector.

Crutchfield's work (1972) is representative of the few early studies that addressed ASL and English. This researcher focused on the count features of both American Sign Language and English (e.g., *much*, *many*, and *few*). If there are differences between the two languages, Crutchfield argued that the initial step is to bring this difference to the student's attention. One of his examples included MUCH BOY LEFT SCHOOL (*Note:* This is the English *gloss* for the ASL-like signs). For ASL users, this signed utterance is not acceptable. One possible correction is: MANY BOY LEFT SCHOOL. However, the English translation (actually, gloss) for this sentence is: *Many boy left school.* (*Note:* Some researchers argue that the English gloss is, *Many boys left school*). After writing this sentence on the board or overhead, it should be pointed out to the students that this sentence, as is, is unacceptable in English. Thus, the next lesson is on the plurality (or count feature) of English.

Crutchfield remarked that the main goal of these lessons is to show similarities of acceptability and unacceptability of utterances in either American Sign Language or English. Consequently, the students can be instructed on how to correct the utterance to make it acceptable in the respective language. As is discussed later, Crutchfield's procedures resemble those of later investigations, which emphasize the use of metalinguistic activities (i.e., teaching students to think and reflect about language items or language itself).

The use of writing as a major mode of teaching English (as a second language) was a major component of a program developed by Goldberg and Bordman (1975). These educators made two modifications in their ESL program. One, they conducted all language lessons in English writing. Two, they attempted to develop procedures that would compel their students to express the concepts in the written language productions. Goldberg and Bordman argued that the written form of English must be utilized so that students can *see* the words that are being used to convey meanings. In their view, the use of sign communication was not explicit enough or did not always reveal the specific words. However, Goldberg and Bordman suggested that it was important to use the sign system or communication mode of the students for the purposes of communication, not instruction.

Goldberg and Bordman also suggested that the emphasis on concepts would address the English structure problems of the students. It was felt that students with hearing impairment did not know what concepts are expressed in English sentences and, in addition, the students might not even know how to use them. These problems are similar to those of other students attempting to learn English as a second language. For example, all ESL students need to be able to differentiate between the following two sentences: *They eat sandwiches* and *They are eating sandwiches*.

Jones (1979) demonstrated that some of the English written language problems of students who are deaf might be due to a misunderstanding of both the manual and nonmanual cues associated with American Sign Language. Manual cues refers to the use of the hands in producing signs. Nonmanual cues refers to non-hand movements associated with the eyes, eyebrows, cheeks, and shoulders (for a detailed discussion, see Wilbur, 1987). In Jones' view, the nonmanual information from ASL is often omitted in the written productions of students who are deaf. Thus, the students might not convey the complete message of the native speaker of English.

To address this situation, it is argued that teachers should enable students to become aware that some signed information has not been represented in their writings. Jones argued that both manual and nonmanual cues are important for conveying a message in American Sign Language. It should be noted that this is quite different from the English-based signed systems in which nonmanual cues play a minor or no role at all. In this case, the nonmanual cues are simply secondary to the message (similar to random gestures that accompany the spoken message in some speakers).

The more recent investigations seem to be variations on a theme. These studies are influenced heavily by the outcomes of contrastive analyses, are focused on the use of English written language only to teach English literacy skills, and are driven by the notion of metacognition as a tool for students to use in analyzing the grammatical elements of both ASL and English. For example, the work of Marbury and Mackinson-Smyth (1986) is typical of these patterns. These researchers employed an ESL technique known as grammar-translation (e.g., see discussion in McLaughlin, 1985). With this technique, the elementary-age ASL-using students who are deaf are required to translate grammatical features of ASL into English. Their attempts become the focus of class discussions. The translations are part of an ASL-signed story in which teachers and students discuss aspects such as characters, events, and actions. Both teacher and students develop a final draft of the ASL-signed story in English written language.

The focus on metalinguistic ability can be seen in several ASL/English instructional projects (Akamatsu & Armour, 1987; Neuroth-Gimbrone & Logiodice, 1992; Strong, 1988b). For example, Akamatsu and Armour (1987) argued that the development of metalinguistic ability might lead to an improvement of the written language ability of students who are deaf. Neuroth-Gimbrone and Logiodice (1992) asserted that the development of proficiency in ASL is a necessary first step in order to maximize the benefits of metalinguistic ability for students who are deaf.

To understand some of the problems of current ASL/English bilingual models, it is important to discuss several other issues: type of student, language goal, and how the

ASL/English situation is similar to or different from other bilingual situations involving two spoken languages such as English/French. For this last issue, it is necessary to include a critique of Cummins' interdependence hypothesis, a discussion of interactive reading theories in light of the research synthesis on second-language learning, and some fundamental requirements for learning the alphabet system of English.

Type of Student and Language Goal

From one perspective, type of student and language goal should be considered together. The language goals might vary with the type of student. Bilingual education programs might be established for a particular type of student, that is, majority-language or minority-language students (e.g., Cummins, 1988). Majority-language students are individuals who speak the majority language of the culture. In the United States, these are individuals who speak English as a first language. Minority-language students are individuals whose first or home language is not the majority language of society. That is, these individuals use a language that is not English, such as French, German, and American Sign Language. Minority-language users are also considered *minimal speakers of English.*

In the United States, majority-language students typically enroll in foreign language or second-language classes. These students are learning a second language for a variety of purposes. However, in Canada, for example, the majority-language students might be enrolled in immersion programs (e.g., Genesee, 1987). Immersion programs are common in areas where there are two respected languages (i.e., English and French). Students in these programs are expected to acquire grammatical, communicative, and academic proficiency in the two languages (e.g., Cummins, 1984, 1988). One of the most common variations of this program model is that students receive instruction in the early grades (i.e., grades 1, 2, and 3) in a language that is not their native language. Thus, French-speaking students would receive instruction in English (grammatical and academic) initially. Instruction begins in their native language after a reasonable level of competency is established in the second language.

It is the types of programs for minority-language students that have caused the most controversy (e.g., see review in Cummins, 1984; Paul & Quigley, 1994b). Cummins (1988) has argued that some programs in the United States fail to make the distinction between majority- and minority-language students. Thus, the type of program recommended for the student might be inappropriate. Typically, the problem is that programs for minority-language students in the United States might be modeled after programs for majority-language students in Canada. The question is, Should minority-language students become competent in both the native language of the home and the majority language of society (i.e., English)? This question is related to the discussion of language goals in the ensuing paragraphs.

Programs for minority-language students in the United States vary from complete submersion in English to 50/50 simultaneous programs to programs that place varying amounts of emphasis on developing both languages (Cummins, 1988; Reich, 1986). As stated previously, the type of program depends on the language goal for the students. There are three broad language goals: shift, maintenance, and enrichment (Reich, 1986).

The goal of language shift is often associated with transitional programs. The minority-language students are expected to shift from the predominant use of the home language to the predominant use of the majority language, or English. In the beginning, the minority language might be employed in the classroom setting; however, the use of the home language diminishes as the students gain proficiency in the majority language. Thus, there is no concerted, systematic plan to maintain or develop further proficiency in the language of the students' home.

The goal of language maintenance is often associated with maintenance bilingual education programs. The intent is to maintain proficiency or prevent the loss of skills in the first language and develop proficiency in the second or majority language. It should be stressed that only the bare minimum is done to maintain the first language. Much of the emphasis, that is, amount of time, resources, and so on, is placed on the development of the majority language. In essence, the best way to teach English is to provide ample and meaningful exposure and instruction in English (e.g., Cummins, 1984, 1988).

The goal of language enrichment is also associated with a maintenance bilingual education program, labeled developmental maintenance (e.g., Cummins, 1988; Otheguy & Otto, 1980). The intent of enrichment is to develop grammatical, communicative, and academic proficiency in both languages, that is, the home language and the majority language of society. Programs that adhere to language enrichment are typically immersion programs and others that employ a 50-50 formula (i.e., half of the school day is in one language and the other half is in the other language). It has been argued that only programs that employed the principle of language enrichment, particularly within a developmental maintenance framework, should be considered bilingual/bicultural. In other words, bilingual/bicultural programs are those that aim to maintain and develop the two languages of the students.

Synthesis of Research

In this section, only a brief summary of research studies is presented. For a more detailed discussion, the reader is referred to Cummins (1984, 1988), Genesee (1987), Swain and Lapkin (1982); for deaf students, see Paul and Quigley (1994a, 1994b). As stated previously, there has been a misinterpretation of the immersion programs in Canada for minority-language students in the United States. This misinterpretation has led to the development of programs that are essentially *submersion* programs (e.g., see discussion in Cummins, 1988). For example, in Canada, the majority-language students might be exposed to or immersed in the minority-language (or a language that is not their first language) for the first few grades. Consequently, research has shown that these students are able to develop grammatical, communicative, and academic proficiency in both languages. These findings have been used to justify the use of English as the first (and perhaps only) language of instruction for *minority-language* students in the United States (e.g., Cummins, 1984, 1988).

Research has not supported the above approach. In order to understand the implications of this research, it is necessary to describe briefly the four types of immersion programs used in the United States: L2 submersion, L2 monolingual immersion, L2 bilingual immersion, and L1 bilingual immersion (also called the minority-language immersion program in Paul, 1990; Paul, Bernhardt, & Gramly, 1992). L2 submersion has been described previously; only English is used with little or no concession to the use of the first language or culture of the minority-language students. L2 monolingual immersion is similar to L2 submersion. However, L2 monolingual immersion proponents do agree that it is necessary to modify and adjust curricular and instructional activities in the second language (typically, grammar and content) in order to facilitate comprehension in the minority-language students. Both L2 and L1 bilingual immersion offer instruction in both languages and cultures of the students. Nevertheless, L1 bilingual immersion places a heavy emphasis on maintaining and developing the first language of the students. In fact, students are often taught to read and write in their native language before they learn literacy skills in the second or majority language.

Cummins (1984, 1988) has reviewed extensively the research on the various program models. He has concluded, as have others (e.g., Genesee, 1987) that minority-language students achieve the highest levels of communicative and academic proficiency in both L1 and L2 immersion programs. The main reason for the effectiveness of these programs is that both types of programs seem to facilitate the transfer from L1 to L2 for the students.

The Notion of Transfer

The nature of this *transfer* has been misinterpreted by many proponents of ASL/English bilingual programs (e.g., see discussions in Mayer & Wells, 1996; Paul & Quigley, 1994a, 1994b; for hearing second-language students, see Grabe, 1988). As mentioned previously, it is often assumed that by acquiring proficiency in one language (e.g., ASL), students who are deaf should be able to acquire proficiency in another language. In addition, Cummins (e.g., 1984) was focused on the reciprocal and concomitant effects of acquiring two languages, especially for minority-language students. Although Cummins' remarks are applicable to the development of literacy in two languages, it should be remembered that he is not, primarily, a literacy theorist/researcher. In addition, based on his conclusions, it cannot be inferred that proficiency in one language, including literacy skills, leads to or is critical for proficiency in a second (or another) language. However, it seems to be evident that progress in a second language is dependent upon the continued development of the first language for students who are considered minority-language students. In one sense, this can be applied to students who are deaf and who know ASL as a first or native language. However, as is discussed later, there are some important differences.

Another theorist, who is quoted frequently by ASL/English bilingual proponents, is Vygotsky (e.g., 1962). Although Vygotsky's principles are important for the acquisition of any language (i.e., first, second, etc.), much of his work highlighted the intricate relationship between language and cognition. This theorist was interested in the development of an internal mediating system (labeled *inner speech*). Within this framework, he remarked that all individuals progress from social speech to egocentric speech (e.g., beginning of representational behavior) to symbolic speech, which mediates thought. In essence, Vygotsky argued that there is an interaction between thought and language; there is no one to one correspondence between these two entities.

More important, in my view, Vygotsky did not specifically or directly address the issue of transfer between two languages. In addition, Vygotsky, similar to Cummins, did not specifically address the issue of developing literacy skills. This does not mean that these theorists have little or nothing to offer on these issues. However, in my view, a better and more direct understanding of second-language literacy has emerged from the research on both first-language and second-language literacy development. Information on first-language literacy was presented in Chapters 2 and 3, and information on second-language literacy (including its relation to first-language literacy) was presented previously in this chapter. The next section addresses the issue of ASL and second-language literacy.

ASL and Second-Language Literacy: Remarks and Future Research

Most proponents of ASL/English bilingualism seem to believe that it is possible to learn to read and write English by (a) using ASL to explain aspects of the English language or culture and (b) requiring that students read or write only English (i.e., manipulate the secondary form only). Thus, in this view, it should be possible to learn the secondary form of a language without manipulating its conversational form (i.e., speech). There does not seem to be much evidence to support this assumption for phonetic-based languages such as English and French for hearing students (e.g., see reviews in Bernhardt, 1991; Grabe, 1988; Paul & Quigley, 1994a).

All readers of English as a second language need to obtain a high level of proficiency in the alphabet system, the system upon which the English written language is based. This knowledge entails phonological and morphological components. Finally, knowledge of the alphabet system assists in the development of rapid word identification skills, which in turn facilitate top-down comprehension processes. Whether this perspective also applies to students with severe to profound hearing impairment needs to be researched further.

There also needs to be additional research on the use of a phonological code in working memory by students with severe to profound hearing impairment. It has been shown that this code is most efficient for processing verbosequential stimuli associated with a phonetic, spoken language such as English. As argued by Quigley and Paul (1994):

> Whether deaf students are reading in English as a first or second language, the central problem remains: the acquisition (cognitive awareness) of the alphabetic system, particularly the internal morphophonological and phonological structures of words, and of other essential components of a language, such as semantics and syntax. . . . the acquisition of a phonetic, spoken language is facilitated by the use of peripheral auditory mechanisms. In the absence of a functioning, peripheral auditory system, other compensatory means need to be developed to aid the short-term working memory processing of verbosequential stimuli associated with a phonetic, spoken language such as English. (pp. 265-266)

Is it possible to bypass phonology and morphology of a phonetic system such as English in order to learn to read and write this language? Even the better ASL readers tend to use a phonological code during reading. How do we explain this situation? Research on the use of ASL to teach English as a second language is limited. In addition, the ASL/English bilingual movement seems to be motivated more by empowerment issues than by research and theoretical effectiveness (e.g., Stuckless, 1991). On the other hand, the strength of this movement is in the assumption that students who are deaf are more likely to acquire a language (i.e., a sign language) at as early an age as possible. This early acquisition is necessary for the subsequent development of literate thought, that is, the ability to engage in critical and reflective thought (e.g., see previous discussion in Chapter 5 of this text).

This brings us back to one of the oldest contentious issues in the field of deafness: the relative ability of the eye to process either spoken or signed languages. Given the importance of establishing a first language as early as possible, this processing issue is a critical area for future research. Whether or not researchers can discover general laws relative to this issue is debatable. For example, is it possible to determine if and when a child should be encouraged to learn a spoken or signed language based on the individual's processing abilities? Thus far, it seems that the eye (without the use of residual hearing) is a relatively poor processor of spoken languages, especially those that are phonetically based or those that "depend heavily on temporal-sequential (verbosequential) input and suprasegmental aspects of speech for correct interpretation" (Quigley & Paul, 1994, p. 267).

A Final Word

The major intent of this chapter was to discuss bilingualism and second-language learning as they apply to children and adolescents who are deaf. The chapter presented some of the major tenets of theories and research on second-language literacy. In essence, it was argued that the acquisition of second-language literacy by students who are deaf is similar to that of first-language learners, especially when considering English.

ASL/English bilingual program models seem to be motivated mainly by sociopolitical goals rather than by educational research. Although sociopolitical goals are important, this might have caused some scholars/researchers to overlook some critical issues relative to the development of literacy for hearing first- and second-language learners. Perhaps the most salient contribution of the lines of research related to ASL/English bilingual programs is the fact that it is essential to develop a first language at as early an age as possible. In addition, as stated previously in Chapter 5, future researchers need to concern themselves with investigating the notion that a high level of English literacy might not be a realistic goal for most students with severe to profound hearing impairment. This does not mean, however, that educators should relinquish this quest. Nevertheless, the development of literate thought, the ability to think critically and reflectively, is of paramount importance. This skill is heavily dependent upon the early development of a first language—perhaps the real goal of most ASL/English bilingual programs.

Further Readings

CHRISTENSEN, K., & DELGADO, G. (Eds.). (1993). *Multicultural issues in deafness.* White Plains, NY: Longman.

DELGADO, G. (Ed.). (1984). *The Hispanic deaf: Issues and challenges in special education.* Washington, DC: Gallaudet University.

GEERTZ, C. (1973). *The interpretation of cultures.* New York: Basic Books.

LONGSTREET, W. (1980). *Aspects of ethnicity: Understanding differences in pluralistic classrooms.* New York: Teachers College.

OGBU, J. (1978). *Minority education and caste.* New York: Academic Press.

PASCOE, E. (1985). *Racial prejudice.* New York: Franklin Watts.

Chapter 7

Instruction and
First-Language Literacy

MARTHA G. GAUSTAD
Bowling Green State University

PETER V. PAUL
The Ohio State University

Theory provides the rationalization for practice, for the reasoned behaviors that give teaching balance and direction. Without theory, teachers become baseless romantics, who know they "do well" in the classroom without understanding how they are accomplishing their work with children so effectively. Educators will have little to say to critics, who may feel they are sentimentalizing curriculum practice, unless teachers understand the hard-headed rationale for motivating students to higher thought and continued learning. When a parent asks a teacher why she is using these "library books instead of basals to teach reading," it is not a rhetorical question; the teacher had better have some sound reasons for teaching as she does (Hedley, 1994, p. 3).

Given the importance of reading to the educational process and the spectacular lack of success in achieving even minimal levels of literacy . . . by most deaf children, it is surprising that (1) relatively little is known about current instructional practices for teaching deaf children to read, and (2) there is little research being conducted to determine the effects of various instructional methods. In sharp contrast, a fairly substantial body of polemic writing is available in which various spokespersons argue for specific approaches and prescribe specific instructional practices which they believe should be used (King & Quigley, 1985, p. 73).

Relative to deafness, the "teaching" of language and literacy is a critical area because it is often stated that most deaf students come to school not knowing *any* social-conventional language and some deaf students know ASL as a first language . . . Thus, the discussion centers on whether English can be "taught" either as a first or second language, either in the primary (speech and/or sign) or secondary form (print) (Paul & Quigley, 1994a, p. 228).

The contents of the three previous passages capture the essence of what is discussed in this chapter on instruction and first-language literacy and how this information should be conceptualized. A portion of the chapter discusses what can be called emerging literacy experiences of good readers/writers prior to their formal schooling period. In illustrating examples of formal literacy instruction, the intent is to provide examples that are related to some conceptual framework, that is, cognitive information-processing, naturalism, or social constructivism or some combination of all three models.

Several remarks should be made here. Firstly, the relationship between theory and practice is not always clear cut and, more often than not, there are bound to be arguments on the interpretation and application of the theory. Secondly, as discussed in Chapter 1, the deeper and more comprehensive the theory, the more difficult it is to derive or develop instructional practices. Thirdly, as mentioned previously, some instructional practices seem to be based on tenets from several theories or frameworks. This resembles what is often called an eclectic approach and is quite common in the education of children who are deaf (e.g., King & Quigley, 1985; Moores, 1987, 1996; Paul & Quigley, 1990). There seem to be some effective ideas using this approach; however, it is often difficult to replicate the situations for the purposes of generalizing the results or principles of instruction.

This issue leads to the fourth and final point, which can be stated as a question: Should practice be grounded in theory? The answer to this question depends on an individual's research bent, for example, empirical, interpretative, or critical. This issue is discussed later as part of the teachability/learnability dichotomy. More interestingly, this notion is related to other issues such as the learning styles of students. For example, in literacy, some scholars argue that visual learners might do better with the whole word or other visual approaches rather than with code-emphasis techniques, which depend on the use of audition (e.g., see discussion in Adams, 1990a).

There are two problems with this assertion. One, as discussed in previous chapters, code-emphasis approaches (particularly the use of the sound system) are important for developing a working understanding of the alphabetic principle, the principle upon which the written English system is based (e.g., Adams, 1990a; Stanovich, 1991, 1992). This applies to students who are deaf and to students learning English as a second language (e.g., Bernhardt, 1991; Paul & Quigley, 1994a). Two, as discussed in Chapter 2, even the effective use of the whole word or sight word approach is related to a good understanding of the morphophonological system of English (e.g., see discussion in Ehri, 1991). Thus, literacy instructional practices based on specific learning styles might need to be reexamined.

The major points raised by the second passage, that is, limited research on instruction and little ongoing instructional research, are still applicable to the present situation, as indicated in Chapters 3 and 4 of this text. One long-standing reason for this dearth of research has been that deafness is a low-incidence condition, which causes difficulty in conducting scientifically sound research. It should be highlighted that this is the case for quantitative researchers, who are mostly interested in product-oriented research, that is, they are interested in attempts to advance knowledge regarding effective methods or the best instructional method.

On the other hand, there has been an increase in qualitative research (i.e., interpretative) in literacy, which is not affected by the size of the sample. This type of research represents what is often called a paradigm shift relative to the advancement of knowledge.

Qualitative researchers argue that there is no such entity as a method or even best method. In fact, there is no separation of the method and the actions of the individual using the method. The focus of this research is on teacher effectiveness, not on product assessment. This type of instruction is often difficult to describe; and, by nature, it depends on the context or situation of the teacher-learner interactions.

Due to the limited research available on students with hearing impairment, many of the techniques described in this chapter are based on research, both quantitative and qualitative, with hearing students. From one perspective, no researcher or theorist, quantitative or qualitative, can specify all the details of instructional practices with literacy. The best that these individuals can do is to provide guidelines, and that is the approach of this chapter. This is even true for qualitative researchers because much of their research is situation- or context-bound and needs to be refined based on the continuing interactions of the teacher and students.

The final major area to discuss briefly is the teachability/learnability issue. This issue has been discussed previously in this text and elsewhere (e.g., Paul & Quigley, 1994a; Quigley & Paul, 1994). From one perspective, it has dominated much of what is known as the whole-language philosophy in literacy. King and Quigley (1985) captured the essence of this issue with the question, can reading be taught or must it be caught? The intent of raising this point here is to express caution for educators of students with hearing impairment. The present authors agree that some aspects of literacy can be taught or, to put it conservatively, presented numerous times with examples and feedback so that students are able to perform the tasks, even in unstructured or different environments. It appears that students can learn these aspects by observing intently the actions of teachers (e.g., modeling, explanations, etc.).

On the contrary, it is not always clear that educators can actually teach or should teach many or all higher-level literacy skills because of the myriad of information needed to perform such skills. This depends on how higher-level skills are defined; nevertheless, it simply is not efficient to teach these skills in a step by step manner. Of course, it is possible to model (think out loud, show problem-solving skills, etc.) your responses; however, this does not necessarily lead to the application of the skill.

A case in point is the answering of script-implicit questions in the Question-Answer Relationship (QAR) framework. As is demonstrated by the examples in this chapter, the answers to all script-implicit QARs require that students have knowledge or information in their heads. To engage in interpretative or critical use of this information is quite complex. It should be recalled that critical theorists argue that there is no best or right interpretation and that all stories are products of personal or social constructions of meanings. These issues should be kept in mind as the reader reviews the literacy examples in the ensuing paragraphs.

Before proceeding to the issues of instruction, a description of the audience for that instruction is in order. The main focus of this chapter is on the acquisition of literacy in English as a first language with respect to learners who are deaf. The chapter takes its perspective from the circumstances of the majority of these students receiving such instruction, that is to say, students with the following demographics: severe to profound sensorineural hearing losses, onset of loss prior to or at age two, average intellectual abilities, residing in homes with hearing parents and siblings, attending day classes with hearing teachers, especially in programs that provide signed communication (most likely some form of manually coded English) along with audiological and speech support services.

General Instructional Issues

The general instructional issues refer to the organization of the classroom, the logistics of the literacy lesson, and the use of materials (for a good discussion on the use and selection of materials, see King & Quigley, 1985). These are important regardless of what philosophical hat educators wear. Some educators disagree; it is not uncommon to find that a literature-based approach is part of the whole-language or naturalistic paradigm, whereas basal readers are not. This is really an oversimplification and needs to be refined. The use of stories in basal readers is not necessarily a cognitive information-processing or naturalistic approach. Rather, it is the activities that accompany the stories that might be classified as belonging to one paradigm or another. In fact, cognitive information-processing scholars advocate the use of children's literature, and some basal readers contain both contrived stories and ecologically written stories by authors who write children's literature.

What are some general instructional issues for teachers of students with hearing impairment? Whether one espouses a cognitive information-processing, naturalistic, or social-constructionist paradigm, there are specific knowledge, skills, and experiences important for novice readers/writers to succeed in acquiring print literacy. These areas are discussed in relation to children with hearing impairment. Our approach in this chapter is to present information based on our interpretation of research and our own professional experiences.

Abilities and experiences that the novice reader/writer should bring to the task of literacy are summarized here (Carnine et al., 1990; Durkin, 1989; Gunning, 1992; Lipson & Wixson, 1991; Mason & Au, 1986).

Physical and mental readiness

- intact cognitive development
- problem-solving strategies
- inferencing abilities
- association abilities
- visual acuity/discrimination

Language and print readiness

- conversational language (communicative and grammatical proficiency whether through oral or signed modalities)
- a broad oral (or signed) vocabulary base
- knowledge of socially based linguistic codes/registers and differences between them
- knowledge of dialogue structure
- knowledge of speaker-listener contracts
- motivation to read/write
- acquaintance with books and other reading materials
- willingness to take risks

Preliteracy experiences

- a wealth of real world activities and associated language
- conversational interaction with many and varied interactors and for many and varied purposes—both successful and unsuccessful experiences
- positive encounters with reading and reading materials
- exposure to a variety of print formats
- models of literacy behavior by significant others
- access to books and writing utensils
- involvement in print literacy activities

If the novice reader/writer does not come to the task of literacy with many of the above skills, then it will be necessary to develop them. In general, the following skills will, most likely, need to be developed by the novice reader/writer:

- alphabetic facility (e.g., letter-sound correspondences)
- decoding strategies
- specific knowledge of linguistic devices/conventions peculiar to the print mode, for example, syntax, morphophonological variants (gonna = going to), semantics (e.g., use of idiomatic and figurative expressions), and pragmatics (e.g., print is impersonal, permanent, formal, and decontextualized)
- metacognitive strategies for interfacing with the print medium

The Emergence of Literacy Skills: Focus on Typical Readers/Writers

The novice reader/writer is not analogous to a computer which, when programmed with the right software, will be able to decipher any piece of text with facility and precision because there is no software sufficient to replicate fully the reading/writing process. This process is neither mechanical nor fully predictable. Rather, it represents an evolving interaction/transaction between the text and person. The reader/writer is a complex, multifaceted entity rich in individuality and interpretation of life experiences and possesses an array of types and levels of competencies, which can be applied to the literacy task.

The first, most fundamental set of abilities that a potential reader/writer brings to literacy tasks follows naturally from intact physical development in an ordinary family (broadly defined), that is, from life experiences and interactions within a social world in the absence of physical or mental impairment. Human beings, from infancy onward, naturally seek perceptual, cognitive, and social stimulation; organize incoming information; deal with ambiguity; and so on.

Children who are deaf are no exception. Anyone who has spent time observing these children can attest to their ability to interact with and manipulate their environment in a purposeful way. The building blocks for discrimination, categorization, association, inferencing, and problem solving are in evidence.

One skill that is controversial, relative to deaf readers/writers, and increasingly tied more substantially by research findings to reading fluency, is the access of the potential reader/writer to a speech-based code. As discussed in Chapter 3, fluent readers (and probably writers) readily decode and mediate via the use of a phonological-based code as the means for accessing information stored in memory. Fluent readers who are deaf seem to utilize speech recoding significantly more often than do less fluent readers.

Recoding to speech theoretically enables a reader to quickly chunk printed stimuli into ever larger bits of information. Given that there is an absolute limit to the number of bits of information that can be processed at any one time (in short-term working memory), this chunking process can and does increase reading fluency. There needs to be attempts to provide more and better access to the speech code for readers/writers who are deaf. As discussed in Chapter 6, this is also true for students who are deaf and who are attempting to learn to read/write English as a second language.

A potential reader/writer should be able to acquire facility with the conversational form of a language, that is, communicative and grammatical competence in a language. The exercise of literacy as a modal variation of human face-to-face communication requires first-hand experience with social and pragmatic aspects of interactions. The potential reader/writer should come to recognize variations in conversational settings, social status, and linguistic registers and should gain facility in code switching among these variations.

Also important is the development of a substantial spoken vocabulary, broadly representative across parts of speech and life experiences. This individual should come to understand that interactions are structured—there are rules about how to have a conversation. Specific awareness should be developed involving the elements of the social contract between speaker and listener regarding the speaker's presuppositions about the listener (e.g., knowledge and motivation about a topic) as well as concerning the process for effectively and efficiently participating in verbal interactions (topic, setting, turn-taking, closing). With the understanding that each conversation is a new adventure, the potential reader/writer should bring to literacy interactions a willingness to experiment, to be creative, all the while accepting the very personal risk of failure to communicate.

In addition to conversational abilities, the potential reader/writer must establish a link to print communication. Some portion of early experiences should ideally have literacy associations. Potential readers/writers need many different encounters with books and other forms of print. They need to see significant adults reading and writing and in every environment be confronted by a variety of print. They should enjoy being read to by people they love, who have intimate knowledge about them. Actual book sharing should be very frequent, personal, and include many different topics and formats of text material. Experiences within books should be related to happenings and knowledge outside of books.

For most hearing prereaders, much learning about literacy takes place before they officially encounter formal elements of literacy instruction (e.g., Adams, 1990a; Anderson et al., 1985; Durkin, 1989; Mason & Au, 1986). They learn how to hold a book, that reading/writing progresses from left to right, and that stories have characters and plots, beginnings and endings. They also learn about humor, mystery, and word play. They learn that it is the relationships between the printed words and the spoken words they know that define how the text is read rather than the appearance of the text (e.g., type, size, arrangement on page). Evidence of these kinds of acquired information can be observed in children's play routines. Preschool children in imaginative play can be heard to introduce their *fairy princess* episode with *once upon a time* or elementary children might introduce a narrative about King Arthur's court with *in the days of old*.

At home, children should have their own easy access to books and writing materials and be encouraged to engage in preliteracy behaviors. Even before they can read, hearing children are also involved in activities that are the forerunners of written communication. Children participate in sending greeting cards for birthdays and holidays, making invitations, creating labels for artwork, making shopping lists or lists for Santa Claus. From these seemingly innocuous activities, hearing children learn important literacy skills. Often they pass through noticeable stages in their acquisition of this knowledge. Parents who have assisted their children in the writing of cards and notes can relate to the humor and frustration of trying to move young writers past the rigid structure of *To* and *From* toward, for example, a more socially appropriate closing for a letter such as *Your Friend*.

Before a child has internalized the relationship between the placement of heading and closing in correspondence to sender and receiver of the communication (print equivalent of the speaker-listener contract), he or she will be reluctant to part with structural markers like *From*, fearing that the receiver will be confused about the sender's identity. Eventually, children acquiesce to closing with *Love* but revert to *To* and *From* when confronted with the need to address a friend. Only later, once instruction on social conventions has been introduced formally with respect to writing, do closings like *Your Friend* appear. Awareness of the purposes of print communication and the usefulness of literacy is essential if a potential reader is to develop the motivation to pursue and sustain the literacy endeavor.

Beginning Literacy and Children Who Are Deaf

The discussion of language exposure and use relative to children who are deaf has been presented in Chapters 5 and 6 of this text and can be found elsewhere (e.g., Luetke-Stahlman & Luckner, 1991; Moores, 1987, 1996; Paul & Quigley, 1994a; Schirmer, 1994; Wilbur, 1987). Although there are legitimate hurdles to providing some experiences for students who are deaf, there are ways to improve their general readiness and experience for literacy learning and growth. The most fundamental issue is the child's exposure to a wide range of meaningful real-world experiences. The cognitive schemata readers/writers bring to text, the scripts they use to interpret content, and the resultant scenarios they build into memory are influenced heavily by their personal knowledge of topics.

To create meaning, children who are deaf must actively participate in the life around them. They must comprehend the language associated with their everyday events and use their knowledge, language, and communication skills to deal with the language and behaviors of others. Within a variety of circumstances, potential readers/writers must have experienced and responded to other people's roles, intents, linguistic idiosyncrasies, and communicative needs.

Research has shown that the world experiences of typical children who are deaf are restricted when compared to their hearing age mates (e.g., see discussions in King &

Quigley, 1985; Moores, 1996; Paul & Jackson, 1993). These restrictions frequently arise neither directly nor of necessity from hearing deficits themselves, but rather from the reactions of adults to the presence of hearing loss. Understandable tendencies toward overprotection results in deaf youngsters not being offered the same kinds of opportunities hearing children have and not benefiting fully from other experiences they do have. For example, they may not spend overnights with grandparents or neighborhood peers, and they may not be encouraged to pay for ice cream from a vendor or handle tickets for amusement park rides. It is especially problematic for caring adults to refrain from interceding in interactions that are rightfully the domain of the child. The child needs to be provided with as much information and practice of skills as possible and then be allowed to proceed as independently as possible.

Children who are deaf need to experience books as hearing preliterate children do, the text as well as the pictures. Because most of these children have obvious problems with conversational English, there is a danger that adults around them underestimate the value of their contacts with text. Parents and preschool teachers might provide books but with the notion that the children will enjoy the pictures, though they are not able to read. Children who are deaf need first-hand experience with many kinds of text, experience that hearing children receive by being read to.

Teachers report that not many parents read books to and with their children who are deaf (e.g., see also, Moores, 1987, 1996). This might be, in part, because large numbers of hearing parents do not sign or not sign fluently enough to read strings of connected text. It might also be due to the awkwardness of the physical arrangements—failing to find a comfortable way to manipulate the child and the book to accomplish satisfactory visual contact for all. When book-sharing does occur between parents and children who are deaf, the character of the interaction is markedly different than that for hearing children. Parents *control* this interaction more with children who are deaf than with hearing children, interrupting and questioning more often (King & Quigley, 1985; Paul & Jackson, 1993). Although they intrude more into the story, they do not use these breaks, as parents of hearing children do, to draw the child's attention to events or information outside the book. Reluctance to move away from the text also might arise from the lack of communicative facility that is necessary to discuss events beyond the here and now.

Similar sources of difficulty, that is, inaccurate evaluation of readiness, communication barriers, and ineffective accommodation to a hearing loss, may also interfere with the child's participation in early writing activities common in the preschool and primary years. Negative expectations of a child's ability to comprehend or contribute may keep hearing parents from even attempting some tasks (for a recent perspective on writing activities, see Albertini & Shannon, 1996). The issue of quality communication among family members, that is, what modes and styles of interactions are used in the home, are of strategic importance here. Preparing a birthday card for Grandma is no simple task if parent and child do not share common symbols for manipulating absent (Grandma) or abstract (birthday) concepts. Even with facile communication, children who will ultimately become successful readers and writers require frequent and repeated experiences with a variety of environmental print (e.g., box labels, street signs, names of people and toys, restaurant menus). Such encounters develop the cognitive routines and structures that lead to literacy.

Instruction: Actions for Meeting Literacy Readiness

An effective preliteracy program for students who are deaf includes frequent contact and correspondence with each child's home. Parents would be in a better position to support literacy endeavors if they were informed of what to do and, particularly, how to engage their child in literacy activities at home (Adams, 1990a; Anderson et al., 1985; Hannon, 1995). Training for parents should include (1) delineation of readiness factors or experiences that normally accompany literacy development, (2) demonstrations of communicative and practical accommodations required by the hearing loss (3) modeling of recommended procedures for accomplishing literacy activities at home, and (4) ongoing consultative interaction for the dual purposes of problem solving and sharing accomplishments related to jointly established objectives.

Real-World/Home Experiences

Teachers can affect positively the home experiences of students who are deaf by helping parents to establish their role as facilitators rather than intermediaries or interpreters for their children. This involves, firstly, communicating accurate expectations for age-appropriate behaviors and activities to the parents. Secondly, it includes devising mutual objectives for specific activities to be accomplished at home with specific support from school. In some cases, it may involve counseling parents as to the value of independence-inducing rather than dependence-inducing parental behavior.

With guidance, parents can be encouraged to broaden the responsibilities given and the roles children are expected to perform. Such activities can be role-played with parents and become a model for their interactions with their children. Possible scenarios include specific scripts that should be representative of the topics, interactions, and language associated with any given situation. Scenario development begins with common everyday occurrences, for example, grocery shopping, and proceeds to ever-widening circles of interactions and situations as the child becomes older (e.g., the dentist office, scout meetings, driving tests). One example of this scenario development is illustrated in Table 7-1.

Links to Literacy: Discussion and Activities

Based on the professional experiences of the present authors, teachers can expand the literacy-promoting capability of the child's time at home by helping parents create functional visual environments in their home (see related discussions in Luetke-Stahlman & Luckner, 1991; Schirmer, 1994). Although it seems common sense to replace the lost hearing acuity with visual input, the means for accomplishing this task might not be so apparent or easily accomplished. Getting the child's attention before communicating, speaking clearly, and so on, are fundamental prerequisites for parent-child communication and will permit interactions involving satisfaction of basic needs during meals, hygiene, and other daily family routines. This level of accommodation to hearing loss is insufficient for engaging in the kinds of activities that promote literacy. Parents might need particular guidelines, perhaps materials, designed to raise the visual quotient of the child's surroundings and interactions.

TABLE 7-1   Parent to deaf child scenario rehearsal script

Problem: Returning a video that was labeled as closed captioned but did not have closed captioning.

Setting/Orientation: When you enter the video store, you will see the large counter. It looks like four counters put together to form a square. The counter closest to the door is for returning videos. The two counters that are on the sides have cash registers, and they are used for checking out videos. The counter that is facing the video shelves is for "customer service." You will need to go to the counter that faces the video shelves.

When you enter the video store, the attendant may ask to take your video. You need to tell him the video did not work correctly, and you need to see the customer service attendant. You will say: "The video that I rented did not work correctly and I wish to see someone in customer service." You do not turn in the video as usual. When you walk through the gates to enter the part of the store that has videos, a buzzer will sound, so you need to let the attendant know that you are bringing a video in. You will walk through the gates and to the counter that faces the video shelves.

You may need to ask for assistance. You need to ask: "May I have some help?" or the person at the desk may ask if you need help: "May I help you?" "What can I do for you?" "What seems to be the problem?" You must explain to the attendant that the video did not have closed captioning. You can say: "I rented this video, and the box is labeled that it has closed captioning. When I watched it at home, the closed captioning did not work."

The attendant may want to view the video to verify that it is not working properly. He will ask for the video: "Let's take a look at it." "May I view here in the store?" Give the attendant the video. The attendant may ask for your receipt: "May I see your receipt?" "I will need proof that you rented it here." The attendant may ask you what you want to do. "Would you like another tape or your money back?" You will have to explain that you want to view the same movie but with closed captioning. If they do not have that, then you want your money back. You would say: "I would like this movie if you have a copy with working closed captioning. If not, then I would like a refund."

The store may have a set rule or policy that says you get a coupon for a free rental. The attendant may say: "Here you go, you can get another video with this coupon." If you choose a different movie or find another of the one you wanted to watch, ask the service attendant to preview it at the store to make sure the closed captioning works. You could say: "Would you please view this quickly to check the closed captioning?" Remember to thank anyone who helps you: "Thank you for your help." If you have a coupon and get another movie, you will need to turn the coupon in to check out the video you choose. When you leave the store, you should have either a video that has working closed captioning or the $5.00 it costs to rent that video.

(Additional suggestions derived from deaf parent-deaf child households can be found in Chapter 8).

That the majority of hearing parents with children who are deaf should be encouraged and supported in the learning of manual communication is a given (or, at least, a strong consideration). Parents can be shown how their addition of visual/manual dimensions to their home communication repertoire will offer specific advantages to their child who is deaf and increase readiness for and participation in literacy instruction at school. For example, parents should be taught how name signs are developed and encouraged and/or helped to locate or create name signs for all significant others in the child's life—relatives, baby-sitters, neighborhood children, and so on. Specific signs should be used to name locations at which events of significance or frequency occur—the mall, the ice cream store, the ice rink, and so on. Likewise other individually important things (e.g., a favorite stuffed animal) or events (e.g., holiday tradition) should be properly identified by specific designation.

Either as a supplement to manual labeling or to spoken communication in oral homes, graphic designators for these people, objects, places, and events should also be devised and routinely employed. Graphic designators might include pictures, symbol designs, stamps, labels, drawings, and so on. These symbolic representations can begin with pictures and progress to printed words and can be the creation of child or parent or a collaborative effort. The list of elements and the descriptions of designator signs and labels can be shared between home and school and periodically updated. Such individual dictionaries are useful in establishing connections to the broader symbolic function of words. They also facilitate parent-child communication during the kinds of literacy-promoting activities advocated for hearing children, such as preparing an invitation for a friend to attend a birthday or bowling party.

Parents can receive training about book-sharing time, the actual process as well as the kinds of information and outcomes that such activities should generate. Table 7-2 contains an outline of basic knowledge about books that young children commonly acquire as a re-

TABLE 7-2   Early book learning concepts

Working Concepts of Text Features

letter
word
sentence
question
dialogue

Vocabulary for Talking About Books

cover
page
story
character
title (name)
author (writer)
illustrator (artist)

How to Manipulate Books

hold right side up
turn pages
where to begin reading
attend to the spaces in text
reading progressions: left to right, top to bottom

Relate Illustration to Text

Knowledge of Book Structures

title page
chapters
table of contents

sult of early experiences and interactions with their parents at home (see also Durkin, 1989; Hannon, 1995). In large part, these are concepts and terminology that enable the child to talk about books.

Parent instruction about literacy at home should include information on how to address the visual needs of the child and how to relate book experiences to the child's life and previous knowledge in a meaningful manner. Models and resources for this activity can be parents who are deaf as well as other hearing parents. As do parents of hearing children, parents of children who are deaf should seat themselves next to rather than in front of the child who is deaf as they read a book together. This permits parents to mark the place in the text as they recite the words of a story or refer to pictures. The arrangement also keeps the text portion in sight of the child while parents sign the story. By presenting a book in this manner, oral, sign, and print components are all simultaneously available, and the child's visual focus can alternate between text and non-text elements. To aid comprehension of hearing children, parents frequently ask questions or relate story elements to things in the child's experience. Parents who are deaf may also use techniques such as signing on the book or miming characters to increase the child's attention or understanding.

As a natural part of this early literacy activity, parents clarify content or vocabulary by providing definitions or meaningful examples known to the child. They highlight novel or important content by drawing the child's attention to it. Conversely, they draw attention away from the text at times, too, to material outside the text that impinges upon the meaning of the text. They ask the child what he or she thinks is going to happen next or how the story will end.

This extended process of book sharing (not just book reading) has implications for higher-order interactions between the child and text. Such overt parental behaviors parallel and model the inferencing, predicting, and other metacognitive strategies and processes that the accomplished reader/writer uses to organize and interpret textual information during independent reading and writing activities. Thus, without a full and frequent book sharing routine, children who are deaf might be missing not just a pleasurable, but critical, component of reading-readiness or emerging literacy experience.

Parents can be shown ways to engage their children who are deaf in expressive print-related activities. They can provide opportunities and materials for practicing letters or doodling with markers or crayons and for creating stories through computer play. More structured and formal routines can also be developed. For example, requiring children to write *thank you notes* (also greetings, invitations, etc.) not only exercises social graces but builds literacy knowledge. This process can begin with dictated content where the child speaks/signs and the parent writes. The final product can be proofread together. Recipients of such correspondence can be drawn into a supportive role by being encouraged to acknowledge the child's message with a return print correspondence. Gradually the child can be moved through stages of copying and then assisted drafting, toward independent composition of increasingly longer and more diverse written products.

Another technique that both requires and elicits cooperation between teachers and parents is the school-home journal. This dialogue activity is a general vehicle for a variety of information sharing, communication, and cooperative endeavors. This procedure is simple and can be coordinated with activities already commonplace in classrooms for children

TABLE 7-3   Description of daily news calendar

Description

The daily news calendar pocket chart is a reusable, manipulative, multipurpose construction. In addition to routine daily instruction, this calendar is designed so that it may be used as an independent activity by children, combined with home-school journal activities, and have its monthly product of cards compiled into a book.

The calendar is made with ten rows of seven pockets (columns) each. The seven columns are headed with labels for days of the week. The odd numbered rows of pockets are used for inserting numerals for the days of the month. Pockets in the even numbered rows will contain calendar cards to represent each day. The numeral cards and daily calendar cards should be approximately 4" by 6", so the pockets must be slightly larger. Daily cards are created to represent some meaningful event or news of the day. These may be prepared ahead of time, as in the case of a field trip or birthday but may also result from an event or news that arises during the morning meeting. As an option, cards for events to happen very late in a month can be placed in the appropriate calendar pocket on the first day of the month and referred to frequently as the day approaches, as a way of utilizing the concept and language of future tense. As each day passes, the cards from earlier days may be used as a meaningful stimulus for utilizing past tense language. At the end of the month, all of the cards can be laminated, punched, placed in order, and held together with rings and added to the class library. These can be checked out to the children's homes as a stimulus for their sharing happenings at school with people at home.

The size and placement of the calendar in an accessible location afford students the opportunity to practice calendar work by removing and replacing the event cards as well as the month set-up cards. Though the days of the week do not change order as do the numerals, it is a good idea also to make this an additional row of pockets with removable cards so as to increase the utility of the calendar as an independent study activity. A regular monthly calendar can be placed nearby as a checking device.

who are deaf, that is, the daily news. The daily news activity can be accomplished utilizing the guidelines provided in Table 7-3.

The end product of the activity is a tag board calendar card with a one sentence statement of the important news for the day along with some graphic depiction of the subject or event. The content of this card is then copied onto a page in each child's journal, a bound composition notebook that travels back and forth to school with the child. As the children leave for the day, they review the signing or reading of the sentence. Upon arrival at home, the child relays this message to the parent either through speech or sign. Sometime later, the parent and child agree upon the most important thing that happened at home during the evening and repeat the process of generating their own sentence and graphic for transmission back to the teacher. The journal can cycle between school and home everyday or every other day and, be more or less the responsibility of the child with increasing age.

The School Environment

Schools must provide extensive and high-quality visual environments for children who are deaf, who are so dependent upon this channel for acquiring knowledge (see related discussions in Moores, 1987, 1996; Paul & Quigley, 1994a, 1994b). Such a classroom might be noticeably different from that of hearing children. For example, one might find graphic or visual representation of all things one would reference in a general education classroom—the pledge of allegiance, work areas of the room, the office, the daily announcements, the speech therapist, and so on.

In this age of technology, there should be a wide range of visual media, that is, a VCR, computer, perhaps a TTY, available in the classroom. Although these technological media are admittedly advantageous and desirable for enhancing the learning of hearing children (arguably, a necessity for some), they are an absolute requirement for accomplishing everyday basic instruction of every student who is deaf. These devices should be as commonplace as the overhead projector.

The effective classroom will also guarantee the visual accessibility of instructional interaction. Most fundamentally, this implies having teachers and/or tutors who are fluent in signed communication, or the provision of appropriately certified interpreters. There is no excuse for poor sign communication in classrooms with students who are deaf. Communication between students and their teachers needs to be facile, fluent, and comprehensible in both directions for any instruction to be successful. This is not to say that only deaf teachers may teach deaf students but, certainly, that only teachers with fluent sign should teach students who are deaf and who use sign.

Provision and Organization of Real World Experiences

Teachers bring tremendous amounts of information into the lives of students who are deaf by setting the proper circumstances for their exposure to greater amounts of appropriate stimulation. The amount of available visual information already packaged in formats that children can manipulate and comprehend has multiplied a thousand-fold during the last decade. Specially-produced topical video materials, videocassettes of broadcast educational programming, cable nature and history channels, captioned television and news all are available to supplement traditional teaching strategies and content. Much of this material can be obtained for classroom use on loan from special education resource centers funded by school districts or collectives, or from public libraries, public television stations, or sometimes for nominal cost from video outlets.

A second visual resource of increasing importance to classroom instruction is the computer. Many of the same resources for video materials can be tapped for computer learning packages. The interactive nature of computers and the potential for individualization make computer materials particularly attractive.

How a classroom is set up to utilize the information children gain from such visual experiences with computers and television is the key to maximizing benefit. The traditional view of the teacher as the source of all instruction has slowly begun to give way to the notion of teacher as facilitator (see discussion in Chapter 1 on reductionism/constructivism). Cooperative learning among heterogeneous groups of children is widely promoted as a positive model for improving both social and intellectual pursuits of a variety of types of students (see reviews in Dixon-Krauss, 1996). Co-teaching and collaboration among special and general education teachers have become a means of providing inclusion experiences for students who are deaf in the general education classroom. All of these developments represent a broadening of the scope of classroom organization and procedures.

Capitalizing on such flexibility provides opportunities for better meeting the individual needs of students who are deaf. The suggestion here is to establish classrooms with more unstructured *flex time* for students to pursue individual as well as group academic objectives. Some time slots can be designated for collective work or instruction such as morning meetings and language arts. Other times are open for independent work on content and material, perhaps procedures, determined during individual meetings with each student at the beginning of each day or week, depending on the age of the student. During open times, when students are working independently, the teacher can work with individuals or small groups of students to accomplish objectives that require direct teacher input (e.g., new content, corrective feedback) or that apply only to one or two students.

Links to Literacy

Evidence of the importance of conversational fluency in a language to the acquisition of literacy by hearing children is well documented. There is also some evidence that has accumulated, correlating conversational fluency in sign to literacy attainment by students who are deaf (e.g., see discussions in Lane et al., 1996; Wilbur, 1987). In addition, there is some research that suggests a relationship between fluency in some manual forms of English and achievement in English literacy (e.g., Luetke-Stahlman, 1988a, 1988b; Moores et al., 1987).

Incomplete and disfluent classroom instruction and interactions can not provide the model or exercise of conversational language required as a prerequisite to literacy. If fluency with printed English is to be a realistic goal of educational programs, it is of paramount importance that teachers improve the quality of the students' conversational English base. To do so, teachers of students who are deaf must reliably encode grammatical features of English, in sign as well as speech, on a regular basis. This is true especially in conjunction with curricular content and activities dealing directly with language and literacy. There is no easily accessible visual substitute for the information contained in the sign encoding of English grammatical morphemes, especially inflections (see related discussions in Luetke-Stahlman, 1988a, 1988b; for another perspective, see Drasgow & Paul, 1995).

Teachers can improve sign English expression and comprehension in classrooms in a number of ways. Persons who are deaf and who use manual systems for signing English (e.g. Signing Exact English; Gustason & Zawolkow, 1993) do so with great fluency and accuracy. Adult signers who are deaf could be engaged by schools to provide instruction and ongoing consultation regarding the classroom use of these systems. Classrooms that require full-time sign communication ideally would have an adult who is deaf present full time (teacher, aide, tutor, or volunteer). More generally, students' sign communication skills can be improved by the formal adoption of sign curricular objectives and content. It is unclear why this aspect of learning, more than others, should be left to chance. Such a curriculum would include all aspects of language, that is, syntax, and pragmatics as well as vocabulary. The ideal sign curriculum would also provide formal instruction on the grammar of American Sign Language as well. (For a more extensive treatment of the role of ASL in the learning of English, see Chapter 8).

Students should profit more from expanded linguistic instruction when the amount and nature of verbal interaction in classrooms is also adjusted (Luetke-Stahlman & Luckner, 1991; McAnally et al., 1994; Schirmer, 1994). A number of studies have revealed very low levels of student expression in classes for students who are deaf. Language is acquired through experimentation during social exchanges for specific purposes in particular situations (e.g., Dixon-Krauss, 1996). If students are not using language, they are losing countless opportunities to learn about it by receiving specific feedback on their evolving structures.

Teacher expansion of students' expressive language has proven to be a very effective method for improving both the content and the grammar of student productions. The amount of expressive language can be increased by altering the proportion of teacher and student controlled time. The independent study classroom structure, mentioned earlier, provides for this kind of adjustment. The potential for student to student interaction is increased. Further, the amount and character of student-teacher communication improves when students have information from non-teacher sources that needs to be shared, questioned, or supplemented. Scheduling of regular discussion-format interaction provides an expected outlet for independent study learning and provides variety in communicative roles for students, as informants and as participant listeners.

In addition to these general strategies for improving underlying linguistic knowledge, there are specific classroom activities that will directly expand the child's readiness for print communication. Some are old standbys whereas others involve the latest technology. By utilizing the traditional practice of labeling (e.g., objects in the room: window, chair, cubby) much sight-word vocabulary can be gained through a child's frequent visual encounters with words as labels. Teachers can make this serendipitous learning more rigorous by periodically stimulating this process. Labels might be moved to wrong objects or places, or replaced with synonymous labels for more advanced students. Children can be challenged to match labels with their proper objects or pictures or timed to see how long it takes to reposition a stack of removed labels.

At the preschool level, classrooms need a reading corner, a place reserved for literacy work. However, it need not be a display area for books or a pseudo rest area. An effective literacy area should contain a wide variety of materials dedicated to the development of visual perception, discrimination, and association as well as to visual-motor coordination and small-motor development. Kits of boxed and labeled materials can be arranged in order of difficulty by topic or skill on shelves that surround a central table and adjacent carpeted space. Similar to the way some Montessori programs are conducted, children can be shown how a particular set of materials is designed to be used and how its container is labeled with graphic symbol, sign, word, and so on.

The literacy center should also house a library of videotaped stories and books. The videos should have either captions or signed accompaniment or both. Such tapes can be found in a variety of formats and levels through educational catalogues. They can also be made with a little assistance using home video cameras. In developing story tapes, the narrator should alternate between the signed story and the book. That is, a segment of text is presented in sign, followed by the printed version along with any accompanying pictures or graphics. A voice-over should accompany the printed text segment. Text segments should be sentence length or shorter for younger students. For older students or longer texts, the segments can be paragraph length so as to maximize the processing of connected text elements. The library of story videos can be loaned between classroom and home.

There it can serve to reinforce school learning as well as become a stimulus for conversation. Additionally, parents can use the videos for sign practice.

Teachers can also affect children's abilities to use information obtained directly from speech. Largely abandoned along with labeling in the signing classroom have been speech-related instructional activities, for example, speechreading and auditory training. At present, such training is conducted almost exclusively in hearing and speech centers or resource rooms in schools. Speechreading and residual hearing might be insufficient for most students who are deaf for purposes of everyday communication. They are, nonetheless, tools that provide the student who can use them, with direct access to spoken English and to any consequent language-processing advantages associated with speech perception.

Instruction for Classroom Development of Literacy Skills

Young and novice readers/writers should encounter meaningful print, that is, print that represents or labels concepts with which they are already familiar. Successful readers need to do much more than translate from sound to print and will utilize many skills and knowledge bases in the process (e.g., Adams, 1990a; Anderson et al., 1985). The most fundamental component of meaningfulness for a reader is his or her information about the world and about human interaction.

Meaningfulness for any particular piece of text can be assured in different ways. First, in selecting reading materials, the teacher can purposely draw upon topics for which students are known to have experience (see also the selection and adaptation of materials as discussed in King & Quigley, 1985). This information can be knowledge the teacher possesses of the student's background or interests, or that is solicited ahead of time from parents or the students themselves. Another way to guarantee familiarity with a topic or to provide the same information for all students is to arrange for collective experiences with specific subject matter, for example, through field trips, guests speakers, classroom activities, experiments, computer activities, or other media.

To augment the language value of such an experience, the teacher can assign or conduct language-oriented preparatory and follow-up activities. As a follow-up, a young class of students might produce a group generated (perhaps dictated) language experience chart story. Older students might engage in a journal expository writing experience. The purpose of these activities is to provide or highlight concepts, vocabulary, figurative language, and other language features that will be encountered in the text the teacher has planned for the students to read. The literature on *whole language* abounds with suggestions on how to provide meaningful language experiences that promote literacy readiness (e.g., see Gunning, 1992; Schirmer, 1994).

To make the most of special activities for purposes of enhancing correlated reading, it is important that such experiences take place *before* students read the assigned text. Special experiences like field trips are expensive in terms of time and resources. Often, teachers plan such events as the culmination of a unit of instruction. Teachers preface a trip or speaker visit with work on important vocabulary and exposure to visuals related to the topic; they read or have the students read a book on the topic, and so on. The aim of these strategies is to maximize the students' readiness to benefit from the information and situations they will encounter through the special event. However, from the standpoint of the goal of promoting literacy, the cart is before the horse. That is, teachers are using language instruction and reading to bolster participation in real life experience rather than just the reverse. If a field trip or special experience is provided before students begin a text, they have personal knowledge to which they can then attach new vocabulary in the text. They have their own notions concerning the elements or sequences of an experience with which they can make sense of the arrangement of events in their reading. Outside experiences also can provide much needed motivation for students to approach reading in the classroom.

Print Vocabulary Building: Sight Words

For many students, some print vocabulary recognition already will be apparent by the time formal reading instruction begins. Some sight recognition can develop incidentally as a result of exposure to classroom labels and the home-school journal mentioned previously. Other words will have become familiar through contact with print in the larger environment (e.g., signs, billboards, cereal boxes) and through observing or participating in functional uses of print in the classroom (e.g., teacher notes, labeled bins and materials, frequently referred to lists of classroom rules).

There are a number of resource lists for sight words, which usually arrange this vocabulary by frequency of use and/or difficulty level (see Johnson & Pearson, 1984). The category of sight vocabulary consists of two classes of important words. First are words that can be identified only by sight because they violate fundamental rules for letter-sound correspondence in English, for example, *is, the, to, they, one*. The second group consists of words for which instant recognition is advantageous either because they occur so frequently or because they are building blocks for longer words, for example, *that, be, will, and, end, or*.

For children who are deaf, building sight vocabulary should begin with the semantically significant (meaningful) words, that is, nouns, verbs, adjectives, adverbs (see research reviews in McAnally et al., 1994; Schirmer, 1994; see also instructional activities presented in Johnson & Pearson, 1984). Once a process has been established and a substantial number of words are recognized automatically, then the list can be broadened to include function words such as articles, pronouns, conjunctions, prepositions, demonstratives, and the verb *to be*. The list of sight words can also include words children will encounter elsewhere or those that are of interest (e.g., *men/women, poison, keep out*). Teachers can individualize each child's list by adding names of family, playmates, pets, and favorite toys.

A very workable sight vocabulary protocol utilizes printed 3x5 file cards, which can be easily manipulated by young children. On each card is printed a single word. Initially the words are printed in lower case manuscript letters because these are the most frequently encountered letters. Later sets can be developed with cursive or capital letter words. The cards can be punched and bound together on a ring, if desired. Optionally, the reverse side of each card might contain the sign or finger spelling of the word or even a picture or graphic for very young children. In this way, a child can self-check understanding during independent practice.

Acquired sight words, along with other words requested by students, should be compiled into a reference dictionary or word bank. Each word should be allocated its own page in a binder. The binder page will contain the word, its finger spelling, meaning, and sign.

Where possible, some graphic or picture would also be appropriate and, perhaps, a sentence using the word as well. Older students might prefer to arrange their practice cards into a file box for reference.

In addition to its usefulness as a reference for spelling and reading, this word bank can be used for sentence building and other language arts activities and especially for creative writing (see related discussions in Johnson & Pearson, 1984; Tompkins, 1990). It is advisable that each child have a sight vocabulary ring/box because it represents a running record of the child's accomplishments, can be taken home for study, and can be used as a personal reference. The word bank reference can also be jointly developed by all class members who contribute words they have mastered and then be shared by all as a classroom resource.

Sight reading practice can be accomplished independently or with a peer once the process has been firmly established with the teacher. Short periods (5 minutes) with a few words each day provide for continuity without excessive frustration. The child is presented with a word and given a few seconds to recognize it. If the child is unsuccessful, the teacher provide the word, and the child is asked to say or sign the word while looking at it. With this process, the goal is to establish an association between the correct word and its corresponding print. Students working independently should be periodically monitored to ensure that they are following the correct procedure.

A word may be considered *mastered* if it is read correctly on five consecutive occasions with a teacher or peer. Once words are mastered they might be removed from the practice set (to the reference area) and replaced with new words. Progress can be recorded in chart form in ways that provide constant feedback and reinforcement to the student. Periodic sessions with the teacher can be used to review mastered words. However, the primary reason for maintaining a sight word repertoire is to have experience reading them in meaningful contexts.

Print Vocabulary Building: Decoding

To comprehend a text completely, a reader has no choice but to at least decode the words on the page. All the advanced preparation, outside information, vocabulary work, and so on, cannot get to the meaning the authors intended for their texts without going through the authors' actual words. Every reader, hearing or deaf, must learn to decode. Decoding is not an equally difficult task for all readers, nor do all readers accomplish the decoding task in the same way. To begin with, decoding is not simple or straightforward and is not accomplished by memorizing a collection of rules for equating printed symbols with sound.

For practical rather than theoretical purposes, let us define decoding as the process of moving from perception of a printed word to the idea (cognitive conceptualization) usually associated with the conversational form of the word (in other words, getting from the page to the reader's head). Decoding is not a single act, nor does it have a single focus. Rather, decoding is a composite of different skills for analyzing various aspects of textual material. These skills include visual and auditory perception and discrimination, identification, classification, sequencing, parsing, association, analysis, memory, prediction, problem solving, all in addition to the vast amounts of topic information a reader must possess. As stated previously in this text, decoding facilitates comprehension and comprehension facilitates decoding (e.g., Adams, 1990a; Anderson et al., 1985; Mason & Au, 1986).

In this chapter, there is no specific discussion of techniques for the training of speechreading and auditory receptive abilities per se. These skills certainly affect an individual's success in working with words; however, each area is a special domain and requires an instructional regimen of its own. Preparation for reading should involve these two elements in conjunction with the spoken (signed), fingerspelled, and printed forms of the language involved.

Even if it is presumed that a child who is deaf will not have access to words through letter-sound relations, every reader needs to be able to distinguish differences among words prior to any further manipulation or learning about individual words. Decoding is a time-critical process. The mechanics of reading as related to time have been explained in detail elsewhere (e.g., Adams, 1990a; Anderson et al., 1985). Most of us have had the experience of reading a piece of text so difficult that, by the time we managed to decode the words and reach the end, we did not know what we had just read. Likely, we would not be able to recall the beginning of the segment. If we decode words too slowly, the first words of a segment will begin to fade from memory by the time we have reached the end of a long sentence (i.e., more than seven words). Elements at the end of a sentence cannot be related to the beginning, if the beginning has already been lost. The same holds true for relations among sentences within a paragraph or among larger segments of text. Thus slow, arduous decoding has severe negative effects upon the construction of meaning. It should be obvious that letter and word recognition need to become automatic (e.g., Adams, 1990a; Anderson et al., 1985).

Letter Identification

Preliminary work for letter recognition can be accomplished long before formal decoding of connected text begins. It begins with perception, discrimination, and identification of all kinds of visual stimuli during the preschool years. Gradually, a variety of materials and opportunities for practice takes the child from work with pictures through drawings and then line graphics to letters. The same developmental process operates with each new kind of stimuli. Children learn to discriminate differences, to compare, contrast, and classify items on the basis of distinct features and, finally, to label the differences in some generally identifiable way. In the process, they need to become sensitive to visual characteristics of the graphic segments that comprise letters, for example:

size	(upper-lower case)
shape	(straight-rounded, open-closed, parallel-intersected)
orientation	*(u-n, b-d)*
sequence	*(n-m).*

The *reading corner* of a preschool or primary classroom should contain many kits of materials designed to develop the necessary visual readiness by leading the novice reader to attend to the characteristics, orientation, and sequential arrangement of graphic figures.

The *alphabet font kit* is an example of one activity kit. It can be used with a teacher initially and later with peers independently. It trains ever finer discriminations of letter forms while providing practice in sorting and letter name association. A sample kit can be constructed easily by making a flashcard form of each letter of multiple fonts from the computer. Fifteen to twenty different fonts will be challenging. Separate sets of upper and lower case letters in each font should be included in the master kit.

The students' response task always is to sort the font flashcards into letter piles with separate piles for As, Bs, Cs, and so on. The teacher selects some subsets of the flashcards for use in the activity. This stimulus subset varies in difficulty with the age and skill of the student. Initially these subsets contain only a few different fonts and the most distinctive letters (see Set 1). The ultimate goal is for students to be able to quickly distinguish letters from various text sources that utilize many different kinds of print. Therefore, the teacher gradually increases the size of the stimulus set, the number of fonts, and the number of letters to discriminate among them, while also reducing the visual contrast of the features of the letters and fonts to be sorted (see Set 2 below). This kit can be designed with self-check notations on the back of each card. Examples of the sets follows.

Sample Font Kit Subsets

Sample Set 1:	o	o	**o**	o				
	1	1	**l**	1				
Sample Set 2:	b	b	b	**b**	b	b	*b*	b
	d	d	d	**d**	d	d	*d*	d
	a	a	a	**a**	a	a	*a*	a

There are a number of other means for building alphabet familiarity and sequence with children who are deaf. Hearing children learn these through familiar songs and rhymes. A unique option for readers who are deaf is sign language resources that focus upon manual alphabet characteristics. There are now videos of ABC stories, signed sequences that tell a story while using in sequence the configurations of the manual alphabet. Some of these also have captioned formats with simultaneous print.

Letter-Sound Association

Learning letter-sound correspondence is obviously a difficult task for students with hearing impairment. Evidence shows this to be true as witnessed by the detrimental effects of chronic otitis media on language and reading development in children (e.g., Kavanaugh, 1986). These children have mild to moderate interference with their hearing on a frequent but intermittent basis. Yet, they can have substantial difficulty acquiring the correct pronunciation and use of common words due to misperception or absence of phonemic sounds. This has ramifications for subsequent acquisition of letter-sound correspondences and for syntactically significant morphemic development, both of which are critical to reading.

It is especially important for students who can do so to be encouraged and supported in their efforts to use the aural/oral system during their processing of print (e.g., see related discussions in Cole & Gregory, 1986). For those students who have usable hearing, time and creativity need to be devoted to providing instruction and practice that enhances their auditory ability to discriminate and identify sounds in relation to print. Students who are deaf have been shown to benefit from instruction that emphasizes speech reading and expressive speech practice as a means to aid their access and use of speech-recoding processing (e.g., see Kelly, 1995; see also, Chapter 3 of this text). Much of this instruction can be directed, if not largely accomplished, by the speech-language therapist, supported by instructional behaviors of the classroom teacher.

One major goal of auditory training is for the student to associate letters or letter combinations with their corresponding speech sounds. Students will move through phases of detecting differences in sounds, comparing and contrasting sounds, on to identifying sounds. Once a sound can be identified auditorily, training for association with its printed form can begin.

Sound discrimination for students with hearing impairment should proceed from discrimination of larger units (more easily discriminated) to smaller units. Full words should be utilized initially, with a move gradually to smaller clusters and eventually to identification of just single sounds. It is recommended that the emphasis should be placed first on learning consonants. Consonant sounds are much more stabile contextually than vowels and also much more visible. The order for consonant recognition instruction should be in initial, then final, then medial position in a word (e.g., Durkin, 1989; Johnson & Pearson, 1984; Mason & Au, 1986). For purposes of planning instruction, classification of sounds and combinations by their level of auditory difficulty can be obtained from the following sources (Carnine et al., 1990; Durkin, 1989; Mason & Au, 1986).

There are also guidelines and programs for development of speechreading skills to visually supplement the auditory identification of letters in words. Such programs emphasize analytical skills and the use of context. When teachers plan auditory or speechreading practice, choices for stimuli should *not* include non-sense syllables or impossible words. Children who are deaf, who spend much of their lives trying to make sense of ambiguous communication, will find nonsense stimuli unnecessarily frustrating and confusing. There is no practical application for such training, and it is therefore not a good use of instructional time.

Whenever possible the students' auditory and/or speechreading practice should include segments of time during each lesson when supplemental visual/manual information is provided (e.g., fingerspelling or cueing). The long-term objective is to withdraw the manual cue gradually as auditory identification alone improves. Visual cues will help students to disambiguate and organize features of the perceived auditory input. The advantage of employing some formal system of manual cues during the speechreading and auditory training sessions is that the student presumably will have additional but unstructured practice with cue-sound associations outside of the training sessions.

The Morphographic Analysis of Words

As mentioned previously, only with great difficulty can students who are deaf utilize information about graphophonemic correspondence for the purpose of decoding text. Some other reliable means for engaging text must be made available to these students. Is there a reasonable substitute for phonics in the word decoding process for those children who are deaf and who cannot accomplish letter-sound correspondence? Either as a supplement or an alternative to sound-based word identification skills, students might be able to utilize meaning-based decoding strategies such as the use of morphological or structural analysis (however, see caveats expressed by Nagy et al., 1994).

A morphograph is a group of letters (aside from whole words) that carries unique meaning, that is, represents a specific letter-meaning relationship. Morphographs include common bound inflectional suffixes like *-ing* and *-ly* and derivational affixes like *pre-* and *-ment*. Included also are word roots and segments of words that always demonstrate the same meaning-print association when they are combined with other morphemes into more complex words. Examples are *struct = to build* or *geo = earth*. There are several arguments in favor of a morphographic emphasis for the reader who is deaf (see also the benefits for hearing readers in Chapter 2 of this text):

1. The raw material for this type of structural word analysis, that is, the relationship of patterns of letters in words or word segments to meanings, is visually mediated and thus available to the reader who is deaf.
2. Morphographic correspondence in English is much more reliable (i.e., consistent and predictable with fewer exceptions) than is graphophonemic correspondence.
3. Ability to apply syntactic knowledge to decoding text is highly correlated with comprehension performance of good readers who are deaf (e.g., Kelly, 1995; see also Chapter 3 of this text).
4. It has been suggested that skilled readers who are deaf pay greater attention to form features of English text than do average deaf readers (e.g., see discussion in Kelly, 1995).
5. Strong evidence exists for the role of a large vocabulary in reading proficiency, and manipulation of morphological forms is critical to development of more advanced vocabulary (see Chapters 2 and 3 of this text).

Relative to curriculum planning, study of the morphology of English has been divided into three phases, which begin in the primary years and extend through the high school years.

Phase 1 The starting point for morphographic training of students is the underlying logic of morphological systems, that is, the notion that there are building blocks of meaning and, in the case of English, the notion of temporal (in print, left to right) sequence in this building process. Fundamental information (though not necessarily the terminology) includes the distinctions between *base*, *compound*, and *complex* words. Discussion of these concepts can be initially developed using basic vocabulary that most young children possess, for example, *fire + truck, pan + cake, balloons, wanted* (for activities with compound words, see Johnson & Pearson, 1984).

Introduction to printed forms can begin with words constructed using early sight vocabulary in combination with each other and with early-acquired (conversational) inflectional suffixes (i.e., *plural -s, -ed,-ing, -er*). The focus is on meaningful clusters of letters; children are constantly being shown and encouraged to parse words into meaningful segments and to identify the meanings associated specifically and consciously with each of these smaller units. The progression of stages should be familiar by now, that is, children will *perceive* the parts as separate morphs, then *discriminate* among them visually, then *identify* the meaning associated with each morphographic representation.

Phase 2 Gradually, the curriculum progresses to include the remaining inflectional suffixes and to introduce common derivational morphemes (prefixes as well as suffixes).

Again, the new morphographs are introduced in combination with the same early sight vocabulary to produce examples like *unhappy, redo, beautiful, useless.* Thereafter, as the students' vocabulary grows, introduction of new morphological information and forms always utilizes the known vocabulary base so that the focus of the students' efforts can be upon the morphemes targeted for instruction.

Phase 3 The most advanced level of morphographic instruction deals with meaningful groups of letters that go beyond the limited set of affixes that attach to base words already in a student's vocabulary. A prime focus here is on word roots.

Evidence has been documented for decades showing that the average high school graduate who is deaf attains less than a fourth grade reading proficiency. There are characteristics of text beyond the fourth grade level that suggest possible stumbling blocks to further reading achievement. One has to do with the level of inference required of readers for comprehension of more advanced text. Another is the expanded use of figurative language, along with idiomatic and colloquial forms. A final characteristic involves the utilization of higher level vocabulary. Some difficult vocabulary results from the utilization of ever more technical and obscure derivational affixes. There is a second aspect of advanced vocabulary that bears noting, namely, the semantic relationships that hold among words that derive from common word roots. Skilled readers have access to this highly generalizable morphographic information. Apparently non-skilled readers may not.

Advanced instruction in morphographic regularities of English is not beyond the resources of students who are deaf. As stated earlier, the morphographic relationships in English are very regular. There is a significant list of morphographs that maintain regular spelling-meaning associations across sets of multimorpheme words that incorporate them (e.g., Dale & O'Rourke, 1971). For example, *script-,* the meaning element *to write,* is incorporated in each of the following words that contains the letter sequence s-c-r-i-p-t: *scripture, transcript. manuscript, inscription, description.* Table 7-4 contains a listing of common morphographs of English along with the meaning(s) with which they are regularly associated.

In some cases, lists of morphographs have been developed and used to improve hearing students' spelling performance. Spelling patterns derived from morphographs are much more predictable. Interestingly enough, though many students who are deaf are not good readers, some may be reasonably good spellers; however, there is a strong relationship between spelling and reading for hearing students (e.g., Adams, 1990a, 1990b). In any case, some students who are deaf are able to use the regularities they notice visually in words to spell them correctly. Teachers need to develop instruction that taps this same knowledge source to enable students to decode words for reading, too. In fact, some scholars advocate using a system involving morphographs as the basis for reading instruction with hearing children because some skilled hearing readers did not seem to use phonic rules to decode English text (however, see the various interpretations of this issue, especially the importance of the sound system in Adams, 1990a, 1990b).

The goals of teaching students who are deaf to decode words by emphasizing morphology are to (1) be able to approach words also from the perspective of meaning units (clusters of letters), not just sound units, and (2) parse words on the basis of meaning-letter cluster associations that will permit students greater access to unknown and more complex words. In both respects, the morphographic system is more stable and reliable

TABLE 7-4   Phases of development for instruction of morphographs and their meanings

Phase 1		
Suffix	*Meaning*	*Example*
-able	capable of being	breakable
-ed	past tense	begged
-er/-or	one who	baker
-es/-s	noun plural	dogs
-en	cause to be or become	awaken
-ing	ongoing action, progressive	swimming
-ly	manner in which, adverb	slowly
-ness	state or quality of	kindness
-s	present indicative singular	runs
-y	condition of, adjective marker	dirty

Phase 2		
Prefix	*Meaning*	*Example*
anti-	against	antiperspirant
de-	from, take away	deport
dis-	apart, away	dislike
il-/im-/in-/ir-	not	irresponsible
mal-	wrong	malnourished
mis-	wrong, bad	misplace

Phase 3		
Root	*Meaning*	*Example*
bio	life	biology
geo	earth	geography
sect	to cut	intersection
dict	to speak	diction
micro	tiny, small	microscope
script	to write	manuscript
phone	sound	telephone
tele	far	telephone
struct	to build	construction
turb	to agitate	disturb

than the sound system. If morphographic analysis improves identification of word segments, it will increase processing speed by reducing the absolute number of units to be decoded.

It is important to recognize, however, that hearing children do not get most of their morphological knowledge from formal instruction (see discussion in Nagy et al., 1994). Their knowledge arises from contact with English morphology during conversational interactions with skilled speakers, through trial and error at both interpreting and expressing meaning. For very many children who are deaf, the greatest volume of conversational interaction with adult models of English may take place in school and through the use of some form of manually coded English (MCE).

Manual English codes (e.g., signed English, Bornstein, Saulnier, & Hamilton, 1983; signing exact English, Gustason & Zawolkow, 1993) have been criticized for failing to represent, at least, the phonological basis of English (e.g., see Drasgow & Paul, 1995). Derived from the regularities of written English, most of the signed systems are considered incomplete and ineffective renditions of conversational English. Perhaps exactly because they avoid the pitfalls of the sound system, such codes might reduce confusion for children who are deaf during reading, producing fewer of the kinds of sounding out errors that phonics produces with unskilled hearing readers. The test of this will be children who are deaf and who truly have had consistent and broad exposure to English through sign. MCE systems provide signs for many affixes, as well as a demonstrated system for extending morphological generalizability through the process of initialization. Unfortunately, much classroom practice falls below the capacity of such manual codes to replicate the English morphological system. Teachers need not sign full English sentences always, but many almost never do. It is paramount that, most of the time and always under certain circumstances, children have reliable and full access through vision to the elements and patterns of English morphology.

How can we improve the implementation of manual English systems for the purpose of teaching English morphology, with an eye toward print literacy? The effort must involve a collaborative effort between school and home. MCE can be daunting to learn, a huge dictionary with many affixes, and so on. Teachers can reduce the strain and likely increase the effectiveness of parent signing if they limit their expectations and establish attainable goals. Parents reasonably can be requested and instructed about how to provide reliable encoding particularly of the English inflectional morphemes and a few derivational ones. It would be of great benefit to the child if mastery of these could be largely facilitated through consistent repetition during familiar situations at home. Responsibility for the remaining affixes would be primarily that of the teacher in the classroom, both to model frequently and appropriately as well as to instruct.

Careful use of manual English codes during language and literacy instruction is essential to the goal of providing students who are deaf with the means to learn English morphology (e.g., see discussion in Gaustad, 1986). This would include complete and correct signing or cueing by the teacher during language emphasis activities like morning meeting/calendar, as well as reading, spelling, and language arts/literature lessons. Of course, the teacher's daily oral book reading would be encoded fully also. Whenever possible, when children who are deaf see printed English, they should also see parallel forms encoded in an appropriate manual format.

Instruction of Morphographs

<u>Sample: Phase 1</u>

Like other types of decoding skills, much of the work with morphographs involves various kinds of exposures and, to a considerable extent, rote memory. The kinds of activities used for sight word learning also can be used to teach the meaning of morphographs. There are ways, however to make morphographic concepts interesting for children who are deaf. Motion visuals are highly useful in transmitting concepts related to verb inflection. Stop motion videos enable the teacher to contrast *The boy will jump* with *The boy is jumping* and both of them with *The boy jumped.* As a general rule, instruction of language concepts is best conducted within a contrast format. Contrast heightens meaning by focusing the child's attention on the language element that changes in conjunction with a noticeable alteration of a stimulus.

The video motion technique can be adapted in many ways, for example, to teach past progressive or perfect forms. If the teacher notes the sequences of the actions on a tape, it is possible to discuss more complex sentences, such as *By the time the boy began to jump, he had rolled already* or *Before the boy was jumping, he was rolling.* Over time these techniques can be used to help students relate inflected forms or complex words to base words, a significant step toward morphographic decoding.

Sample: Phase 2

For more advanced lessons with derivational morphemes, the following activities might be of benefit. The teacher needs to develop creative exercises that are catered to the individual needs of the students. The activities below are based on the work of Dale and O'Rourke (1971).

The first exercise concerns prefixes that deal with number. The goal is to facilitate the learning of words that can often be put into logical groupings based on roots, prefixes, and suffixes. One such logical grouping is that of number. Examples of number prefixes are *mono* and *uni* (one); *bi* and *di* (two); *tri* (three); and so on. The student should be led to the notion that these prefixes and their associated meanings are part of numerous words, for example, *mono* is present in *monocle, monoplane, monogram, monorail,* and *monotonous.* The prefix *bi* can be found in *bicycle, binocular, bisect, bigamy,* and so on.

As an exercise (or two or three), the teacher might display on the chalkboard or overhead projector the following prefixes: *uni (1) mono (1) bi (2) tri (3) quad (4) pent (5) sex (6) sept (7) oct (8) novem (9) dec (10) cent* (100). Using these prefixes, the students are asked to write as many words as they can. First, students can use a dictionary to locate words and, then can be encouraged to create and define their own words.

Sample: Phase 3

Yet another exercise of this type utilizes word roots in combination with the number prefixes. This combination alters the meaning of the root, for example, the root *gamy* means marriage. From this root, there are words such as *monogamy, bigamy, trigamy.* Some of these words are difficult, but the more difficult words can be used to challenge students. Younger students might be able to work with words such as *uni + cycle, bi + cycle, tri + cycle; bi + weekly, bi + monthly, bi + yearly, tri + weekly, tri + monthly, tri + angle.*

All students might be surprised about the number of additional words that can be formed from number prefixes. Consider the following examples.

From **mono** *(one):*

monarch (one ruler)
monk (one who lives alone)
montheism (belief in one God)
monotone (one tone)
monoxide (has one oxygen atom)

From **uni** *(one):*

unique (only one of its kind)
unison (blend together to make one sound)
unite (become one)
univalve (one-shelled animal)
unifoliate (having one leaf)
unicorn (one-horned animal)

From **bi** *(two):*

bicorn (two-horned animal)
biannual (twice a year)
bicuspid (two-pointed tooth)
bifocal (having two focuses)
bisect (to cut in two)
bivalve (two-shelled animal)
bifoliate (have two leaves)
bipolar (having two poles)

From **di** *(two):*

dioxide (has two oxygen atoms)
diphthong (two vowels with one sound)
duet (two singers)
duplicate (two copies)

From **tri** *(three):*

trident (three-pronged fork)
trifocal (having three focuses)
trio (group of three)
triple (three-base hit)
triplets (three of similar age)
triplicate (three copies)
tripod (three legged)

From **quad** *(four):*

quadrangle (having four angles)
quadrilateral (four-sided)

quadruped (four-legged)
quart (one-fourth of a gallon)

***From* quint *(five)*, sex *(six)*, sept *(seven)*, octo *(eight)*, novem *(nine)*, deca *(ten)*:**

quintet (group of five)
sextet (group of six)
septet (group of seven)
octet (group of eight)
November (Roman ninth month)
decade (ten years)
decathalon (ten contests)
December (Roman tenth month)

***From* cent *(one hundred)*:**

century (100 years)
centipede (hundred-legged)
centennial (100 anniversary)
centenarian (person who is 100 years old)

The types of exercises that can be developed are limited by the imagination of the teacher. Consider Activity 1.

Activity 1

How many feet?
  a. unipod
  b. biped
  c. tripod
  d. quadruped
  e. hexapod
  f. octopod (as in octopus)

For another activity, the teacher can display a base word, for example, *cycle*, with *wheel* in parentheses, on the chalkboard or overhead, then provide prefixes: *uni-*, *bi*, and *tri-*, and so on. Students are required to combine a prefix with *cycle* and discuss the meaning of the complex word that results, such as *unicycle*, *bicycle*, and *tricycle*. Again, the concept can be expanded creatively by encouraging students to explain or draw their own versions, for example, *octacycle*.

Another, more difficult, activity is to display a prefix with multiple word or root selections to which it can be affixed. For example, the prefix *tri* can be placed on the left side of the page with other words or word parts on the right side such as *angle*, *cycle*, *logy*, *plet*, and *pod*. The students are required to create complex words and discuss the meanings, *triangle*, *tricycle*, *trilogy*, *triplet*, and *tripod*.

After students acquire a good working knowledge of words and word parts, they might be ready for the next activity; Table of Combining Parts (adapted from Dale &

O'Rourke, 1971). The placement of the Xs indicates which word parts across the top (e.g., *gon*, *ton*) can be combined with the word parts on the side of the page (e.g., *mono*, *bi*).

Example of a Table of Combining Parts

	A gon (angle)	B ton (pitch)	C cycl (wheel)	D gam (marriage)	E angul/angle (angle)	F ped/pod (foot)	G enni/annus (year)
mono (1)		X	X	X		X	
bi, di (2)	X		X	X	X	X	X
tri (3)	X		X	X	X	X	X
oct (8)	X				X	X	
dec (10)	X					X	X
poly (many)	X	X	X	X	X		

Subsequently, the student can use the Table of Combining Parts to complete the following matching exercises.

Activity A

1. monotonous
2. monocycle
3. monogamy
4. polygamy
5. bigonial
6. bicycle
7. bigamist

_____ **a.** having two angles
_____ **b.** having only one husband or wife
_____ **c.** marrying several persons
_____ **d.** having two wives at once
_____ **e.** always the same
_____ **f.** one-wheeled vehicle
_____ **g.** two-wheeled vehicle

Activity B

1. biannual
2. quadricycle
3. biangular
4. tricycle
5. trigamist
6. triangle
7. triennial

_____ **a.** three-angled figure
_____ **b.** every third year
_____ **c.** three-wheeled vehicle
_____ **d.** having two angles
_____ **e.** three wives at once
_____ **f.** happens twice a year
_____ **g.** four-wheeled cycle

Activity C

1. monopode
2. biped
3. decapod
4. hexapod
5. tripod
6. octopus
7. quadruped

_____ **a.** a horse
_____ **b.** three-legged stand
_____ **c.** has eight feet (tentacles)
_____ **d.** a man
_____ **e.** an insect (has six legs)
_____ **f.** having one foot
_____ **g.** lobster or crayfish (has 10 legs)

For variety, additional practice with vocabulary development can include activities such as word maps and even semantic feature analyses (discussed previously in the text). Additional examples of these activities are discussed in Chapter 8.

General Notes on Decoding Instruction

Instruction designed to teach the decoding of words should take place outside of reading comprehension instruction, that is, a child's public reading should not be interrupted for purposes of correcting or demonstrating decoding strategies. There are three important reasons why separate instruction is appropriate. First, the purpose of decoding is to speed the reading process in order to facilitate comprehension. Consequently, teaching the child to focus on correcting each word is counterproductive. Over a period of time, it will instill bad habits, which will be extremely difficult to break. Second, interruptions disrupt the flow of meaning and interfere with the reader's ability to make sense of the text. This, in turn, produces frustration and distaste for reading. Third, motivation to read derives from satisfaction and success. Interruption during reading publicly conveys a message of incompetence, which produces discouragement and unwillingness to risk attempting difficult vocabulary.

Decoding activities usually should involve text that is very familiar to the reader, not just the content but the actual language. It is no less valid or beneficial to decode or recognize familiar words than unfamiliar ones. Each decoding experience, each success, practices principles that will fine tune the efficiency of the reading process. Repeated reading of books at home and at school will provide textual familiarity, which the teacher can use to improve decoding practice.

We end this section with a list of guidelines for teachers in making decisions on what words to emphasize in a particular story.

Vocabulary Guidelines

1. First, read through the passages in the text that the students will be reading in class. Note which words in the story have more than one meaning or which are prominent in the story.
2. Estimate the importance of key multimeaning words and other important words (e.g., technical words, etc.). Which words are crucial to students' comprehension of the story? Does a given word appear frequently throughout the story and the rest of the text? Is this an important word at the reading grade level of the student?
3. Decide how likely students are to derive the meanings of these words from context. Is the context elaborate enough to reveal the particular meaning of the word?
4. Next, decide what aspects of these words need to be emphasized. Is it necessary for students to know several meanings of a word? Should they know other nuances or related concepts such as idiomatic or metaphoric usage? Will this knowledge contribute to an understanding of important concepts in this piece and subsequent reading?
5. Finally, find out how much students know about these words. Use techniques such as semantic maps, word maps, and semantic feature analyses to enhance and activate their knowledge.
6. Design vocabulary instruction to meet specific uncovered needs.

Use of Higher-Level Comprehension Skills

As discussed in Chapter 2, there are other skills important for the reading process, specifically, higher-level comprehension skills. Such skills enable the student to construct an overall model of text meaning as well as to more quickly identify an unknown word. Novice readers must learn to pursue and interpret many sources of meaning that lie within the text but beyond the word level. Clues to meaning can be garnered from the interaction of semantic, lexical, syntactic, and pragmatic aspects of the text. This narrowing process is perhaps best understood by following a reader through the process.

For example, imagine that a reader comes upon an unfamiliar word in a story. *It was a dangerous situation for the l_ _ _ _ _ _ _ _ _, being surrounded by giants with no means of escape.* The reader is unable, initially, to decode the word. He or she needs supplemental information by which to narrow the possibilities. A logical starting place is the kind of book the reader has chosen. The kind of book sets expectations for many aspects of text. If the reader has a book of fairy tales, he or she might conjure up visions of armies of giants. If it is a book on Irish culture, the perspective on the giants might diminish somewhat. Our mystery book happens to be about archaeology.

Comprehension skills also involve the use and understanding of English language features, competencies that are part of the intuitive linguistic knowledge of typically hearing individuals. For example, the search for the meaning of a word can be narrowed further by determining the part of speech of the target word. This can be accomplished by the syntactic examination of the surrounding sentence. In our example above, there are multiple clues to use. First, the unknown word is preceded by the article *the*. This narrows the choices for part of speech to two. It is either a noun or an adjective. The second clue to the nature of the word is its role in the sentence. In this case, the unknown word is also the object of the preposition *for,* which we are able to determine because it is the last word of the phrase, and it is followed by a comma. So far we have concluded that our unknown word is a noun that is at least somewhat related to archaeology.

What more can be determined about the meaning of the word? To determine the semantic nature of the unknown word, again, there are multiple clues to be found in the surrounding text. The portion of text preceding any difficult word and the semantic context within which the unknown word is embedded are of significant importance to the reader in unraveling its meaning. What evidence for resolving the mystery is contained close by in the sample text? We know from the immediate sentence that our word names something, and we know that the something is in danger. If we know the principles for applying lexical features in text, we can determine that our noun is an animate being because it, at least, has the capability to escape. Suppose we know, from previous information in the text, that the setting for the scene in question is an arrangement of ancient stone columns from an Egyptian ruin. Suppose the immediately preceding sentence is *As the man strained to see the detail of the huge pillar, the ground began to shake violently beneath his feet.*

Once the reader has gathered all of this contextual data, he or she has already established much of the meaning of the sentence; that is, the man examining the ruins is in immediate danger from an earthquake because he is standing among unstable huge stone structures with no protection and not enough time to get free of them. What is left for the reader to determine is who the man is. What type of person has an interest in stone carving? Do we know anything else that would help to identify the particular man? There is one last piece of evidence for decoding the word on the page. For this evidence we must look again at the word itself. What is the beginning letter of the mystery word? Answer, the letter *l*. What kind of person associated with stone carving has a label that begins with *l*? Our unknown word is *lapidarist*.

Any one reader will not use all of the above clues; nor would the detective work necessarily proceed in the sequence delineated above. This example demonstrates how all aspects of text interact to determine meaning and, therefore, are components in comprehending the message of the text as a whole. Similarly, instruction for the purpose of teaching readers to decode efficiently must involve multiple aspects of linguistic knowledge as well as practice with strategies to use when decoding fails. The higher-order variables of interest here are advance organizers (e.g., prior knowledge skills), context analysis, interpretation of figurative language, making predictions, inferencing (e.g., asking and answering questions such as QARs), and metacognitive skills.

Advanced Organizers for Reading

As preparation for reading any text, the teacher should activate and enhance knowledge that the reader/writer has about the particular topic (see Chapter 2 of this text). A starting point for this activity is the cover of the book. What can be determined about what's inside a book from the cover? Obviously, this includes perusal of the title and any external graphics, but for more experienced readers, important clues can also come from knowing the author and sometimes from the size or shape of a book. Depending on the students and the extended plan for instruction, the teacher might at this time offer glimpses into the book, specifically the table of contents or visuals. The introduction should be an extended activity with the purpose of eliciting as much relevant information as possible. Specifically, the teacher will want to lead the students to significant vocabulary and concepts to be found in the text and, also, to elicit any experiences that the children might have with the topic or the particular type of book. The collective knowledge of a group can add significantly to each individual's store of relevant information and the vocabulary used to express it.

The introductory session concludes with the teacher contributing important missing information while providing an overview of the book. This includes establishing the type of book, topic, and structure. For example, let's suppose that children are looking at a book about volcanoes. The teacher might say, "This book about volcanoes includes chapters on the science and geography of volcanoes and it has a special chapter called Little Known Facts About Volcanoes."

Context Analysis

Skills in analysis of context will aid students in determining the meanings of individual words in text but will also lead them to understand the unity among features of text, which determines meaning for an entire passage. Context analysis isolates individual words or structures as a means to demonstrate or evaluate their relationship to other elements in a text.

The basic format of this instruction is to remove from view one element of a piece of text (letter, word, phrase, or even sentence) and then have students identify the missing element. One by one, students can be taught to use various kinds of information. Strategies for identifying missing elements can involve semantic, syntactic, morphological, graphic, and pragmatic cues. The instruction builds over time across multiple dimensions, gradually progressing from simple cues (e.g., word order, the __) to more obscure or technical sources of information (e.g., morphology, *-ist*) and from work with individual words to progressively more complex and/or longer segments.

Among other competencies, context analysis targets an important deficit in the students' knowledge of English sentence grammar, that is, comprehension and expression of relationships among sentence components. For example:

- Work with noun phrases highlights the importance of word order.
- Certain kinds of verbs determine the number and relations of nouns in a sentence.
- Pronoun selection (i.e., case) indicates relations of noun elements to verbs and other nouns. Further, pronouns highlight the interplay between sentences when students must explain how they selected a particular form of pronoun.
- Prepositions indicate relations between actions and objects and in relation to locations.

Relationships derived from passive constructions, possession, cause-effect, and temporal sequencing are examples of semantics, which can be demonstrated during context analysis instruction. The only limitation is the creativity of the teacher.

The practical mechanics of context exercises can be accomplished in many different ways, which is a major reason it is such a useful technique. With young children, chart stories developed for other purposes during language arts or other curricular activities can be the stimulus for this activity. For beginning experiences, the teacher may choose to read the piece once with the children first. Then the word is covered by the teacher and the students must identify it. Older students can complete many variations on this theme with paper and pencil tasks. They may enjoy creating mystery work pages for each other. It is fairly easy to provide printed answer keys for context worksheets. In one variation, students may be given choices from which to select the missing element. Actually, rather than making the procedure simpler, and seemingly less useful, this technique offers opportunities to increase the value of the instruction because students must evaluate and explain the pros and cons of the various options. Effective materials, therefore, carefully manipulate the stimulus choices as well as the type of student response required.

The goal of context analysis, beyond more efficient word identification, is familiarity with the processes and information sources used to accomplish it. This knowledge will evolve from the discussions surrounding group context analysis activities. As the targets of instruction move from word order to different parts of speech and so on, interactions between the semantic and syntactic elements of text and among various segments of text can be addressed.

Semantic Webbing

As the introduction proceeds, the teacher records on the overhead or chart paper the vocabulary and concepts that arise during discussion. This written record is available to be used during the second preparatory session, which is devoted to the activity of semantic mapping. Semantic webbing or mapping refers to the organization or relationship that exists among concepts or language elements (see Gunning, 1992; Heimlich & Pittelman,

1986). Once an extended list of words or concepts for the book is elicited, the teacher can prompt students to organize them in meaningful ways.

There are a number of possible semantic orientations for structuring this activity. Elements can be related characteristically (two-legged, four-legged), functionally (eating utensils, gardening tools), sequentially (first, second, third base), hierarchically (fish, guppy), by cause-effect (disease→symptoms), part-whole (car, axle), contrast (antonyms), and so on. By guiding students to create and examine multiple arrangements for an identified set of elements, the teacher can stimulate cognitive breadth and flexibility (Mason & Au, 1986; Pearson & Johnson, 1978). In this way, the activity affords a greater likelihood that each student will discover ways in which his or her information will apply to the text during reading. Over time, such demonstrations also encourage the formation of reading habits whereby a reader will search beyond an initial interpretation of text to possible alternatives. See Figure 2-2 in Chapter 2 for examples of a semantic map or web.

Figurative Language

An area of reading and writing that causes great consternation among teachers of students who are deaf is figurative language (see also Chapter 3). Figurative language refers to a word or cluster of words that do not mean what they appear to mean, in other words, they are unrelated to the literal or regular meanings associated with the words in a sequence. For purposes of this discussion, we include in the category of figurative language the following forms: multiple meaning words, idioms, colloquial expressions, and figures of speech such as metaphor and simile. Hearing readers may have an advantage with regard to figurative language because the meaninglessness of these forms, when taken literally, is more likely to be noticed compared to these students' other language and reading experiences. In contrast, for students who are deaf, confused language input is commonplace and they are constantly faced with communicative ambiguity. Thus, the necessity of applying special comprehension strategies in the case of figurative language forms may not be so apparent to them.

With some figurative forms, a general translation strategy can be provided for arriving at a proper interpretation. Once a reader knows to compare the elements stated in a simile, for example, *He ran like the wind,* the problem is on the way to being solved as long as the logic of the analogy is obvious. At the other end of the continuum of explicitness, there is no hope, only memorization. In the case of most fixed idioms, there is no or little direct connection between any words in the idiomatic phrase and the meaning of the structure, *It's raining cats and dogs.* The only way to learn to interpret them correctly is to memorize the meaning association. This is accomplished in the same fashion as sight vocabulary and morphographs, that is, with a variety of creative word exercises and exposures.

A realistic objective of instruction regarding figurative language is to enable children who are deaf to detect at least these forms of expressions. Then the student can implement necessary interpretative strategies. One general suggestion, for the visually oriented students, is to pay special attention any time the words of a text create an implausible (humorous) picture in their minds. *He ate like a horse, Your eyes are bigger than your stomach.* This visual orientation also can be used to make memorization exercises more fun. Students can produce visual images corresponding to the idiom or metaphor. These can be placed on the reverse side of a flashcard containing the figurative phrase. A second flash card contains the proper interpretation of the expression. If identical puzzle-fit notches are placed on both edges of the original card, either side may be used as the stimulus cue until the linguistic equation is mastered. Students can be encouraged to use their creativity to create new figurative expressions for notions they communicate frequently.

Each classroom for students who are deaf should also have a dictionary of figurative language examples because even when the students recognize one in text, it is not possible to locate meanings in a standard dictionary. This special dictionary can be organized alphabetically by the first letter of the first major word so that a dictionary protocol can be used. Graphics generated by students can accompany the entries.

Instruction for multiple meaning words is an extension of the work on using context. Students can be shown how to use surrounding text to select among alternative interpretations or modify the interpretation of a problematic word. Shades of meanings, associated with some words, can be demonstrated in a sequence along a continuum anchored by the two most extreme expressions of a concept. This technique can easily be adapted for self-study, also with puzzle notches, to link a sequence of cards. For example:

---

annoyed || perturbed || irritated || upset || angry || enraged || rabid

---

Word sets for synonyms and shades of meaning can be developed for use even with very young children to introduce them to the flexibility and precision of language. Instruction devoted to reading and interpreting such words should be undertaken in conjunction with applications of this information to creative expressions. Students can be given practice in recasting words, phrases, and even sentences using different words but retaining the general meaning of the original.

Making Predictions
Once information has been developed and organized, students can be encouraged to make evidence-based predictions about many aspects of the content of the book. Do you expect this book to tell a story or provide information? How will the book begin? What kinds of people or characters will the book talk about? As a group or individually, students should compile a list of questions to be answered by reading the book. The kinds and topics of questions, and the information sought, will depend on the type of book. The idea is that as students read a book they will monitor what they read with the questions in mind, that is, the questions can help to pinpoint important details in the text. Over many book experiences, students can be led to realize that books of a certain type involve similar kinds of questions (e.g., see Gunning, 1992; Lipson & Wixson, 1991; Mason & Au, 1986).

Initially, the question development process will be a more conscious and teacher-directed activity. Eventually, it needs to become internalized, with the students automatically noting information rather than searching for facts. Otherwise, the monitoring process can interfere with overall comprehension of the material (for more details on the importance of questions, see Mason & Au, 1986; Pearson & Johnson, 1978).

Preparatory activities in advance of encountering a text should not be reserved only for material that students will read independently. The processes of semantic mapping, predicting, and prequestioning text can be useful when preparing a story to be read to students as well. While being read to, students can complete monitoring practice and other activities under what might be an easier format (watching or listening), that is, without the added demands of having to simultaneously decode the text. This type of activity might also be of benefit for deaf students who are learning English as a second language (see Chapter 8 of this text).

Inferencing

Inference requires a reader to go beyond ideas expressed explicitly in the words on a page to ideas that are only implied by the actual text. Instruction for developing inferential readers has both objective and subjective components. The *objective* component involves training in the skills of interpretation and evaluation, among others. The notion here is not to teach meaning per se or the individual values that underlie evaluation but, rather, to develop the strategies or skills for engaging in these cognitive processes. They require the student to push past the obvious conclusion from first glance at the text to see other possible *readings* of a text. Necessarily, this will involve multiple readings, something many students are not accustomed to doing.

Inference requires the reader to hold multiple bits of information from text in memory for various kinds of manipulation. The means to improving memory for text is through exposure to long sequences of text. Much of inference concerns relationships between portions of text, for example, issues of cause and effect, analysis of components, and implications of sequences. For this reason, a cornerstone of learning to infer is experience with efficient and comprehensible processing of textual information. The answer to both memory and text experience is students being read to by skilled readers. Listening to (watching) someone read eliminates the obstacles of print processing while providing the benefits of exposure to print structures and language. It is a valid instructional enterprise that should continue throughout the schooling of students who are deaf (and probably hearing students). The students' focus can then be entirely upon comprehension and thinking about text content.

To encourage the kinds of cognitive and linguistic flexibility and analysis that facilitate inferencing, students need much practice with examination and manipulation of text components. Interpretation is a multidimensional enterprise. Practice with interpreting pictures and picture sequences is a good place to start with young children even before they can read. Matching pictures with appropriate language is a variation on this approach. Students can create stories for pictures or sequences. Later when students are working with text, they can perform similar tasks, some of which require more analysis. Examples include matching main ideas to paragraphs or adding information to a story (e.g. character, scene) that would be consonant with elements already included, even providing a different title or ending.

Students can be provided with specific training in question-answer relationships (see review in Chapter 2) that will help them to identify certain kinds of information in the text. Such practice can be applied to discussions of the main idea or to summarizing text and other exercises in which they are able to identify specific text information that supports their answers.

A more nebulous aspect of inference is what can be labeled as subjective inference. This aspect refers to the interpretations, conclusions, hypotheses, analyses, and so on, that use as their data base the personal knowledge and experience of the reader. The text is the springboard for meaning, but the final resolution depends heavily upon variables in the reader's background.

Consider the following example. The text reads: *This birthday was one to remember.* There are few readers for whom this sentence will awaken no significant memory. The example is purposely vivid to demonstrate how text activates expectations in a reader, which influences further reactions to the text that follows. If there are good past birthday experiences, the reader should infer that positive things are about to happen when the next sentence reads: *All her life she had wished for a surprise party.* If there are bad past birthday experiences, the reader might find the second sentence a prelude to impending disaster. When the final sentence reads, *All things considered, it was not a bad party!,* two readers might have very different opinions regarding the interpretation of that evaluation. The differences will not have arisen in the text, itself, but within the readers.

To help students understand and deal with the concept and process of inference, they must have certain kinds of experiences as well as the language to discuss them. They need a variety of cause-effect experiences that range from physical and observable to social and private. Both types must be probed for the reactions they stimulate in the student. Students who are deaf miss much vicarious exposure to life events. Hearing children grow up overhearing life; they share Aunt Gertrude's terror of driving on the freeway or the neighbor's grief over a lost ring. Without effort, they discover the commonalties among human experience as well as the realization that not everyone thinks as they do about everything. It is a frustrating, and in many respects, unnoticed outcome of deafness that the student frequently does not know himself (through the reflection of others) as hearing students may.

Readers who are deaf need direct practice in being walked through events and their explicit and implicit ramifications. When confronted by an event in text, teachers can supply inferential probes. *Has something like that ever happened to you? How did you feel? What did you do about it? What happened as a result?* With students who are deaf it is important to probe even further to demonstrate that effects are long-lasting and cumulative and may be distorted with time, for example, *How do you feel about it now? What have you learned from your experience?*

Many deaf students approach text events without information critical to the inferencing task (e.g., see reviews in McAnally et al., 1994; Paul & Quigley, 1994a; see also Chapter 3): (1) they are missing data about the unseen aspects of an event or character, and (2) they are missing the vocabulary and interpretative language necessary to analyze, categorize, and express inferential responses—to make inferences about feelings, motives, rationales, and potential reactions. Teachers can use non-threatening and impersonal experiences with books to provide this personal-social-linguistic facility to students who are deaf.

Each of these areas has been referred to in this chapter with respect to teacher or parent behavior in relation to providing preparation or instruction for reading/writing. However, strategies for accomplishing these objectives can be addressed specifically in the literacy curriculum for students who are deaf. Instructional planning should include opportunities for guided practice in using the techniques and for purposes of individualizing the details to suit the reader's age and personal style (see discussions in Luetke-Stahlman & Luckner, 1991; McAnally et al., 1994).

Comprehension is commonly thought of as the outcome of some experience, whether real events or text. Much reading time and effort is expended measuring students' comprehension of what they have read. Unfortunately, comparatively little time is spent teaching students how to comprehend. A number of straightforward techniques and resources can be provided to students that will enable them to improve their comprehension with each piece of text they read.

Learning to Comprehend: The Use of Predictable Books

At the same time as children acquire skills and facility with the elements and processes of decoding, they need to encounter words, grammatical structures, morphographs, and so on, in connected text. Working with words in context is easier than in isolation and presents the reader with realistic trial-and-error practice. Unfortunately, the texts of many basal reading series and some children's literature do not reflect the global process that is contextual reading. Typical reading series, which focus upon phonic approaches to decoding, are designed to create cumulative structured practice in identifying phonetic units. These texts frequently utilize rhyming or alliterative mechanisms to highlight specific sounds or combinations. With a need to control vocabulary, the contrived content of such texts often becomes very unnatural, resulting in reading that is devoid of meaningfulness. Under these circumstances, reading can be boring, or worse, confusing. Problems arise when a novice reader attempts to derive a sense of story from text that is not focused on story-like construction and that has no purposeful context. By removing decoding from meaningful context, such texts actually undermine the acquisition of many text-based and extra-text inferencing skills, which a proficient reader needs to learn to use. Novice readers who are deaf, who make use of phonics information with great effort, require early reading experiences that highlight and begin to integrate the variety of higher-level information sources available to assist a reader in decoding any piece of text. *Predictable* books afford such opportunities for novice readers.

Predictable books reflect the fundamental notion that the task of decoding any unit in text (i.e., word, phrase) is made easier if the number of possible alternatives is reduced. This is accomplished by using other information in the text to make a good guess about the unidentified unit; a reader then needs only to make the orthographic comparisons necessary to determine whether the actual print represents the expected word. If a correct guess has been made, then many other orthographic comparisons (i.e., of the word in the text to other irrelevant possibilities) are eliminated. In this way, prediction saves considerable processing time, which can then be devoted to higher-level aspects of comprehension.

Predictable books utilize a number of different devices or patterns to guide a reader to correctly identify words in the text. These include sound (rhyme), repetitive phrasing, use of the same content elements, syntactic structure ("and then the mama bear said . . ."), cumulative sequences, use of multiple items from a conceptual category, sequence (parts of the body, times of day), and common cultural patterns (alphabet, numbers, songs). Generous, but careful, use of pictures or accompanying graphics also enhances the predictability of the printed words. Table 7-5 contains examples of text devices that enhance prediction

TABLE 7-5 Predictable book patterns and examples

Patterned Sound (rhyme or repetition)
- *Is Your Mama a Llama?* Deborah Guarino
- *Goodnight Moon* Margaret Wise Brown
- *More Spaghetti, I say!* Rita Golden Gelman

Patterned Phrasing (exact repetition of word or phrase)
- *I Was So Mad* Mercer Mayer
- *Three Billy-Goats Gruff* Illustrator: Ellen Appleby
- *Who Spilled the Milk?* Harriet Ziefert

Patterned Syntax (repeated structure, e.g., prepositional phrases or structural arrangement; question-answer)
- *In a Dark, Dark Wood* June Melser and Joy Cowley
- *If You Give a Mouse a Cookie* Laura Joffe Numeroff
- *Cookie's Week* Cindy Ward

Plot Pattern (repeated plot elements, e.g., actions-consequences)
- *Once a Mouse . . .* Marcia Brown
- *Alexander and the Terrible, Horrible, No Good, Very Bad Day* Judith Viorst
- *The Big Red Blanket* Harriet Ziefert
- *Can I Keep Him?* Steven Kellogg

Category Pattern (vocabulary related within a conceptual category)
- *Mud* Wendy Cheyette Lewison
- *A House Is a House For Me* Mary Ann Hoberman
- *Too Many Balloons* Catherine Matthias

Sequence Pattern (temporal or event)
- *Love You Forever* Robert Munsch
- *The Ball Game* David Packard
- *The Very Hungry Caterpillar* Eric Carle

Cultural Pattern (familiar verbal routines, e.g., numbers, alphabet, holiday expressions)
- *Move Over* Harriet Ziefert
- *Q Is for Duck* Mary Elting and Michael Folsom
- *Six Creepy Sheep* Judith Ross Enderle and Stephanie Gordon Tessler

Cumulative Pattern (a verbal string is developed by repetition with addition)
- *Buzz Said the Bee* Wendy Cheyette Lewison
- *The Little Old Lady Who Was Not Afraid of Anything* Linda Williams
- *There Was an Old Lady Who Swallowed a Fly* Illustrator: Pam Adams

Note: References for the picture books.

Brown, M. (1947). *Goodnight Moon.* Harper & Row.
Brown, M. (1961). *Once a Mouse . . .* New York: Macmillan.
Carle, E. (1987). *The Very Hungry Caterpillar.* New York: Scholastic.
Elting, M., & Folsom, M. (1980). *Q Is for Duck.* New York: Clarion Books.
Enderle, J., & Tessler, S. (1992). *Six Creepy Sheep.* New York: Puffin Books.
Gelman, R. (1977). *More Spaghetti, I Say!* New York: Scholastic.
Guarino, D. (1989). *Is Your Mama a Llama?* New York: Scholastic.
Hoberman, M. (1978). *A House Is a House for Me.* New York: The Viking Press.
Kellogg, S. (1971). *Can I Keep Him?* New York: Dial Books for Young Readers.
Lewison, W. (1990). *Mud.* New York: Random House.
Lewison, W. (1992). *Buzz Said the Bee.* New York: Scholastic.
Matthias, C. (1982). *Too Many Balloons.* Regensteiner Publishing Enterprises.
Mayer, M. (1983). *I Was So Mad.* Wisconsin: Western Publishing Company.
Melser, J., & Cowley, J. (1980). *In a Dark, Dark Wood.* Shortland Publications Limited.
Munsch, R. (1986). *Love You Forever.* Ontario, Canada: Firefly Books.
Numeroff, L. (1985). *If You Give a Mouse a Cookie.* New York: Scholastic.
Packard, D. (1973). *There Was and Old Lady Who Swallowed a Fly.* Child's Play (International) Ltd.
Packard, D. (1984). *The Three Billy-Goats Gruff.* New York: Scholastic.
Packard, D. (1993). *The Ball Game.* New York: Scholastic.
Viorst, J. (1972). *Alexander and the Terrible, Horrible, No Good, Very Bad Day.* New York: Scholastic.
Ward, C. (1988). *Cookie's Week.* New York: G.P. Putnam's Sons.
Williams, L. (1986). *The Little Old Lady Who Was Not Afraid of Anything.* New York: Harper Trophy.
Ziefert, H. (1991). *Move Over.* New York: HarperCollins.
Ziefert, H. (1992). *The Big, Red Blanket.* New York: HarperCollins.
Ziefert, H. (1992). *Who Spilled the Milk?* New York: HarperCollins.

Note: Additional references for picture books and other types of books can be found in Appendix B.

and also provides titles of children's books that utilize each type of device. Some predictable books employ only one device, some use multiple cues simultaneously.

For younger students, instruction with predictable books may involve only how to search out, recognize, and employ the various kinds of device(s) used in such texts. The principle objective here is an introduction to how contextual decoding works, how clues to meaning are to be found in other places beyond the letters of the word being decoded. Older students may be provided with instruction aimed at analyzing these text devices, in order to understand why they are so effective. This analysis would further students' conceptualization of the discourse, syntactic, semantic, and inferential aspects of text as well as how relationships among these impact successful comprehension. Examples of various kinds of predictable books can be used in conjunction with the context analysis instruction mentioned previously.

A second, but no less important, reason for using predictable books in beginning reading is to guarantee the novice reader who is deaf success in his or her early attempts to read. Precisely because they make decoding the words easier, predictable books should be a basic text source during the process of *learning* to comprehend (as opposed to using already mastered comprehension skills).

In the early phase, once a text has been selected for students to read, the teacher may want to begin by reading the book to the students. A single reading can provide opportunities for the student to exercise emerging analytical skills while not providing sufficient exposure to make the decoding process any less valid. Each word in the text still will be encountered as an unknown entity. The teacher can utilize this presentation to highlight important aspects of the particular book. Phrasing, pauses, and exaggeration in sign and voice can be used to highlight the particular predictable features of the book, for example, the patterned language or syntactic devices. If the teacher has preceded this reading with semantic mapping instruction regarding categories or sequencing, the patterns will be much more salient for the listener/reader.

The heart of early reading comprehension instruction for students who are deaf must be individualization. Consideration must be given to the background, the ability, linguistic skills, and learning characteristics of each learner. Only with closely guided instruction can the teacher maximize the specificity of his or her responses to the nature of a child's attempts and direct application of the student's previous learning and experience to contextual reading. Two procedures will be especially useful in conducting individualized reading sessions: the Request Procedure and Miscue Analysis.

Request Procedure

This procedure, developed by Manzo (1969), utilizes reciprocal reading to develop students' comprehension skills. It was designed to provide students with models of good text-based questions by the teacher as well as with opportunities to formulate and receive feedback about their own questions. The procedure involves the teacher and student moving through a text, one passage at a time, while alternating roles as reader and questioner. For example, the teacher might read one sentence, and the student would have a turn to ask questions about what the teacher read. For the next sentence the roles would be reversed.

In addition to answering the student's questions, the teacher also can offer feedback on the nature and adequacy of the questions themselves—the form and clarity of the question, the logic behind asking a particular question, the likelihood of a particular question eliciting the information the student desires, and so on. During the teacher's turn as questioner, there is an opportunity to model correct form for questions a student has not yet mastered as well as to introduce new question forms or to demonstrate how variety in questioning can improve the breadth and quality of information the reader obtains. As the Request Procedure was originally designed, once a student evidences comprehension of the text and knowledge of what to expect in the remaining text, he or she can be directed to complete the reading silently. This would be followed by summary comprehension assessment.

It should be apparent that, if well planned and executed, this form of reciprocal reading procedure can offer instruction for many skills that positively affect comprehension. Not only can the teacher improve comprehension of the text at hand but also can begin to develop students' metacognitive skills that apply to reading more generally. By walking the student through the comprehension process, the teacher can demonstrate the purposes and concepts of organizing information while reading, monitoring ongoing comprehension, and predicting subsequent content in the text.

There are many possible variations on this procedure. Alterations may be necessitated by the age or ability of the students, as a means to offer variety or to arrange the instructional context to accomplish specific objectives. Teachers can vary the length of the passage read before changing roles, vary the numbers of questions permitted per turn, or vary the number of students in the reading group. In the beginning, or with very young readers, a teacher may want to help students develop a set of starter questions from which to choose. In this way, each reader has material from which to create a plan and can experience satisfaction as a questioner during the early stages of learning how to comprehend.

Miscue Analysis

To develop appropriate reading instruction, teachers must know what strategies a student is using when confronted with new text. As a means of assessing an individual student's strengths, weaknesses, or habits while decoding text, teachers can use a process called miscue analysis (see discussions in Goodman, 1976, 1985; see also examples in King & Quigley, 1985, and McCormick, 1987). This is a system for noting both the frequency and types of errors students make while reading. The errors are illustrative in that they reveal the way in which the child approaches unfamiliar text. Does the student decode letter by letter regardless of context? If so, misread words are likely to be similar in form to the actual text (e.g. *ben* for *den*). Does the student take a guess at a word that fits the meaning of the sentence? If so, the erroneous attempts will likely fit the same part of speech and conceptual category as the target word but may not even start with the correct first letter. Because the teacher can then compare the strategies the child is using with ones that would be more successful in context, the results of miscue analysis are useful for instituting specific corrective measures. Miscue analysis will also help to discover strategies the reader may not understand how to use so that supplemental instruction (perhaps group instruction) can be planned.

Formal miscue analysis can be conducted with recorded student readings, and the results plotted as a means to record reading progress. However, over time a teacher can become so familiar with the system that it can be used on the spot as a guide for the teacher while reading with an individual child. Miscue analysis is considered a teacher's evaluation tool, but there is no reason it also cannot be an instructional tool. With more advanced readers, teacher and student can join to evaluate a sample of the student's reading performance, discuss alternative strategies, and formulate appropriate practice assignments.

The design and conduct of early reading instruction is important not only for the specific skills that may be developed, but also for the patterns of text behavior it helps to develop in the new reader. Habits of reading letter by letter or of rereading to assure the correctness of every word will impede a reader's progress and, if uncorrected, negatively affect achievement and reading enjoyment for a lifetime. A general text strategy (actually, metacognitive strategies; see Mason & Au, 1986) to encourage novice readers who are deaf might be the following:

- Turn the page.
- Look at the pictures or graphics.
- Attempt to read the text.
- When faced with an unfamiliar word, ignore it or make a guess based on context information and the first letter of the word.
- Keep going and see if the text makes sense (if so, continue reading).
- If the text no longer makes sense, reread the questionable section using more deliberate, analytical strategies.

More on Comprehension Activities

In this section are guidelines for constructing additional, more advanced comprehension activities and for developing comprehension questions. Examples of the activities are related to two contrived stories, for example, *Bats* and *The Birth of the Universe*. The guidelines can be used with any story, most especially if the teacher decides to use trade books or children's literature.

The first issue for the teacher to decide is how to measure comprehension. The major choices are the use of questions or the use of retelling techniques (e.g., see discussion in Mason & Au, 1986; Pearson & Johnson, 1978). With respect to questions, the teacher can generate a set of prior knowledge questions that can be asked prior to and after the story selection. Two broad types of prior knowledge questions are passage-specific and topic-specific. Passage-specific questions are those that can be answered by reading the story; typically, these are text-explicit (i.e., literal) and text-implicit (i.e., inferential) questions (see examples in the ensuing paragraphs). Topic-specific questions focus on certain topics and are not answered by the information in the story. Other questions require the students to relate information from the passage to their own experiences. For example, in the story on bats, a passage-specific question that can be answered by the information in the story is: Are bats large or small? In the story, there is a discussion of both large and small bats. A topic-specific question might be: What other animals are mammals like bats? or How do people feel about bats? The answers to these questions are not in this story about bats.

After asking the questions, either the teacher or the students can provide answers both verbally (speech and/or sign) and written (this, of course, depends on the skills of the students). After the selection has been read, the questions can be discussed again. It should be noted that the answers (guesses) to passage-specific questions can be rechecked after the selection has been read. It is important to follow with another similar story on the same topic or a nearly similar topic. This provides experience with cumulative background building and utilization.

It is also important to assess children's reasoning and critical thinking skills. They can be required to explain information from the story, evaluate the information, or justify their answers to the comprehension questions (after reading or listening to the story selection). As stated previously, the teacher will need to decide when to begin the end-of-reading questions, that is, after one paragraph, one page, or the whole story.

There are several methods to use in asking comprehension questions, for example, retelling, short-answer or fill-in-the-blank, sentence verification, true-false, and multiple choice. Though these formats may be familiar, we would like to highlight some of them.

Retelling is one of the most interesting techniques, and most educators are probably not aware that this is a high-level metacognitive activity (e.g., see discussion in Mason & Au, 1986; Pearson & Fielding, 1991; Pearson & Johnson, 1978). In fact, all question-answering activities involve the use of metacognitive skills (see discussion of metacognition in Chapter 2). In retelling, children are asked to write or tell what they remember after reading a text selection. This activity is performed with no look back or rereading (i.e., books are closed). What children relay provides information about their organization of stored information. In addition, it tells teachers what they (children) thought was important, and it suggests how they interpreted it. This activity is useful for evaluating children's understanding of the whole story or of specific parts of the story. The teacher might determine whether children are paying attention to the sequence of information or are able to pick out initiating events and resolutions in narratives or the important ideas in an expository story. If the teacher wants the children to focus on certain aspects in the retelling activity, she or he needs to construct guiding questions.

Another interesting activity that can be attempted is sentence verification (or true/false or yes/maybe/no). For this task, the teacher can list a set of sentences—some taken directly from the story, some changed a little, and some unrelated to the story—and ask students to circle those they think will appear (prior to reading) or appeared (after reading) in the story. The following examples pertain to a story about *Blue Jeans*. After students give their answers, the teacher and students should engage in a discussion on why each answer was given. Answers may vary from student to student, depending on their background knowledge. The answers to these questions can be discussed again after the students have read the story.

Blue Jeans

Today you are going to read a story like the stories you read at school. This story is about Levi, the man who invented blue jeans in 1849. Think about what life was like during the gold rush of California in the 1850s and how blue jeans were made. Think about why gold miners and other people needed strong pants like blue jeans.

Below are several ideas. For each idea, decide whether or not you might find it in the story. Circle the best answer. Your choices are:

Yes   =   *The idea would be in this story.*
Maybe =   *The idea might be in this story.*
No   =   *The idea would not be in this story.*

1. Gold was discovered in California.   Yes   Maybe   No.
2. People traveled to California in the 1850s by bus.   Yes   Maybe   No.
3. Levi was a miner.   Yes   Maybe   No.
4. Levi went to Kmart to find material for his jeans.   Yes   Maybe   No.
5. This story happened in France.   Yes   Maybe   No.
6. Gold miners used their pockets to hold gold.   Yes   Maybe   No.
7. Gold miners liked blue jeans because they needed
strong pants.   Yes   Maybe   No.
8. People who went to California to find gold decided to
stay there.   Yes   Maybe   No.
9. Levi put rivets on the pockets of the blue jeans so that
the pockets would be stronger.   Yes   Maybe   No.
10. Levi became famous because he invented socks.   Yes   Maybe   No.

As another example, consider the construction of prereading questions for an expository story entitled *Bats*.

Bats—Prereading Questions

1. This is a story about animals called bats. Have you ever seen a live bat? A picture of a bat? Tell me about it. What do you think this story will tell us?
2. Tell me what you know about bats. What do they look like? Are they big or small or both? Are bats different from birds? Why or why not? Are bats similar to birds? Why or why not?
3. What is a mammal? Are bats mammals? How do you know that? What other animals are mammals? What is a reptile? An amphibian? How are mammals different from reptiles? How are mammals and reptiles similar? Compare mammals and amphibians. Tell me about the differences. The similarities.
4. What do bats do during the day? At night?
5. Where do bats live? Why do they live in these places?
6. Do bats fly in the dark? How do bats fly in the dark? Do bats fly during the daytime? How do they do that?
7. What do bats eat? How do bats catch their food?
8. How do people feel about bats? Why? How do you feel about bats? Are bats dangerous? How do you know that?

If students are reading a narrative story, the prereading questions might be different. Suppose students are to read a story about Jill, a 15-year-old girl whose parents are going away for a weekend. Jill can stay in the house but must check in with the neighbors next door. As part of a deal for staying home, Jill's parents have given her chores to do. Here are some sample questions and directions for the teacher.

Jill and the Weekend

1. Select several major ideas or points concerning the protagonist's situations or actions.
2. Ask students a set of questions that could be related to their background experiences.
   a. What are chores?
   b. Do you like to do chores? Why or why not?
   c. Why is it important to do chores?
   d. Have your parents ever given you chores that you did not like to do? Name some of them. What did you do?
3. Ask the students: If you had a choice between going to the movies or mowing the lawn, what would you do? Why? Is it possible to do both actions?
4. Jill, the main character in our story, is home alone for the weekend. She is being watched by her neighbors. Jill did not want to go on a trip with her parents. Her parents agreed to let Jill stay home, providing she completed chores around the house. Do you think Jill will do her chores? Why or why not? What do you think will happen in this story?
5. Ask the students: What would Jill's parents say or do if she decides not to any chores? Do you think Jill's parents will let her stay home alone again?
6. After students read the story, have them compare their own predictions about Jill's actions with the actual outcomes of the story. As a creative bent, the students can suggest changes in the story and create a different ending.

Question-Answer Relationships (QARs)

The three levels of question-answer relationships with examples were described in Chapter 2. Following the story *Bats* are five questions that have been answered and labeled to define the question-answer relationship.

Bats

This is a story about bats. We will learn how bats fly, hunt for food, and sleep. Bats look like birds; however, bats are different from birds. Birds have feathers on their bodies. Bats have fur on their bodies, not feathers. Their wings and tails are made of skin, which is leathery and stretched across thin bones.

Bats are different from birds in other ways. Bats do not lay eggs, as birds do. Baby bats are born alive. In this way, baby bats are like baby kittens. Mother bats nurse their babies with their own milk. That is why bats, like mice, cats, cows, and people, are called mammals. Of all mammals, bats are the only ones that can truly fly.

Most small bats are awake at night. They sleep during the day. Just about the time the sun goes down, they wake up and flutter around their roosting places. These places may be in old houses and caves or in other dark places. At night, they fly out to hunt for food. At daybreak, they return.

Sample Postreading Questions: QARs

1. Bats have fur on their bodies not _____.
   a. wings   b. tails
   c. feathers   d. skin
   Answer is *c* ; the QAR is labeled text-explicit.

2. Which animals are mammals?

   a. cats   **b.** bats

   c. cows   **d.** butterflies

Answers are *a, b,* and *c;* the QAR is labeled script-implicit.

3. What do bats do at daybreak?

   a. eat insects   **b.** return to their roosting places

   c. hunt for food **d.** lay eggs

Answer is *b;* the QAR is labeled text-implicit.

4. Mother bats have babies in the same way as mother _____.

   a. ducks   **b.** birds

   c. cats   **d.** frogs

Answer is *c;* the QAR is labeled script-implicit.

5. Bats are in a special class of animals. Other animals in this class could be

  a _____.

   a. cow   **b.** turtle

   c. bird   **d.** horse

Answers are *a* and *d;* the QAR is labeled script-implicit.

Consider the following story for another activity involving QARs. This time, we will let you provide the answers and the QAR labels!

Birth of the Universe

Prior to the 1960s, the thinking of cosmologists on the creation of the universe was heavily influenced by a theory called steady state. Succinctly put, steady-state theorists argued that this world has no beginning and no end. Because matter is neither created nor destroyed, the universe will go on forever and ever. Philosophically, this notion appealed to the atheists, but it was despised somewhat by the theologians. The joy of the atheists, however, was short-lived.

Evidence collected during the late 1960s and early 1970s suggested that the universe came into being with a big bang. Some big bang theorists argued that the universe had a beginning and will come to an end as a result of its expansion. The theologians interpreted this as evidence for Judgment Day, whereas the atheists simply ignored this view. The cosmologists labeled it the open-universe big bang theory.

Although the open-universe theory is in vogue, some theorists argued that it is still possible for the world to fall back upon itself, producing a big crunch. This view is known as the close-universe big bang theory. This idea still makes the theologians happy and the atheists uncomfortable. The opposite would be true if there is enough evidence for an oscillating-universe big bang theory. In this view, the universe is said to begin with a big bang, end with a big crunch, and then begin all over again with another big bang. All knowledge of the previous universe disappears with each big bang.

Future theorists might construct yet another theory regarding the beginning and end of the universe. In fact, there is an argument for a theory in an area called plasma cosmology. In some respects, this theory is similar to the steady-state idea. Specifically, some plasma cosmologists believe that the universe has no beginning and might have no ending. Soon, the theologians and the atheists will be arguing again. In addition, big bang proponents will argue with plasma cosmologists. The big bang theorists insist that no informed person can dispute the fact that the universe began with a big bang. The problem is how the universe will end. Although some plasma cosmologists disagree, they admit that much of the available evidence still favors an open universe.

So, on and on it goes. Atheists versus theologians. Philosophers versus scientists. Open universe versus close universe. Big bang versus plasma cosmology. At one point, nearly everyone agreed that the steady-state theory was dead.

How do you feel about all this? Perhaps you feel the same way that Walt Whitman felt:

When I heard the learned astronomer,
When the proofs, the figures, were ranged in columns before me,
When I was shown the charts and diagrams, to add, divide, and measure
them,
When I sitting heard the astronomer where he lectured with much applause
in the lecture room.
How soon unaccountable, I became tired and sick,
Till rising and gliding out I wander'd off by myself,
In the mythical moist night air, and from time to time,
Look'd up in perfect silence at the stars.   (Whitman, 1980, p. 226)

Label the following questions as TE (text-explicit), TI (text-implicit), or SI (script-implicit).

1. Why do atheists and theologians argue?
2. Prior to the 1960s, the thinking of cosmologists on the creation of the universe was heavily influenced by a theory called _____.
3. The steady-state theory appealed to the atheists. True or false?
4. What do cosmologists do?
5. What are the names of the three big bang theories?
6. How do atheists feel about the concept of God?
7. Which big bang theory is in vogue?
8. Are theologians happy with the oscillating big bang theory?
9. Would agnostics like the steady-state theory?
10. If plasma cosmology is similar to steady state, would atheists like the theory?
11. Which of the theories do you think Walt Whitman would have agreed with?

Another challenging, postreading activity is as follows. The story is about a prolific inventor named Garret Morgan. The teacher should read the directions to the students and ensure that they understand them.

Directions: Read the first and second paragraphs on page X (a specific page of the story). For each of the following questions, check YES if the answer is in these paragraphs. Check NO if the answer is not in these paragraphs. If you checked YES, find the answer and underline it in the paragraph.

1. What did Garrett start?   YES ___   NO ___
2. A car and a _____ had crashed into each other.   YES ___   NO ___
3. Who searched for an answer to stopping the smoke and
   gas and still letting a person breathe?   YES ___   NO ___

4. Garrett's answer to saving fire fighters was
the _____.   YES ___   NO ___
5. Garrett Morgan's safety hood helped fire fighters.   YES ___   NO ___
6. Garrett Morgan's safety hood covered a fire
fighter's _____.   YES ___   NO ___

Whatever format is chosen for comprehension practice, a fundamental goal must always be to enhance the learning of comprehension skills, not just the answers to today's questions. Teachers should remember that students can learn as much from errors as from correct answers. With appropriate feedback and with guided discussion, students can be led to acquire a process as well as the content.

Metacognitive Activities

Metacognition was discussed in Chapter 2. Some of the metacognitive activities that seem to be important for reading are (1) clarifying the purpose for reading, (2) identifying the important components or ideas in a message or story, (3) self-checking to see if learning or comprehension is occurring, and (4) using productive strategies when a comprehension failure or breakdown occurs (e.g., see discussion in Mason & Au, 1986). Appropriate strategies, ranging from least to most disruptive of overall comprehension are (1) ignore the problem and continue to read, (2) put off a judgment temporarily, (3) make a guess using the information from the story, (4) reread parts, starting with the sentence, previous paragraph, previous page, and so on, and (5) go to a reliable source for assistance.

There are a number of instructional activities that can be constructed by the imaginative teacher to develop metacognitive skills and habits. Here is the Bat story again, followed by sample exercises.

Bats

This is a story about bats. We will learn how bats fly, hunt for food, and sleep. Bats look like birds; however, bats are different from birds. Birds have feathers on their bodies. Bats have fur on their bodies, not feathers. Their wings and tails are made of skin, which is leathery and stretched across thin bones.

Bats are different from birds in other ways. Bats do not lay eggs, as birds do. Baby bats are born alive. In this way, baby bats are like baby kittens. Mother bats nurse their babies with their own milk. That is why bats, like mice, cats, cows, and people, are called mammals. Of all mammals, bats are the only ones that can truly fly.

Most small bats are awake at night. They sleep during the day. Just about the time the sun goes down, they wake up and flutter around their roosting places. These places may be in old houses and caves or in other dark places. At night, they fly out to hunt for food. At daybreak, they return.

Activity 1

Say to the student; You have just read a story about bats, but your friends have not read it yet. Imagine that you want to tell them what the story is mainly about. There are two choices for student responses.

A. You have one minute to tell your friend what this story is mainly about.

B. You must tell what this story is about in 25 words or less.

For the next variation, students are required to select the best response.

C. This story is mainly about. . . .
   1. The different kinds of bats used in baseball games.
   2. The eating, hunting, and flying habits of different kinds of bats.
   3. The eating, hunting, and flying habits of different kinds of animals.

Another similar example: This story is mainly about.
   1. How bats are different from birds.
   2. Why bats are mammals like cats, cows, and people.
   3. What bats look like and how they hunt and fly.

If students are having difficulty with this activity for the whole story, variations that can be used are:

This page is mainly about . . .
This paragraph is mainly about . . .

   The purpose of this activity is to help students identify and evaluate the components or relationships in a passage. These basic activities can be followed with discussions of how one determines what is important. As another alternative, the teacher could have two students conduct the story sharing activity. Then, the class can evaluate which student had better comprehension of the passage and why.

   For some questions, students may say that they know the answers, even though the answers are not on the specified page or in the specified paragraphs. This can lend itself to a discussion of how they know this answer or how they got this information. The point, here, is that when we read, some information is in our heads, not on the page, and that it is a good idea to use information in your head to interpret text and to answer questions.

   Another similar metacognitive activity is as follows.

Activity 2

   You want to tell your friend what the story is mainly about. How much will it help to say to him or her that . . .

   1. It is about the eating, hunting, and flying habits of different kinds of bats.
      a. This will help a lot.
      b. This might help a little bit.
      c. This will not help at all.
   2. It is about the ways that bats are different from birds.
      a. This will help a lot.
      b. This might help a little bit.
      c. This will not help at all.
   3. It is about the way bats see in the dark.
      a. This will help a lot.
      b. This might help a little bit.
      c. This will not help at all.

Similar to the lessons on vocabulary variables, there are guidelines for the teacher to consider in the development of comprehension activities.

Comprehension Checklist

1. Have I written an adequate list of prereading questions that specifically focus on activating and enriching prior knowledge experiences?
2. Have I used a variety of formats to assess prior knowledge, for example, yes/no and *wh-* questions, true/false and sentence verification techniques, and others?
3. Have I written prediction-related questions?
4. Have I established a purpose for reading? Have I listed some major points or topics that I want the reader to pay attention to? Have I reminded the readers that I may ask questions about these topics after they read the story? Have I reminded the readers that I may ask them to retell the story, emphasizing some of the major points that we discussed earlier?
5. Have I written an adequate list of postreading (or guided reading) questions? Have I asked questions on three levels, that is, text explicit, text implicit, and script implicit? Have I asked questions related to the main idea, vocabulary, sequence, and evaluation or ones that require creative responses?
6. Have I used a variety of formats to assess comprehension of postreading (or guided reading) questions, for example, yes/no and *wh-*questions, true/false, sentence verification techniques, and others?
7. Do some of my postreading or guided reading questions relate to some of my prior knowledge and other prereading questions?
8. Have I developed additional metacognitive activities (i.e., in addition to developing comprehension questions).

Learning to Write: The Use of Journals

Earlier in this chapter, we discussed the school-home journal as a means for developing interactions with parents and fostering in young children who are deaf an idea of how print communication works. Later, as formal instruction in literacy begins, the journal concept can be refocused to engage students directly in written exchanges with the teacher.

Teacher-student dialogue journals have multiple advantages for instruction of writing with students who are deaf (see also the discussion in Albertini & Shannon, 1996). They are relatively simple to use, time effective, and adaptable to a variety of purposes. Importantly, they are also motivating for students; so, if for no other reason, they have positive effects on student literacy achievement (e.g., Luetke-Stahlman & Luckner, 1991; Tompkins, 1990).

Dialogue journals are a reciprocal writing activity, with the journal passing between student and teacher, preferably on a daily or every-other-day cycle. The journal itself can be of almost any style, but should be fairly sturdy so that the collection of writings will stay together throughout the school year. Students enjoy personalizing the journals by creating special covers, and so on. The dialogue process begins with the student writing on a topic of his or her choice, then returning the journal to the teacher for a response. The teacher reads the entry and provides a prompt response. Then, it is the student's turn again. The second student turn may continue the same topic by responding to the teacher's comments, but, especially in the beginning, student entries tend to be unrelated to previous ones.

There are ground rules for this conversation in writing. Foremost, students should be informed that, like any personal exchange, the journal will be considered private communication. Its contents will not be shared with others without their permission. Second, journal writing is a class requirement, but the topic of each entry will be student controlled. Students should be given three alternatives each day for writing journal entries: write on any topic of their choosing, write on a topic provided each day by the teacher, or spend the allocated time writing I do not choose to write today. (This last option is rarely selected and almost never for more than one day, even by the most reluctant writers). A teacher should plan to begin the journal as a standard part of classroom activities from the beginning of the school year. Initiating the procedure with the most positive writers and treating the journal as a *special* activity will motivate the remaining students.

The character of the teacher's response is critical to the success of the journal procedure. It affects both the quality and quantity of the students' entries. The teacher must respond to each student entry in the journal. It is very important that, in replying to the content of the entry, the teacher be careful never to correct the journal writing as in a language assignment (i.e., spelling, grammar, vocabulary usage, handwriting). It is true that the journal can be an excellent vehicle for identifying student writing problems. Yet, the teacher will address these needs or errors more effectively by finding instances in drafting the reply to model exactly the forms or vocabulary that the student omitted or misused in the preceding entry. For example, if a student, in referring to his brother's skiing accident wrote *My brother don't hurt hisself too bad,* the teacher could reply *I'm really glad that your brother didn't hurt himself too badly* (see more detailed examples in Gaustad & Messenheimer-Young, 1991).

It is also important for the teacher to model a variety of language and communication forms in creating journal responses. Two characteristics of good teacher entries are to be personal and to ask questions. Ritualized responses like *nice writing* or *that's interesting* are communication dead ends. Replying in a personal fashion and by relating the student's experience to similar ones the teacher may have experienced provide an avenue to reuse specific language for correction or modeling purposes. Further, it serves to validate or provide an alternative view for a student's observations, feelings, or problems. It can also be a stimulus for warmer, more open, and trusting relationships with students. Teachers can use creative writing snippets as a way to devise replies. If a student wrote *My favorite car is a Thunderbird.* the teacher could reply, *If someone asked me to design a new kind of car, this is what it would be like,* and continue with use of multifaceted descriptive characterizations (e.g., design, handling, etc.,) using a broad and varied vocabulary.

Effective teacher journals also prod students to think, question, and include more detail in their writing. In addition to carefully constructed content, the teacher should direct probes that sometimes may target information and sometimes the student's use of specific language forms. This can be accomplished by including explicit questions or requests for expansion on some aspect of a topic the student has mentioned. Requests can range from asking for omitted facts to soliciting opinions. Relaying to the student that an idea was miscommunicated initially should be followed by specific questions or guidelines that will enable the student to construct a successful reply. Over time, this strategy will instill a sensitivity to the needs of the reader and prompt constructive forethought about drafting clearer writing. With younger students, the teacher might simply rephrase the student's statement with *Did you mean _____?* Both modeling and questioning processes take time to result in noticeable changes in the student's writing. Frequent repetitions of question types on multiple occasions, with reference to varied topics, will probably be necessary before students attempt new strategies or begin asking questions themselves. With regard to the latter, students are far more likely to ask questions of a teacher who has established a pattern of offering personal detail or shared thinking during previous journal exchanges.

Although journals are not meant to be language lessons per se, they are useful for assessing a student's writing skills, evaluating progress, and planning instruction. When a teacher notes repeated difficulties with particular forms or vocabulary in a student's writing or the same problem in multiple students' journals, this information can be the springboard for constructing formal lessons that target linguistic competencies for which the students have shown a need or readiness.

Journal entries can also lead to instruction of different forms of writing outside the journal context. Beginning writers will find it easier to write about the here and now, about concrete things they can experience first hand, and about topics with which they are familiar. Writing must be a meaningful activity. Gradually, writing can move to topics distant in location or time, more abstract and objective. With encouragement and experience, students will also gain the confidence to move from largely descriptive writing to expository and creative endeavors. The necessary experience can come from the everyday exercises and feedback of journal writing.

Some Final Points on Writing Activities

Throughout this chapter, we have provided some examples of how reading and writing instruction can be connected. In this section, we would like to highlight briefly some additional aspects of the writing process. Our bias is that we favor the cognitive-interactive, composing model of Tierney and Pearson (1983) within a framework for providing a balance in dealing with both the lower-level and higher-levels skills of writing (e.g., see discussion in Tompkins, 1990).

This focus has several aspects. Firstly, as argued by Tierney and Pearson (1983), both reading and writing entail complex interactions between the student and the text from which the student is trying to construct a model of meaning. Readers construct a meaning model of existing texts whereas writers construct meaning by composing texts. In this sense, writing develops as a result of, and in tandem with, reading.

Secondly, in order for the reading and writing interaction to proceed smoothly, students need to have automatic, fluent lower-level (i.e. decoding/encoding) skills so that they can concentrate on the construction of meaning via the use of higher-level processes. In other words, teachers need to emphasize comprehension and other higher-level skills such as organization, intent, and audience along with meeting needs for lower-level skills such as grammar, spelling, and punctuation. Some educators would argue that grammar and spelling are not necessarily lower-level skills for students who are deaf (e.g., Paul & Quigley, 1990).

The third and final point to be made here is that the writing process can be conceptualized as consisting of five stages: planning or prewriting, drafting or composing, revising, editing, and sharing (e.g., Tierney & Pearson, 1983; Tompkins, 1990). The activities during the planning or prewriting stage are similar to those used during the prereading stage to facilitate meaningfulness and organization. For example, students need to select topics based on their experiences, identify their audience, establish their purpose for writing on this topic, and develop a plan or outline. The teacher might need to enrich and activate the prior knowledge of the students relative to their topics. This can be done by the use of probing questions or semantic elaboration techniques, as described in this chapter.

The second stage involves drafting or composing. In essence, the students produce a first draft, called a rough draft, of their paper. They should be able to use their outline or semantic map as a guideline for developing the main idea, introductory paragraph, supporting details, and so on. Teachers should provide supportive comments such as *This is a nice first draft. You have used almost all of the information on your outline or semantic map. Have you had any more ideas while you were writing? Do you want to add anything to the outline or your paper?* Students might wish to solicit some preliminary comments from their peers on this rough draft. In addition, students might ask for assistance with spelling, word choice, or other mechanics. Mechanics aside, the students' primary focus should be on the overall content of the paper.

During the revising stage, the writer becomes a very active reader. That is, students participate in the evaluation of their own composition as well as those of others in the class. During this stage, the students might attempt to alter, expand, and clarify their products based on the comments of the teacher and other students. The teacher might decide to assist the student with any problems that arose in use of the lower-level mechanics. It might be necessary to provide supplemental instruction in these troublesome areas. During this phase, both the teacher and student should be involved in individual conferences to discuss and evaluate the compositions.

In the editing stage, the students attempt to proofread their compositions and those of other students in the class. There should be an attempt to correct most, if not all, of the lower-level errors. Strictly speaking, the editing stage should not involve any major rewriting of sections of the paper. However, it is possible that students might want to engage in some substantive revisions. In this sense, they are returning to the revising stage or, as argued by Tierney and Pearson (1983), students can proceed back and forth between stages or perform the tasks in two or more stages in a concurrent fashion.

The final stage is considered the formal sharing stage. Here the students attempt to publish or display their work or share it with an audience for discussion purposes.

Given a process-oriented approach to writing, there are two additional parameters for writing instruction with students who are deaf: frequency and integration. We have emphasized the reciprocal nature of reading and writing. There is another level at which interrelationships may be developed and that occurs within the general curriculum. Reading and writing instruction need not and, probably should not, take place separately from other curriculum content. Integrated instruction is a matter of efficiency as well as transfer. Children can practice inference and metacognitive skills with material from content area texts just as well or perhaps more purposefully than with reading books. The various types of written productions are also well suited to the nature and topics of particular subject matter areas; for example, descriptive writing in conjunction with units on poetry or adjectives, expository writing in conjunction with investigation in science, and narrative writing in conjunction with history reports. Integrating literacy instruction across the curriculum makes the best use of student time and provides a sense of cohesiveness and interplay between widely divergent topics and skills.

A Final Word

The main intent of this chapter was to provide some general guidelines and discussion with regard to issues on instruction and first-language literacy. As much as possible, there was an attempt to provide instructional examples that could be related to the three broad literacy paradigms: cognitive information processing, naturalism, and social constructionism. However, the authors revealed that their bias was toward cognitive information-processing models, particularly interactive ones.

It was emphasized that the instructional activities should be viewed as guidelines. It is almost always necessary for the teacher to modify them in order to meet the individual needs of the students. This is an issue that will be reiterated in Chapter 8, and that chapter covers some basic principles of instruction and second-language literacy.

Much of what is known about instruction and literacy is based on theories and research on hearing students. It was argued that the bulk of this information is applicable to students who are deaf, mainly because of the assumption that the development of literacy is the same for both children and adolescents who are deaf and who are hearing. After presenting some basic information about the emerging literacy situation involving both the home and school, the rest of the chapter illustrated instructional exercises that addressed both lower-level and higher-level skills in reading and writing.

Further Readings

DECHANT, E. (1991). *Understanding and teaching reading: An interactive model.* Hillsdale, NJ: Erlbaum.

MAY, F. (1990). *Reading as communication: An interactive approach* (3rd ed.). Columbus, OH: Merrill.

PIKE, K., COMPAIN, R., & MUMPER, J. (1994). *New connections: An integrated approach to literacy.* New York: HarperCollins.

STRICKLAND, K. (1995). *Literacy not labels: Celebrating students' strengths through whole language.* Portsmouth, NH: Boynton/Cook.

VACCA, J., VACCA, R., & GOVE, M. (1991). *Reading and learning to read* (2nd ed.). New York: HarperCollins.

WISEMAN, D. (1992). *Learning to read with literature.* Boston, MA: Allyn & Bacon.

Chapter 8

Instruction and
Second-Language Literacy

PETER V. PAUL
The Ohio State University

MARTHA G. GAUSTAD
Bowling Green State University

It has become apparent that children from minority-language groups differ greatly in their English ability, and a number of educators have advocated programs that are more tailored to the needs of individuals. In fact, emphasis on what is called "Individualized Instruction" dates back to the 1970s, when experience with the audio-lingual method in FLES classrooms taught educators that children learned at different rates and were receptive to different methods. Many children lacked the skills to sustain themselves for long periods without adult support and assistance, although others had no difficulty in doing so. Furthermore, children reacted differently to the teacher: some children responded to praise, others to embarrassment; some needed encouragement, others needed to be left alone. Teachers have to know the students well on a personal basis. They can then adjust their goals somewhat more realistically to student needs, interests, and capabilities (McLaughlin, 1985, p. 113).

There is no doubt that developments in ESL composition have been influenced by and, to a certain extent, are parallel to developments in the teaching of writing to native speakers of English. However, the unique context of ESL composition has necessitated somewhat distinct perspectives, models, and practices (Silva, 1990, p. 11).

The above quotes are interesting for a number of reasons, some of which will become clear throughout this chapter. The need for individualized instruction is one of the major tenets for teaching children with special needs in traditional special-education programs. Because of differential experiences, learning styles, and learning rates of second-language learners, this has also become an important need for children in bilingual and second-language programs. As discussed in the previous chapter, the best that can be done here is to provide guidelines for the development of instructional activities in bilingual or second-language learning situations. Most of these guidelines are similar to those that have been presented for students learning literacy in English as a first language; a few depend on the unique situations of ESL (English as a second language) students (e.g., nature of the first language, age at which student begins program, and so on).

Chapter 6 provided the theoretical and research support for establishing bilingual and second-language learning programs for children and adolescents with severe to profound hearing impairment, especially those who know American Sign Language (ASL) as a first language. There was also a discussion of the most effective type of program, based on the research on typical hearing students. Because establishing bilingual/bicultural and second-language literacy programs is in its infancy for students who are deaf, there is not much research information available. Even more surprising is the fact that several programs have been implemented without much thought to the theoretical and research foundations for establishing them (see Paul & Quigley, 1994a; Paul & Quigley, 1994b). This is especially true for the manner in which some programs advocate the teaching of English literacy skills.

This chapter provides information on several methods and procedures that have been used, mostly with hearing second-language learners. There is some documentation for the use of methods with deaf second-language or bilingual learners. Some discussion in this area centers on the use of ASL or the use of certain features of ASL to teach English literacy skills. The reader should keep in mind that much of the information in Chapter 7 is also applicable to students with hearing impairment who are learning English as a second language and, also, for those students who have not learned English as a first language. This point has been underscored by numerous second-language theorists and researchers (e.g., Bernhardt, 1991; McLaughlin, 1987). As aptly stated by McLaughlin (1985, p. 113):

> ... the most important influence on second-language teaching has been research on first-language acquisition and the growing conviction of many educators that understanding the process of first-language learning has critical implications for second-language teaching.

According to Grabe (1988, 1991), second-language literacy has proceeded through stages that are somewhat similar to those of first-language literacy. For example, the audio-lingual approaches were influenced primarily by behaviorism and the notion that literacy can be subdivided into various components, similar to bottom-up approaches to reading. Goodman's psycholinguistic-transactional approach has had a tremendous impact on second-language learning and literacy, as exemplified by the work of Krashen (1981, 1982, 1985).

The inadequacies of the psycholinguistic approach paved the way for cognitive information-processing approaches, particularly interactive models (e.g., Bernhardt, 1991; Grabe, 1988) and social-cognitive models (e.g., Bernhardt, 1991). The field has also felt the impact of research on writing, especially reading-writing connections (e.g., Kroll, 1990; Raimes, 1983). As discussed for first-language literacy, there seems to be some consensus that both word identification and comprehension are important for the task of reading in ESL and that lower-level (e.g., mechanics) and higher-level (e.g., intent) skills are critical for writing in ESL. However, in a similar manner, there is continuing debate on the manner in which to develop second-language literacy.

Much of the attention on bilingual education and ESL for students who are deaf has been devoted to the establishment of ASL/English programs. This underemphasizes the need for bilingual programs for students who are both hearing-impaired/deaf and members of another language-minority group such as Spanish and German. In any case, much of the focus in this chapter is on instructional methods and procedures that can be used with ASL/English students who are deaf or students who are deaf and who are limited users of English. Additional topics to be covered are the selection of the students and teachers and instructional and curricular issues.

As discussed in Chapter 6, most second-language literacy models emphasize two broad points:

1. Initially, second-language students are dependent on their first-language skills, particularly their first-language literacy skills (e.g., see reviews in Bernhardt, 1991; Grabe, 1988; 1991). That is, second-language students use knowledge of their native language to make sense of the text. It is suspected that they even force their native phonological system upon the orthography of English. As they acquire communicative and grammatical proficiency in English, they tend to utilize the rule system of English, in part, to make sense of English text. This leads to the assumption that transfer skills are, in part, strategies based on the acquisition of the first-language literacy. In addition, first-language literacy skills might be of benefit in understanding and developing second-language literacy skills (e.g., see reviews in Bernhardt, 1991; Friedlander, 1990).

2. Eventually, there needs to be a reciprocal relationship between the conversational and written forms of the second language (e.g., see Brady & Shankweiler, 1991; Shankweiler & Liberman, 1989). This does not mean that second-language students have no need or do not rely on their native language, especially for mediation or clarification purposes. It does imply, however, that it is necessary to possess both bottom-up and top-down skills of literacy and to understand the alphabetic code, the code upon which the English written language system is based. Knowledge of the alphabetic code requires, at least, a good working knowledge of the morphophonological system of English. In other words, second-language readers/writers experience problems that are somewhat similar to those of poor first-language readers/writers of English. In addition, it can be implied that high-levels of English literacy are difficult to reach if students are dependent predominantly on the conversational mode of their native language in order to make sense of the phoneme-grapheme rule system of English.

A failure to consider these two points above might have contributed to the misinterpretation of prominent theories and models by several proponents and developers of ASL/English bilingual/bicultural programs (e.g., see Mayer & Wells, 1996). Part of the neglect might also be due to the fact that ASL-using students do not have access to a written component in their language. That is, a literate component, similar to reading and writing printed materials, does not exist or is not applicable to ASL. In this sense, it is difficult to discuss the application of skills in ASL to the learning of literacy skills in English as a second language.

Nevertheless, as demonstrated later, it is important to bank on the visual language processing of most students with severe to profound hearing impairment. As a visual-gestural language, ASL is most suited to instructional activities that emphasize certain visual aspects for demonstrating grammatical features of English. This approach can be used to teach English as a first or second language.

The use of ASL features notwithstanding, many of the suggestions in this chapter, although based on their use with hearing students, have been influenced by methods and strategies for teaching first-language students to read and write. This seems to support the notion, as suggested by McLaughlin (1984, 1985), that second-language learning is generally similar to first-language learning, especially when viewed from a cognitive developmental perspective. Again, these general *similarities* should be considered as guidelines in developing and implementing instructional methods and materials. It is still necessary to modify and adapt these activities (i.e., individualize them) based on the teacher-student interactions in classroom settings.

Selection of Students and Teachers

One of the most controversial issues in the establishment of bilingual and second-language programs is the selection of the students and teachers. Who should participate? Assuming that such programs are acceptable to the parents and community, a strong case can be made for students with hearing impairment who reside in homes in which English is not the first language or culture.

In the field of deafness, there seems to be a line of thinking that all students who are deaf (from moderate to profound levels of hearing impairment) should be placed in bilingual and second-language programs, especially ASL/English programs (e.g., see discussions in Johnson, Liddell, & Erting, 1989; Paul, 1991; Paul & Quigley, 1994a; see also the point of view in Lane et al., 1996). Basically, there are two strong arguments for such an assertion, both of which were mentioned briefly in Chapter 6. One argument centers on the notion of a first language. It is remarked that most students who are deaf and who begin formal schooling with a proficiency in a language are most likely to know ASL. These students are equipped with well-developed cognitive and linguistic foundations and are ready to engage in the academic language of school. It is also implied that using or teaching English as a first language is not beneficial for the overwhelming majority of students who are deaf. It is averred that most of these students will eventually become members of the Deaf culture in which ASL is the major means of communication.

The second argument revolves around the use of negative data. That is, it is reasoned that ASL should be the first language for most students who are deaf because of the limited merits and relative ineffectiveness of current programs and methods. It is presumed that most students will achieve a higher level of English literacy and academic achievement via the use of ASL. In other words, ASL-using students should have an easier time learning English as a second language than non-ASL-using students.

This all-encompassing point of view is counterproductive because it assumes that there is one best approach for all children with severe to profound hearing impairment. This seems to be contrary to the explicit doctrine of individualized education in the field of special education. Most important, it does not consider the needs of the child who is deaf within a family system as opposed to only soliciting the opinions of experts such as members of the Deaf community or professionals in the field of deafness. Decisions on the use of ASL in a bilingual program cannot be based solely or predominantly upon theory and research. Ultimately, it is a decision that needs to be made by parents or caretakers who have considered their child's needs and interests as well as the opinions of professionals and other interested persons.

Similar to other areas, there seem to be acrimonious debates regarding the characteristics of teachers and other professionals in bilingual and/or second-language learning programs (e.g., see discussions in Lane et al., 1996; Johnson et al., 1989). If the focus is on ASL/English programs, then there is no question that teachers need to be bilingual, that is, they need to be proficient in the use of ASL and English. This should be the case even though some classes might be conducted via the use of only one language, depending on the program model that is adopted. Bilingual teachers provide the necessary role models for language proficiency.

It seems perfunctory to state that a considerable number of teachers should be, take your choice of words, Deaf, deaf, or hearing-impaired. Teachers who are Deaf or members of the Deaf culture can serve as role models and can provide a bilingual/bicultural environment. It needs to be emphasized that these teachers also need to be bilingual (ASL and English) because the language role model is equally as important.

Curricular and Instructional Issues

As implied in the quote at the beginning of this chapter, there is no substantial empirical data in support of *one* specific instructional method for bilingual or second-language education programs (e.g., Cook, 1991; McLaughlin, 1985; Prabhu, 1990). Nevertheless, depending on the program model, bilingual programs involving English as the target language typically aim for proficiency in the two languages, in both the conversational (oral) and written form (reading, writing). Even in second-language programs involving English, a certain level of proficiency in the conversational form is a desirable, and necessary, goal, especially for the subsequent development of literacy (e.g., see also the discussion in Mayer & Wells, 1996).

The language-teaching approach is pervasively influenced by the position of individuals regarding the similarity/difference hypothesis of first- and second-language learning (see Chapter 6 for details; see also, Cook, 1991; McLaughlin, 1985). That is, the focus is on whether first-language acquisition is similar to or different from second-language acquisition of the same language. In this chapter, the position is that they are developmentally similar, thus the reason for depending on and applying knowledge of English first-language literacy to the development of English second-language literacy. A list of implications related to the similarity/difference hypothesis is delineated in Table 8-1.

Despite the proliferation of methods used, the trend is toward an eclectic approach that focuses on the individual needs of the students. This process has been called *pragmatic eclecticism* or *methodological pluralism* (e.g., Baily, 1983; Scovel, 1988). This has also led to a questioning of the issue of best method, which has mostly been the domain of re-

TABLE 8-1   Implications related to the similarity/difference hypothesis

Focus on Similarities

- Development is essentially similar to L1, that is, L2 learners proceed through stages, make errors, and use strategies that are similar to L1 learners for the same language.
- The focus is on communicative proficiency; learners are not expected to speak grammatically.
- There is an increased tolerance for production errors.
- The emphasis is on the discovery of patterns; some structured activities are also acceptable.

Focus on Differences

- L2 acquisition is different from L1 and is influenced predominantly by the language structures in L1.
- L2 learners are required to speak in a grammatical manner; in fact, instruction is geared to accomplish this purpose right from the inception of the program.
- There is a focus on the correction of production errors.
- The use of systematic, structured lessons is desirable, especially with an emphasis on repetition and reinforcement.

Source: Based on the discussions in Cook, 1991 and McLaughlin, 1985.

searchers doing quantitative studies (i.e., group comparisons) (Prabhu, 1990). Researchers who focus on qualitative analyses do not believe that there is a separation of the method and the teacher or even a separation of the method and the classroom situation in which it is used (e.g., Prabhu, 1990). In other words, teaching or learning is a context-specific phenomenon, influenced by myriad interactions between and among teachers and students in the classroom setting. Thus, the instructional procedures recommended in this chapter are guidelines based on descriptive reports of classroom research, research findings on literacy, and common sense and experience (e.g., see also Scovel, 1988).

In focusing on individualized instruction, the teacher needs to consider several factors, for example, how students (1) perceive the learning process, (2) interpret goals and expectations, (3) react to incentives, and (4) develop self-confidence and motivation. Of paramount importance is the modification of instructional techniques, materials, and pace to suit the needs of students. Individualized instruction can be conceptualized in several ways, three of which are (1) the assignment of different goals to learners, (2) the assignment of the same goals accomplished with the use of different instructional approaches, and (3) the assignment of the same goals accomplished at different rates (e.g., Heward & Orlansky, 1992; Politzer, 1971).

It should be added that not all or even most instructional activities should be so individualized that a particular student has little or no interaction with peers. Within a constructivist paradigm (see Chapter 1 of this text), it is argued that school is a socialization process whereby learning occurs as a result of social interactions (e.g., spontaneous, mediated) between students and students and between teachers and students (e.g., Dixon-Krauss, 1996; Scott, Hiebert, & Anderson, 1994). This does not denigrate the benefits of direct instruction, even on an individualized level, although more research is needed in this area. Nevertheless, neither direct instruction nor individualized instruction can account for all or even most of language and literacy development in children (Paul & Quigley, 1994a; Scott et al., 1994).

Use of ASL in Teaching English

Relative to students who are deaf, the research literature contains descriptions of ASL/English bilingual programs, particularly with a focus on methods used to teach English as a second language or, rather, English literacy skills (e.g., Neuroth-Gimbrone & Logiodice, 1992; Paul & Quigley, 1994b; Strong, 1988a, 1988b). Most of the existing programs attempt to use what is often called a metalinguistic approach. That is, students are exposed to both ASL and English and are guided by the teacher in a discussion of similarities and differences. In some cases, it is proposed that students learn ASL as a first language prior to learning English as a second language. As stated in Chapter 6, the foundation of many of these approaches seems to be based on the earlier concept of contrastive analyses. Two examples of instructional approaches are discussed in the ensuing paragraphs.

Strong (1988b) described a program in which ASL is to be developed as a first language or enhanced further as the first language (i.e., expanded, elaborated, etc.). Subsequently, ASL can be used as an instructional tool to teach English as a second language. Another major goal is to ensure that both ASL and English are perceived as equal but separate entities. In addition, the students need to develop the ability to recognize similarities and differences between the two languages.

Strong and his colleagues developed a bilingual program for children between the ages of 4 and 7 years, inclusive, who are deaf. They constructed culturally appropriate activities such as the use of TTY, not a telephone, and watching conversations, rather than overhearing them. There were stories in ASL, which were presented either live or on videotape. Later, there were lessons that focused on similarities and differences between ASL and English.

An example of the latter follows:

> Stories are presented on videotape, first in ASL and then in a strict manual version of English . . . Children are encouraged to look for differences in the two versions, with the teacher guiding them toward those that pertain to the theme of the particular unit. . . . the goal is to introduce English and to show some of the ways in which it differs from ASL . . . (p. 122)

This strong metalinguistic component can been found in several other programs (e.g., Akamatsu & Armour, 1987; Neuroth-Gimbrone & Logiodice, 1992). For example, Neuroth-Gimbrone and Logiodice (1992) described their metalinguistic activity as a translation process in which students engaged in "attaching labels in a different language (English) to knowledge, concepts, thoughts or ideas they already had in their first language" (p. 83). One of the major goals was to enable the students to translate into and comprehend English sentences. Relative to the reading activity, the focus was on fluency initially, then clarity, and finally grammatical correctness. Students were expected to develop adequate metalinguistic skills in both ASL and English.

As discussed in Chapter 6, many of these programs seem to adopt approaches in which the use and development of the conversational form of English (i.e., speech and/or signs) are bypassed. This neglects what we have learned about first-language literacy. In addition, it fails to capitalize on using the visual-motor aspects of ASL as an important means for conveying information, including specific grammatical information about English. At the surface level, this implies that students who are deaf are visual learners and the visual mode is paramount. This seemingly simple concept has not been fully realized in the education of these students, particularly in the teaching of English. The ensuing sections provide some theoretical and research background and the resultant instructional strategies for this concept.

Clarification of Terminology

To begin, let us define communication as the act of transmitting a message, some symbol or idea, request, and so on, between a sender and a receiver. A message is encoded symbolically in some way by a sender, transmitted in some way, and decoded by the receiver. Successful communication presumes that the message received was the same message the sender intended. A communication breakdown occurs when the two messages differ. Failure can occur in the faithfulness of encoding the message, precision in transmitting the message, or conventionality in decoding the transmitted symbols. The fundamental components here are *message, sender,* and *receiver.*

In human communication, there are many ways in which messages (symbols) can be transmitted. These means frequently are defined by the situation or the particular individuals engaging in the communication. Modes can be sound based, visually based, motoric, graphic, and so on, and the symbols (messages) transmitted range from very general to very precise. Examples include Morse code, mime, flag signals on ships, international road signs, quarterback signals, police traffic control gestures, and of course signed, spoken, or printed words. The fundamental concepts here are *mode* and *transmission.*

The vast amount of human communication takes place through language, a structured cultural phenomenon. Language can be defined as the rule-governed use of a system of arbitrary symbols whose definition and usage are agreed upon by the community of users (e.g., Bloom & Lahey, 1978). Languages of all varieties share the properties of arbitrariness and grammatical constraint and *evidence* semantic, syntactic, phonological, morphological, and pragmatic aspects. The fundamental concepts here are the *arbitrariness* of symbols, *rules* of grammar, and a *community* of users.

The terms *communication*, *modality,* and *language* are not interchangeable. For example, speech and language are not the same entity. Speech is one modality by which language may be transmitted. The use of language does not guarantee communication and so on.

As applied to the education of students who are deaf, these definitions explicate some important distinctions. For example, sign and speech are different modalities for communication. ASL and English are different languages. ASL is a language in the visual-motor modality, which does not occur in auditory-oral or print modes. Oral and printed English are basically the same language in two different modalities. Manually Coded English systems (e.g., signed English, Seeing Essential English) were designed to provide yet another visual mode, one that represents English manually.

The modality through which a language is expressed has linguistic, social, and some say, cognitive implications. Mason and Allen (1986) explained differences between written and conversational forms of language in terms of physical, situational, functional, and structural parameters. Someone listening to a speech or conversation cannot control the rate at which they must receive information whereas a reader can and may do so. Written language is more formal and permanent (e.g., Adams, 1990a, 1990b). Compared to the interactive nature of conversation, it provides minimal context and, therefore, can be much more ambiguous. Suprasegmental features and nonverbal accompaniments to language, which carry much meaning in conversation, are not encoded specifically in print thus rendering print more rigid and more prone to misinterpretation. From a structural standpoint, there are forms that are more highly associated with the impersonal nature of print than conversational language. For example, conversation relies largely upon active voice agent-action-object structures whereas in print, passive voice object-action-agent constructions are commonplace. In addition, conversational language has been characterized as having narrative-like or topic-comment, organization, whereas written language demonstrates more logical or analytical organization.

This discussion of the relationship between communication mode and language is relevant to the analysis of the possible roles or functions of English and ASL in the education of students with hearing impairment. If print literacy is a goal in educating students who are deaf, then we are necessarily implying an instructional design predicated upon mastery of English printed language conventions. The mode of instruction is not inherently specified by the goal statement per se. Rather, it is *determined* by the communication needs of students and the parameters of the subject matter and instructional context.

As implied in Chapter 6, there have been persistent and emotionally charged discussions of bilingual/bicultural education for students who are deaf. A notion for consideration here is that the instructional issue for the majority of children who are deaf, with hearing parents, really is not a question of language or culture but, more fundamentally, one of modality. Whether their native language is ASL or English, whether they are from birth members of the Deaf or hearing cultures, individuals with severe to profound hearing impairment rely on vision to learn about and interact with the world. We could argue that their native modality is vision.

This notion of the nativeness of the visual modality should not be taken lightly. In the absence of a functional auditory system, the importance of vision as a source of information seems obvious. The development of keen visual perception, conscious attention to eye contact, instinctive reactions to variations in visual environment or light conditions are logical outcomes of reliance on vision for survival as well as for convenience. However, if educators are to appreciate the full potency of this modality, they need to develop a broader perspective, that is, not only recognize passive reliance on visual input, but also active manipulation of features of this modality must be addressed and understood.

The central characteristic of the visual mode is the three-dimensional nature of physical space. Its significance is enhanced in combination with simultaneity along the temporal dimension. In a visual presentation, one can represent objects spatially as well as temporally. In addition, it is possible for two visual stimuli to occur at once and both be perceived, whereas simultaneous auditory phenomena tend to overlap and distort or interfere with one another.

Besides depending upon vision, individuals who are deaf use visually-based devices in many ways for many purposes. There is much evidence in support of this notion (e.g., see Lane et al., 1996; Wilbur, 1987). The classic example is the work of Goldin-Meadow (e.g., see Goldin-Meadow & Feldman, 1975), who described the creation of signed communication systems by deaf children of hearing parents. Her subjects were preschool-aged (18 months to 4 years) children, apparently enrolled in oral educational programs, whose parents did not use sign with them. The discussion focused on the development of gestural communication in the children, beginning with single-unit, non-specific natural gestures such as points or the offering of an open palm to gain *more* of a desired item. Sign development then progressed to the creation of specific lexical elements, which reflected the visually recognizable characteristics of referents, for example, children who are deaf symbolize actions or objects acted upon in particular ways by using action gestures. In later stages, the youngsters used sign combinations to denote semantic relations.

An important analysis, which served to determine the origin of the signs, revealed that the types and usage of signs by the children's parents were delayed and less sophisticated compared to that of the children. In other words, the parents were adopting the gestures first used by the children. Goldin-Meadow and her collaborators suggested that, in developing sign forms, these very young children were relying upon features (e.g., motoric aspects) of their experiences in interacting with objects in their environment.

In sum, it can be argued that individuals who are deaf, especially those deaf from birth, are intimately and inextricably bound to the visual modality and come to develop extraordinary sensitivity to the parameters of this modality. This sensitivity and the resulting competence in physical manipulation of these modal parameters permit highly creative and idiosyncratic use of this modality. In the absence of a functional auditory system, the human drive to interact motivates these individuals to use the raw materials at their disposal, namely their eyes, hands, and spatial expertise to construct visual-manual communication systems. These systems take account (1) of the visual nature of the referent or situation, (2) of the physical parameters for manipulating space, and (3) of possibilities for encoding information clearly and easily with the hands and body.

ASL and the Visual Modality

Previously, some basic parameters of the visual-manual modality were introduced, namely three-dimensional space and simultaneity in the perception of visually presented stimuli. Here ASL is examined with regard to the utilization of these features in a linguistic way. Linguists have documented many formational devices that capitalize on various aspects of visual perception, for example, form, location, direction, repetition, sequence, size, manner, and indexing (e.g., Baker & Cokely, 1980; Wilbur, 1987). This presentation is not meant to be a comprehensive nor detailed linguistic analysis of ASL. Rather, it is meant to provide an understanding of how modality can influence linguistic expression and how aspects of the visual mode are and can be used to heighten clarity in the communication of deaf persons (for detailed discussions, see Baker & Cokely, 1980; Klima & Bellugi, 1979; Wilbur, 1987).

The Use of Space
ASL relies upon the dimension of space to encode and transmit grammatical information. Space is used to illustrate and visualize relationships of various kinds among elements of

the propositions to be communicated. These include relationships among the nouns associated with a particular verb in a single proposition, as well as relationships among multiple propositions. In the former instance, the English representation of relationships results in a simple sentence with multiple nouns filling the positions of subject and various object slots such as direct object, indirect object, and object(s) of a preposition. In the latter instance, the resulting English sentence would be a compound or complex sentence with some propositions embedded as subordinate clauses.

ASL utilizes location of objects in space and the execution of verbs in relation to those locations as means to clarify the logical relations among elements in the expression of propositions. The signer's space always represents the position of the speaker, or first person reference (I, me, mine). The space directly opposite the speaker is used to represent the receiver, or second person reference (you, your). The space to either side of the signer is used to represent entities spoken about or third person reference (he, she, it, they, their, etc.). When a signer wishes to discuss interactions among people or objects, these elements are identified in sign and then placed in the appropriate locations. Thereafter, any reference to them is accompanied by reference to the established location. In this way, spatial reference serves to augment the sign words used for communication to provide precision regarding conversational referents. Relationships may be clarified even further in ASL by variations in how the ASL verb is executed. This leads to discussion of another visual-motor device utilized in ASL, which is modulation of signed elements.

Modulation of Signs

Modulation refers to alteration in the production of a signed element from the citation or dictionary form of the sign. These production differences serve a number of types of grammatical functions. In the case of verbs and their objects, alteration in the directional component of a verb indicates the direct versus indirect objects of that verb. Other manipulations in the movement or manner with which signs are executed can specifically alter the resulting interpretation of the sign, the kind of inflectional and derivational processes apparent in spoken languages.

Some defined movement patterns in ASL have a specific semantic association. Examples of this effect are *iterative* or *continuous* aspects applied to the movement production of a sign. Production of quick repeated movements instead of a singular movement for a sign such as <u>sick</u> would be interpreted as *often sick*. Circular or elliptical movements, rather than the normally straight movement for the same sign, would be interpreted as *continuously sick* or *sick for a long time*. Iterative, durational, and continuous modulations retain the same general interpretation when they are applied to alter other signs, for example, *often funny*, or *searching for a long time*.

Other production variations have less prescribed semantic effects. Klima and Bellugi (1979) have described dimensions of sign production, including the manner and size of movements. The signer's concept of the relative size of a house can be indicated by enlarging or reducing the spatial dimensions of the outline produced in signing <u>house</u>. A sign such as <u>happy</u>, when produced with hands that are comparatively tense or motions that are restrained, would bring into question or reduce the interpreted degree of happiness communicated by the signer, much as a speaker might through an accompanying sarcastic tone of voice.

Nonverbal Aspects of Sign

Interpretation of ASL, especially of inflectional and derivational processes, is further clarified or extended by nonverbal features that accompany the manual productions. In some instances, nonverbal behaviors have very specific grammatical functions, whereas, in others, the information reinforces or clarifies rather than alters the existing interpretation. Three examples will be presented that demonstrate major aspects of nonlexical production in ASL: facial expression, eye gaze, and body position.

The visual center or focus during signed interaction is the signer's face. Like tone in vocal communication, expression in a signer's face carries tremendous amounts of information. Even in the communication of hearing persons, facial expression lends credence, intensity, and so on, to a speaker's words. Various manipulations of mouth, eyes, and brows along with head nods and shakes can signal disagreement, skepticism, disgust, and so on. In ASL, facial expressions have been utilized more formally to serve grammatical functions. For example, raised eyebrows indicate that a yes–no question is being asked, whereas furrowed eyebrows signal *wh*-questions. Other such behaviors may impart information regarding the relationship of propositions to each other, for example, subordination.

Features of eye gaze, specifically, serve a variety of purposes in sign communication. Foremost, the establishment of eye contact between interactors ensures an avenue for communication. So, in ASL, a shift in gaze or eye contact can signify turn-taking between interactors. It can also indicate a shift in the conversational topic. Direction of gaze can be used to focus the receiver's attention in some way as well as to supplement the signer's presentation of a narrative or to clarify elements of a dialogue. When retelling a conversation between an adult and a child, a signer might look down when presenting the adults dialogue and look up when presenting the language of the child. In this example, a signer might also use body language to make the point more precisely.

Signers can use the natural postures of the body and the forms it can assume to communicate information. Classifiers in ASL are generic gestures that represent a class of objects or shapes. These body articulations can be large (involving the whole body) or small (just a finger). They either supplement or replace specific lexical signs in an ASL sentence. In the dialogue example above, the signer might further clarify which participant was speaking by using the orientation of his body to represent turn-taking, that is, facing slightly left across the midline of the body to indicate the adult dialogue, then facing slightly right across the midline to indicate that the child was speaking.

In the following example, a hand classifier is used in place of a sign. To explain the design of a vase, a signer might use one hand to outline the shape of the vase and then, while holding that hand configuration in view, use the other hand to indicate locations on the vase about which other information is given. As with other components of ASL grammar, some classifiers are associated with specific semantics, for example, *vehicle, person, disc, box*. However, in much classifier use, the forms or combinations of forms depicted by body, arm(s), hand(s), finger(s), and so on, are unique and impromptu, much as a mime would create.

Simultaneity

The example of the vase above illustrates yet another capability of signed communication. That is, that multiple bits of information can be communicated simultaneously. As with the vase, the receiver can keep the object in mind as the description of it is presented. Two hands can sign the same thing at the same time to lend clarity, intensity, or the notion of multiplicity to the proposition being communicated. Or, each hand may present different information; for example, with one hand, the signer produces *please open,* whereas the other hand indexes the window the signer wishes to have opened. Obviously, this capability is important to considerations of efficiency and effectiveness in signed communication.

The Visual Modality and Conversational Language

In this section, the concern is with the development of a conversation language via visual modality. As with hearing children, during the early phases of development, the attainment of successful communication is the goal. The focus is on the message rather than the linguistic nature of it. Parent and child must come to understand one another. In addition to form, the child acquires knowledge about language use with different interactors and in different situations. Most important, the child takes in information about the world and about meaning and learns how to use language to encode meaning.

When hearing parents communicate with children who are deaf, they must be careful to encode content visually. This means more than the use of hands and signs. The establishment of eye contact is critical to initiating and maintaining communication. Mothers of very young infants who are deaf ensure that the child attends visually during interaction by gently cupping or turning the baby's head (see discussion in Moores, 1987, 1996). Tapping the child or the floor, table, and so on, are also ways to get visual attention to communication. However, eye contact need not always mean eye-to-eye. It is the source of information that must be within the child's gaze. This is the kind of visual fact that people who are deaf realize but that hearing people may not. As a result, hearing parents and some teachers may insist upon establishing eye contact before beginning to sign to children who are deaf. Mather (1990) reported that people who are deaf feel no such constraint and will begin to sign, just making sure the signs are within the child's line of sight. As a further means to help young children to focus on the topic as they receive communication, people who are deaf will frequently sign on the objects about which they are communicating or hold an object in view while they sign.

The extent of the signing space may also be a developmental issue. Researchers have noted that young children who are deaf may require a reduced signing space or smaller signs as they learn to function within visual constraints (Gaustad, 1986; Mather, 1990). Smaller signs accommodate more intimate communication. This sort of flexibility in normal sign behavior, especially of adults who are deaf, is apparent in other ways, too. In addition to sign space, the actual formational parameters of signs may be manipulated in communication with children who are deaf in ways not used in signing with adults. The direction of signs, onset or offset locations, placement, orientation, number of repetitions, and so on, may be adjusted to affect noticeability and clarity for the child (Mather, 1990). The dimension of adult signing least likely to be altered in such a way is handshape (Gaustad, 1984). (The notable exception is the intentional use of *baby signs* with toddlers who are deaf.) This strong constraint on handshape may be due to the fact that handshape is the feature most often manipulated in producing new and distinct signs.

Another avenue for early communication with children who are deaf is nonsign gestures and other forms of body language. The basic principles underlying mime and classifiers are not difficult to comprehend but can offer means for communication when words or signs fail on either side of the interaction. Much of children's early communication revolves around common routines. Generic gestures can be the beginning of language routines for setting the table, getting ready for bed, or for a car ride, or for gym or the audiologist. Children who are deaf can be encouraged to dialogue about these routines, to pretend, to play with the gestures in unusual and funny ways. Over many repetitions, standard lexical items can be introduced in conjunction with the mime (as the participant's sign skills permit). Retellings of stories (from events or books) can be accomplished in a similar fashion. An atmosphere open to the creative use of gesture and sign broadens the visual possibilities for the child's reception and production of communication.

Beyond increasing the use and flexibility of visual/sign communication of adults with youngsters who are deaf is the need to provide more opportunities for the children to communicate. Compared with hearing children, children who are deaf are not asked as often for information or to make choices or to create language in play. Studies have shown the dominance in classroom communication of teacher talk. And it has been reported that parents and teachers of hearing children ask more *wh*-questions than do parents of deaf children, who tend to frame their inquiries in terms that require only yes–no responses (Mather, 1990). Although these behaviors may be intended to prevent communication errors, they have the detrimental effect of eliminating opportunities for youngsters to encode meanings and to receive feedback on the adequacy of their language attempts. The development of concepts related to inquiry and choice, for example, the relationships between questions and answers, are also inhibited. If children are communicating, they should be expected to clarify, expand, or explain their communications. They are often asked to repeat, but this generally is not very satisfying on either side. The use of gesture and sign in developing questions, choices, dialogue, and creative uses of language can further develop as adults read to children who are deaf.

The Visual Modality and Early Reading

The Use of Multiple Readings

There is accumulating evidence that repeated exposure to the same text, while being read to, is not only pleasurable for a child but also serves to provide additional opportunities for gaining different kinds of information about the particular text and about printed language in general. Such information will include insights into the nature of printed language, the structure of books, and the relationship of textual content to real life.

Repeated reading also has its parallel in the process by which children acquire conversational language. Through repeated verbal interactions with familiar characters in the child's environment, usually the parents, a child becomes intimate with the structure, function, and content of the primary caregiver's language patterns. This knowledge serves as a means of linguistic introduction to the rest of the world. Repeated exposure to the same book makes possible a multifaceted analysis of the text: in-depth (seemingly personal) knowledge of the characters, the plot sequences, and even the actual language in the text. This kind of familiarity leads the reader eventually to the point of being able to conjecture new or alternative events that might feasibly occur or language one would expect these characters to use.

What happens over multiple readings is that the child listener is given the opportunity to focus alternatively on different aspects of the text; one time the voices, the next time the order of events, yet another time on the pragmatics of situations that occur. In this way, the reader comes to conceptualize not only the meaning of the text but also the ways in which text is similar to and different from conversational language, for example, how dialogue is fashioned, how a plot is developed, and how the physical book is organized. The behavior of adult readers impacts the kinds of understanding a child will take away from the experience. Recent investigations of deaf parents and teachers with deaf children have provided insights into effective book-sharing techniques that take into account the visual needs of a child who is deaf (Schleper, 1995). This literature provides strategies for manipulating the book itself, descriptions of reading behaviors that include acting-out story segments and dialogue, and even suggestions for helping the child to follow the English text and the signs for it simultaneously. Table 8-2 provides some general guidelines for book-sharing with students who are deaf.

Parents should maintain the practice of reading to children long after they begin formal reading themselves. Again, there is a useful parallel in the development of conversational language. The literature on language acquisition reveals that, in communicating with children, caregivers utilize vocabulary and sentence structures that are slightly ahead of those being used by the child at that time. In this way, the immediate communication probably can be understood, but it also serves as a stimulus for more advanced language forms.

Parents should increase both the variety and difficulty of the texts they select to read with their children. Some features of the experience are maintained, including multiple readings of selections. With advanced texts, children can be introduced to more sophisticated vocabulary as well as to more complex sentence and discourse structures. In this way, children preview and abstract information about new and more difficult elements in the context of fluent reading. That is, delivery of text by a competent reader, who skillfully

TABLE 8-2   Procedures deaf adults use when reading with deaf children

List of Procedures

Use sign as much as possible.
Keep both the English text and sign visible to the child at the same time.
Don't limit the story to text only, use the illustrations to expound on the meaning of the text.
Move from telling a story with elaboration to a closer rendition of the text with consecutive readings.
Let the child direct the pace of the story and the level at which it is told, allow time for the child to look at illustrations.
Adjust sign placement and style to fit the story, signs may be made on the book or even on the child.
Relate story to child's own experiences or to references the child can use.
Use effective yet gentle and subtle strategies to maintain attention such as a light nudge or shifting the book.
Use eye gaze to elicit participation.
Provide a positive environment, allow the child to make observations and interpretations without corrections

Note: Adapted from Schleper (1995).

parses the text into appropriate chunks, demonstrates at once how to parse larger bits of text for comprehension purposes, and indicates structural and semantic interrelationships among portions of text. The child develops a conceptual structure for material he or she will soon encounter in independent reading.

Teachers can continue and expand on this advantage by including in the everyday classroom schedule a story time followed by a short discussion time. The teacher's reading selections may be more systematic than those of parents, however. Teachers can identify text selections so as to provide the basis for specific goals and activities planned for upcoming reading instruction: historical selections for work on story sequence, poetry for lessons on figurative language, and mysteries for introduction of discussion regarding inference.

Multiple reading is a means for coordinating instruction on metacognitive aspects of reading (discussed in Chapter 7). Students can be directed, over repeated readings, to search for specific content or process features of text, for example:

first reading	always for fun or story retelling
second reading	answer comprehension questions
additional reading(s)	locate main ideas and supporting detail
or	find text segments that don't mean exactly what they say (idioms, metaphors)
or	make an outline or time line of events in the story
or	locate places where you read between the lines

Storytelling and Retelling

Retellings of stories and books are a productive way for students who are deaf to examine and experiment with the features of both the visual mode and language. This general process can be used with students from very young ages through high school. In addition to developing reading and language skills, the process is adaptable for assessment purposes. Storytellings and retelling are behaviors that derive from experiences with stories and books. Both are techniques for engaging students actively in using and creating language. Students experience language in either a conversational or text-based mode. Then, they are required to retell or recreate the story. Initially, this can be a meaning-based retelling with the goal of providing the main elements of the story, characters, setting, plot, and conclusion. At higher levels or later in a particular unit of work with one story, students might be required to provide a version with greater attention to the language used to tell the story. Students might be queried or prompted about actual vocabulary and style, What words did this author use to talk about that event? Retelling activities increases concentration on story structure as well as language. The students' ability to recall the story gives an indication of how they are processing stories and decoding the language within them. As an alternate strategy, students can be required to retell the story to someone who truly is unfamiliar with it, followed by questions that will provide feedback as to the completeness and quality of the student's version.

Students also may be involved in other kinds of activities based upon story reading, which will reinforce storytelling and retelling abilities. These activities can vary from role-playing to creative recastings or expansions of the story. Variety is an important component in both the instructional experiences and the reading materials. Story retelling and multiple readings should also be integrated with writing instruction. Younger students can periodically conduct their retelling in a written format or react to an experience in a journal entry. For advanced students, once a piece of text has become very familiar, they can be instructed to devise alternate text segments and describe or analyze why their piece is representative of the original text's language or structure or why their creation is a feasible outcome of story lines.

The goal of bringing readers to an ever increasing understanding of the detail and language in a text can be integrated with the goal of relating students' facility with ASL and English. Multiple reading is a process ready-made for moving between known and less-known languages. For many students who are deaf, this will mean using ASL knowledge as a means to gain facility with conventions of English print. This is a practical concept for multiple readings, both at school and home. Recently, authors of qualitative studies have described the reading practices of families with children who are deaf (Ewoldt, 1994; Maxwell, 1984, Schleper, 1995). Schleper (1995) has discussed a method used by deaf parents with deaf children. In this description, the adult reader introduces the book to the child through ASL in more of a storytelling mode, that is, taking on the nonverbal features of the characters, acting out scenes, and improvising dialogue. Gradually, with repeated readings of the same story over time, this same adult moves closer and closer to the specificity of the actual words in the text. This is a move from the comfortable more conversational tone of ASL to the formal and sequential nature of presentation in English print. Spatial and animated features of ASL signing give way to the prescribed order and complexity of the printed language. During classroom instruction, teachers can extend this idea in a more deliberate comparison of the language devices used in visual and spoken languages to accomplish various communication and literacy objectives.

Visual Techniques for Teaching English Structures

In this section, we provide suggestions on how properties or features of visual communication might be incorporated into English language/reading instruction. Lessons can be learned from ASL as a means to improve the conceptualizations of students who are deaf for linguistic and literacy principles.

In the circumstances of deaf children with deaf parents or of deaf teachers, the development of visual sensitivity and the sharing of visual-manual linguistic insight from parent or teacher to deaf child is automatic and casual. In the majority of situations, deaf children with hearing parents and teachers, the suggestions will have to be instituted with more formalized training, perhaps under the guidance of adults who are deaf.

Brown (1973) and various of his protégés, in their work with young hearing children, have documented the relative difficulty and order of acquisition for basic features of English. Along with this developmental sequence, they have provided explanations of the perceptual or linguistic parameters underlying the observed difficulties. An order of difficulty for many of these same basic structures for young children who are deaf can be found in Gaustad (1986), who has provided a careful outline and logic underlying the difficulty of many complex structures and grammatical relationships in and between English sentences. Her research examined the competencies of hearing students, but the results and explanations hold as a very succinct explanation for the problems of older deaf users of English as well (for additional details and references, see Moores, 1987, 1996; Quigley & Kretschmer, 1982).

Direct and Indirect Objects

The word order of English, as an indicator of grammatical relations, is not problematic in the expression of most simple sentence relationships. The predominant English word order of subject-verb-object coincides with the physical or logical relationships that exist among the referent elements in the world, that is, the agent-action-recipient of the action.

Consider these sentences:

1. The mother kissed her newborn baby.
2. The mother gave the baby a bottle of juice.

Mastery of word order regularities probably is not required for comprehension of these sentences. The receiver of these sentences is not likely to misinterpret that the baby kissed the mother. The same holds true for the relationship between nouns and modifying prepositional phrases. In the case of sentence 2, one is not likely to misinterpret that the juice was made of bottles.

Correct interpretation is more tenuous when word order disagrees with real world expectations or when more than one relationship among the elements of a proposition is possible. Consider these sentences:

3. The student drew the teacher a picture of a square around some trees.
4. The dog kissed the child.
5. The child was kissed by the dog.

With the elements of sentence 3, different logical relationships are possible so reliance upon expressed word order is necessary for correct comprehension of the intended meaning. A picture of a square around some trees is very different than a picture of some trees around a square. Similar problems occur when word order disagrees with expectations as in the case of passive voice, when the word order of subject-verb-object represents a reversal of semantic relations, that is, recipient-action-agent. With sentence 5, word order leads one to misinterpretation.

In signing constructions like these for students who are deaf, adults can make the relationships clear by using locations in space and the direction of verbs to specify the nature of the actions or arrangements of objects. One can actually place a referent in space as it is mentioned and then relate other signs to that object's location. Another technique is to use body language so as to clarify the location of referents. Consider these sentences:

The raggedy old woman watched the man buy a hot dog from the vendor parked at the corner. The man told the vendor to give her a hot dog, too.
To produce an unambiguous rendering, a signer could:

- lean slightly right and nearby or point to that space while referring to
  The raggedy old woman.
- direct the sign verb *watch* toward the man's location, away and in front of the woman, while producing
  watched the man.

- direct the sign verb *buy* from the man's location toward the location of the vendor, away and on the left of the man, while producing
  buy a hot dog from the vendor.
- pull back toward neutral position while encoding the description of the vendor.

Once these positions are established, the signer can continue in the same fashion using direction from the man to the vendor for the verb *told* and from the vendor to the old woman for the verb *give.*

Passive Voice

Sometimes, the addition of nonverbal cues will clarify the verbal meaning. For passive constructions, body leaning to show the agent-recipient relationship or the use of mime may eliminate the confusion. Although ASL may not have passive constructions per se, paralinguistic and nonverbal cues can encode this meaning. In sentence 4 presented previously, the meaning of the dog kissing the child likely will be transmitted without special supplements. In sentence 5, however, the fact of the child being kissed will likely be misinterpreted (actually reversed) unless other means are used because (1) the word order is reversed and (2) of the two possible events, the dog being the kisser is the least likely conceptually. To clarify this sentence, while signing the verb toward the girl's location (right side), a signer might pull his or her head back as if receiving the kiss. For verbs with a directional component, a signer might restrain or alter production of the verb, for example, not really pushing the verb *push* forward while, at the same time, miming an appropriate body response, for example, *jerking* the shoulder forward as if pushed from behind.

Progressive and Indicative Verbs

Modulation of verbs can also be used to contrast difficult forms. Indicative forms are particularly hard for children who are deaf to master because they are not widely used in conversation and because they require agreement between the subject and the verb. The verb form itself can be made more distinct by signing it in a style clearly different from more common forms. As mentioned earlier, the notion of *continuous* is accomplished in ASL by inflecting the verb with an elliptical motion. English signing requires the addition of the affix -ING (e.g., as in signed English, Signing Exact English). But many verbs lend themselves to expression of a progressive form by physically extending the parameters of the sign's execution, for example, *walk*, in which alternate stepping motions of the hands can move continuously forward as the affix is added to create *walking*. The contrasting indicative form is restrained by comparison, appearing very much like the unmarked citation or dictionary form.

Verb Tenses

Additional clarification of verb tense can be accomplished by utilizing the conceptual frame found in ASL, that is, past is behind the signer, present along the plane in which the signer stands, and future ahead of the signer. The tense forms of many motion verbs can be made more distinctive by directing the movement either slightly forward or behind the signer. An alternative would be, again, to lean the body forward or back while executing the full verb signs with *ed, past,* or *will.*

Adverbials

Either when directly adding adverbs to the verb phrase or when executing verbs that imply adverbial modification, the signer can usually enhance the perception of these constructions by the manner in which the verbs themselves are executed. Directional and motion verbs are particularly amenable to this kind of manipulation (e.g., walked fast, gingerly, or heavy footed). If a sentence includes the adverbial notion of speed, the verb should be signed quickly. If tentativeness is implied in the sentence, the verb can be executed hesitantly (slowly and with pauses). Synonyms that imply motion differences can be conveyed in this manner, incorporating mimetic features, for example, stagger, prance, waddle, tiptoe. Of course, many times such signing will be enhanced by the addition of appropriate facial expressions, too.

Complex Sentences

It is important to examine the issue of advanced sentence construction in English and how this might be clarified through visual means. With the exceptions of some basic adverbial clauses, usually at the end of sentences, complex sentences in English are difficult for students who are deaf to comprehend as well as to produce. Medial subordinate clauses, for example, relative clauses modifying the subject, are particularly problematic because they interrupt the flow of the main clause and blur the relationships among sentence elements. Another factor causing processing difficulties is the sheer length of complex sentences. Especially in signed format, they surpass the capability of the visual system as an input mechanism. All of the sentence information may not be input before the memory trace of the sentence begins to deteriorate. There is some research to indicate, that while still not the best of all worlds, chunking sentence segments meaningfully aids processing (for research on chunking and deafness, see King & Quigley, 1985).

Paralinguistic features of signing can be useful in helping students to separate and process clause information correctly. Along with instruction regarding the meaning of punctuation, students can be shown how to parse sentences. For the sake of visual processing, consider the main clause of a sentence as occupying the center of the signing space as it runs left to right in front of the signer. Any break or deviation from the main clause will be indicated by a shift in location away from that plane at a point in accordance with the portion of the sentence to which the clause refers or that it modifies.

Consider this sentence:

The valet to whom I gave my keys was not on duty when I left the building.
A linear depiction of the encoding of this sentence might look as follows:

The valet   was not on duty
    to whom I gave my keys   when I left the building.

As a further means to set off subordinate clauses, one might sign them smaller or in a more confined space (less freely) than an independent clause. Given that relative clauses are designed to provide detail or specification to the receiver, they could sometimes amusingly be treated as if representing secret knowledge known only to the signer.

Clauses containing *before* and *after* are particularly vexsome to all learners of English. For good reason, the words *before* and *after* refer to the placement in time of the independent clause, not to the dependent clause in which the word appears. Consider this sentence:

The actor went to bed after he became ill.

What happened *after* or last was that the actor went to bed. Perhaps comprehension of this relationship could be accomplished by visualizing the structure spatially. If students understand that the first event in time is closest to the signer, the rule for demonstrating such sentences would be this: If the word *before* appears in a clause, place signing of the other clause closer to the signer (i.e., mimicking the movement within the sign for *before*). For clauses with *after*, the placement of the other (independent) clause would be farther from the signer (mimicking the movement for *after*). Then, comprehension of the order of events indicated by the sentence would always begin with the event closest to the signer.

Considerations

These kinds of visual techniques (i.e., verb modulation, exaggerated body language) will not work for every English construction nor in every situation. They will work less well with more advanced vocabulary where there is less iconicity in the phonology of the verb as in *establish* or *wonder*. This should not be a problem.

First, it is not intended that every sentence produced in sign should be rendered in this fashion. This type of visualization is meant to be a supplemental tool, an informative variant. It will prove especially useful with younger children because it will increase the cues available for perceiving signed information so that the content of it can be learned. The addition of mimes and facial expressions will make signed English communication more interesting, which will only heighten students' visual attention.

Second, such visual-manual manipulation will be especially useful during classroom language instruction. Remember, it is here that the teacher should make the greatest effort to encode English faithfully. There must be sufficient, good, and varied examples to use for instructional purposes. And there are: Signs for most of a child's early vocabulary provide adequate resources for demonstration. Beyond instruction, these visual devices serve the purpose of enhancing the visual presentation of language, in this case English. They will come into play depending upon the situation, the audience, and the purpose of the communication. The more ambiguous or difficult the communication, the greater the need for visual support.

A cautionary note is required concerning deaf children of deaf parents, who may be accustomed to more formalized usage of ASL modulations and other features. Although hearing parents can be encouraged to add gestures generally to their signing without interfering with the child's comprehension, classroom personnel will need to take account of the special needs of deaf students of deaf parents to avoid confusion for them. Some of these concerns can be addressed with specific ASL to English instruction (see following section). Teachers will require sufficient sign facility to accommodate all of the children's needs.

ASL/English: Some Selected Points

Teachers can facilitate the learning of English through the child's knowledge of ASL. These students will likely be very aware of the kinds of visual techniques discussed previously. In addition, they will possess linguistic structures for concepts that English encodes differently but for which a direct explanation might be more efficient than incidental exposure to the language. Following are some suggestions for specific aspects of English structures and the corresponding ASL features that could be used to clarify them.

Structure of English Sentences

The topic-comment orientation of some ASL conversation can be used as the basis for explaining the subject–predicate arrangement of the common English sentence order. It can also be the basis for a discussion or demonstration of the relationship of relative clauses to their main clause referents.

Modifier Relationships

The practice of incorporating adjectival elements into the signing of nouns, and adverbial information into the signing of adjectives, in ASL might be an introduction to the structure of adjective phrases in English. The necessity in a language for a linguistic means to express differences between phrases like *infinitely small* or *incredibly large* could be the lead in to explaining this type of word order constraint in English. Using the modulation of ASL verbs as the reference point, a similar rationale could be applied to the relationship of verbs and adverbs in verb phrases like those in the following sentences: *The worker was sick constantly* or *The child interrupted repeatedly*.

Vocabulary Development

There are numerous ways in which vocabulary instruction can be conducted in a bilingual program (see also later sections of this chapter). There are two principles, however, that if understood, could provide the basis for a broader conceptualization of fundamental concepts of vocabulary building. These are principles of iconicity in ASL and the use of initialization in the development of signed English vocabulary.

More advanced students can be informed directly about the principle of iconicity, how the iconic nature of some signs represents the reverse of the property of symbols to be arbitrary. This play with the relationship of meaning to words can be extended by activities in which children create their own iconic signs for a deaf Star Fleet Captain to use with aliens.

The principle of initialization can be taught in much the same way. Initialization is an extension of the concept of families of morphologically related signs in ASL. For example, in ASL many signs for meanings with a *male* component are made at the same location, with the hand at or near the top half of the signer's head (boy, man, uncle, son, grandfather). Many signs with a feeling component are made using the same handshape, which happens to look like the number eight (e.g., *like, hate, touch, sympathize, excite*). In Signing Exact English (Gustason & Zawolkow, 1993), initialization creates a family of morphologically related signs by systematically varying the handshape component of the same base sign, for example, sign for FRIEND + N handshape = *neighbor;* FRIEND+ R handshape = *relation*. Students can examine and compare selected sets of sign words to reveal the underlying generalities of the process. Then they can practice using the knowledge they discover to create real signs for special or personal things for which they may not already have a sign. Helping older students to understand the principle underlying initialization will provide a meaningful introduction to the notion of word roots. That is, it is not the whole sign form that is the same across members of a related set, but some significant portion of it, and that portion always carries the same or a very similar fragment of meaning.

Summary

It is hoped that this general visual approach to English instruction for children who are deaf, without early exposure to ASL, could lead to some greater consensus about the role of ASL in the instruction of these students. In the present context, the idea of bilingual education is not transfer, per se, from first to second language, as is usually conceived. Instead, we would like to suggest the concepts of parallel acquisition and shared dominance, each language lending its special aspects to the overall linguistic competence of the student who are deaf. If not ideal, at least it takes practical advantage of the realities in the lives of these students.

ASL/English Bilingual Education: Some Considerations

In a previous publication (Paul & Quigley, 1994b), the first author of this chapter has illustrated some general techniques and principles that should be considered in an ASL/English bilingual program. These are discussed in the ensuing paragraphs and are based on the examples in texts on hearing students in second-language programs and on a minority-language immersion model discussed and developed by Paul and Quigley (1994b). The first area addresses the enhancement and further development of ASL.

Language Proficiency: Communicative and Academic

In any bilingual program, students who are deaf, similar to other bilingual students, will have a range of proficiency in the two languages, in our case, ASL and English. If students are from only ASL-using homes, then the majority of communicative and instructional activities should be in ASL initially. If students are from ASL/English-using homes, then the relative proficiency in each language should be assessed prior to determining a program model (e.g., see discussion in Luetke-Stahlman & Luckner, 1991).

Regardless of the program model, it is critical for students to develop both communicative and academic proficiency in one language as early as possible. Communicative proficiency refers to the use of the language for ordinary everyday purposes—sharing information, asking for directions or clarification, and engaging in conversations during mealtimes and other social events (e.g., Bowen, Madsen, & Hilferty, 1985; McLaughlin, 1985; Scovel, 1982, 1988). These interactions, structured and spontaneous (or mediated natural interactions, see Dixon-Krauss, 1996), should enable the students to develop or further enhance grammatical knowledge of their language.

Depending on the age and ability level of the students, the teacher can construct activities and topics that are meaningful and interesting such as show and tell, storytelling, games such as *Twenty Questions* or *Animal-Vegetable-Mineral*, and problem-solving tasks (see also, the early language/literacy discussion in Chapter 7). The point here is that a certain level of communicative proficiency is necessary prior to dealing with so-called academic topics as presented in school texts. This is analogous to typical first-language students who attend schools with reasonably developed skills and knowledge of their cultures via the use of their first or home languages. Subsequently, these students are expected to learn about subject matter or academic content, which refers to the development of academic proficiency.

If ASL is the first language used, then all instructional activities and materials need to be presented and conducted via the use of ASL (see also, Paul & Quigley, 1994b). This requires, at least, the use of visual media such as videotapes, films, and interactive video. These media might contain English captions; however, no formal instruction in English literacy should be planned until after proficiency in ASL has been demonstrated at a reasonable level. Students should be exposed to print incidentally, similar to first-language learners.

It is important to emphasize the visual component, or what can be called the access issue relative to the use of ASL, which does not have a written, literary component. All of the printed materials, for example, academic texts, library books, magazines, newsletters, children's literature, and so on, should be made available on videotapes (or other visual media) via the use of ASL on the grade or ability level of the students. Students should have opportunities to check out or utilize, for example, a videotape or compact disk on a particular topic and interact with this medium in the same manner as another student would interact with a book or other printed material.

In essence, students who are deaf should have visual access to all information provided for typical students at a particular grade or age level in school. The length of this process, 3, 5, or 12 school years, depends on the bilingual education model. In our view, bilingualism in schools means accessibility in both languages.

Relative to language/communication development, it should be remembered that students with a level of proficiency in ASL and attempting to learn a second language might engage in learning activities similar to other second-language learners (Bernhardt, 1991; McLaughlin, 1984, 1985; Taylor, 1990). For example, ASL-using students might attempt to substitute an ASL item for its English equivalent. Or, they might alter the English sign equivalent to fit the morphology of ASL. This phenomenon has been observed, for different reasons, by signing students who are deaf (e.g., see discussions in Drasgow & Paul, 1995; see also, the detailed discussion in Paul & Quigley, 1994a). Finally, students might guess at an English sign based on its similarity to an ASL-using sign.

The foregoing discussion highlights the importance of translation, particularly as a metacognitive strategy. In addition, it supports the necessity and acceptability of oscillating between the two languages to provide clarification in usage, meaning, and understanding of the English words and concepts. The teacher needs to be sophisticated enough to notice these subtle responses by the students and to engage them in a discussion or demonstration of differences. Simply showing the students the *correct* way to use the English sign might not be productive or useful.

In the literature on bilingualism and second-language learning, several language-teaching approaches have been described. Some of them are appropriate for the ASL/English situation or for working with ASL as a first language, for example, the natural ap-

TABLE 8-3   Guidelines for assessing/determining language/communication needs

Guidelines Using a Functional Approach

- An assessment should be made of the language/communication skills that are needed to function in classes in which only English is used. This assessment should cover instructional methods, materials, and the types of tests used in the English classroom settings (e.g., English language classes, literacy, mathematics, science, etc.).
- Instruction should be individualized and should be catered to the language/communication needs of the students. The concept of individualized instruction allows for the use of different instructional methods, materials, and goals and for different rates of instructional delivery.
- The decision to enroll students in a predominantly English-using classroom should be based on a comprehensive assessment of their conversational and written language skills in English.

Source: Based on the work of Chamot (1983).

proach (e.g., Krashen, 1981, 1982, 1985) and the functional approach (e.g., Chamot, 1983). The natural approach is similar to what has been used with students who are deaf and learning English as a first or second language (e.g., McAnally et al., 1994). In assessing and determining the language and communication needs of students who are deaf in an ASL/English bilingual program, some guidelines from the functional approach might be useful. These guidelines are presented in Table 8-3.

Conversational Language Proficiency in English: Issues

Within the framework of a minority-language immersion program or a developmental maintenance program (see Chapter 6), the majority language, English, is introduced after a reasonable development and use of ASL as the language of instruction and communication. Issues concerning the amount of time for each language have been discussed elsewhere (e.g., Paul & Quigley, 1994b). The point to stress here is that students need to be able to manipulate English in the conversational mode (e.g., speech or sign) in order to develop the reciprocal relationship between the conversational and written forms of English.

Developing communicative and academic proficiency in English has been an enduring problematic concern for educators of children and adolescents who are deaf (e.g., Moores, 1987, 1996). It is no less of a concern for teaching English as a second language, especially if one of the goals is the development of English literacy skills. The problem in this area is related to the ongoing debates with regard to the use of sign communication, particularly with respect to English-based signed systems.

An in-depth discussion of the problems associated with the use of signed systems can be found elsewhere (e.g., Drasgow & Paul, 1995; Paul & Quigley, 1994a; Wilbur, 1987). The selection of a particular signed system for use in a bilingual/bicultural program is debatable, with most educators holding the belief that there is not a sufficient amount of data available to make an informed decision (however, cf., Luetke-Stahlman, 1988a, 1988b). As argued elsewhere (e.g., Paul & Quigley, 1994a), most signed systems are not used exclusively in a consistent or systematic manner in educational programs for students with severe to profound hearing impairment. There seems to be limited evidence that communicative or academic proficiency in English is even possible via the use of these systems with many students with severe to profound hearing impairment.

Of course, it needs to be remembered that the use of a signed system is not an all-encompassing issue in the development of English language and literacy skills. Much more is needed for English development than the use of signs in a systematic and consistent manner. However, the two major issues in the use of the signed systems are accessibility and completeness (e.g., see Dragsow & Paul, 1995; Paul & Quigley, 1994a).

English language development is dependent upon reasonable access into all components, that is, phonology, morphology, syntax, and semantics. Without the adequate perception of speech by students who are deaf, the use of the signed systems in a simultaneous fashion (i.e., speech and sign simultaneously) does not provide complete access to phonology. Even more interesting is the importance of the perception of suprasegmentals (e.g., intonation, pitch, pause) on the development of the morphophonological system of English and English literacy (e.g., Brady & Shankweiler, 1991; Shankweiler & Liberman, 1989). Finally, even with attempts to completely represent English via signed systems, students who are deaf are not necessarily understanding or perceiving connected English features, for example, derivational or inflectional morphology (see discussions in Dragsow & Paul, 1995; Paul & Quigley, 1994a).

The foregoing discussion emphasizes, in part, the difficulty of developing English as a first or second language in students with severe to profound hearing impairment. If English is to be developed as a second language, then educators and researchers need to find more efficient ways to enable students with hearing impairment to access the morphophonological system. Most of the methods in the ensuing paragraphs are based on research and practice with hearing students. Whether they are beneficial for students with hearing impairment is an open debate; however, they should be considered guidelines, especially if the goal is communicative and academic proficiency in English.

Language Proficiency in English: Communicative and Academic

By now, it should be clear that it is critical to develop proficiency in both the conversational and written forms of English and that proficiency in the written form is enhanced or facilitated by proficiency in the conversational form. A number of procedures and techniques are available in various sources (e.g., Bowen et al., 1985; Clark, 1982; Cook, 1991). To reiterate: Depending on the bilingual/bicultural model, the teacher might need to alternate instruction in ASL and English. At times, it might be necessary to start with instruction in English and move to explanations or clarifications in ASL.

Activities that focus on English communicative proficiency, similar to those for ASL communicative proficiency, should include a wide variety of conversational issues, such as asking questions for clarification, for directions, and for information. These issues should be meaningful to the students, that is, similar to real-life experiences. However, it is also possible to engage in metalinguistic discussions with regard to the grammar of English; this time, the discussion is in English as much as possible.

Obviously, it is not possible to jump into English at this level with young children with severe to profound impairment. Nevertheless, with a focus on communicative proficiency, the goal is to enable the students to use conversational English either via signs and/or speech. Useful techniques include (again) sharing activities such as show-and-tell, dialogues, discussing field trips, and so on. These can be organized around themes. A perspective on these activities has been described elsewhere (Paul & Quigley, 1994b):

> Tasks at the simple end of the continuum require students to respond in a physical manner—that is, sit, stand, jump and so on . . . Examples include the following: Sit down at your desk; Walk to the window; Please open the door; and Walk around the table. Teachers should take care to use signs or words that help students to understand certain classroom rules and procedures. An example of a series of more complex listening or watching tasks (especially in the academic content area) is (a) Take out your reading book; (b) Open it to page one; (c) Find the second paragraph; (d) Look at the first line; (e) Find the third word; and (f) Tell (speak or sign) me what it is (adapted from Bowen et al., 1985). These commands can be administered and completed one at a time or all at once. Teachers can then proceed to activities that require limited responses, such as (a) Tell me your name; (b) Do you live in a house? (c) Do you live in an apartment? and (d) Do you live with your family? Teachers can tell a story and ask questions. To designate this as a listening or watching activity, not a memory one, the questions should be simple. Higher level questions and those requiring more demands on memory should be reserved for reading and the other academic content areas. (pp. 247–248)

At some point during these instructional periods, it might be necessary for the teacher to expend some time on specific grammatical and vocabulary features of English. This should not be construed as an either/or situation, that is, a natural versus a structural approach because there is no substantial evidence for the superiority of either broad approach (e.g., see discussions in McAnally et al., 1994; Quigley & Paul, 1994). Given the fact that many students who are deaf have problems with specific structures in print, it is critical for the students to be exposed to these structures in the conversational mode. In addition, the students need to manipulate (i.e., use) the structures as part of their interactions. Thus, it might be necessary for teachers to create or structure some classroom activities so that students are encouraged to utilize specific structures. For example, a student can be required to discuss with the rest of the class one topic in the past tense. The teacher can give the students a few verbs, both regular and irregular, to use in their presentations. Again, the level of this activity, including the number and kind of verbs, varies according to the ability of students. Consider the following example:

<u>Topic</u>:   Baseball game between the Cleveland Indians and the New York Yankees

<u>Words to be used</u>: attend, hit, see, run, slide, pitch, throw

It might be possible to combine conversational and reading/writing activities. As discussed in Chapter 4, it is not necessary to wait until a high level of proficiency in the conversational mode is developed prior to the introduction of literacy activities. In the ensuing sections, there are examples for addressing specific features, similar to those discussed in Chapter 7, vocabulary and comprehension.

Vocabulary: Instructional Issues

Not surprisingly, the instruction of vocabulary has been neglected in both foreign-language and second-language teaching (e.g., see discussions in Richards, 1976; Taylor, 1990). It is important to repeat here that students might need some structured activities that enable them to increase their awareness of the sound system of English, particularly phonology and morphology. Some examples of lessons in morphology were presented in Chapter 7. The use of phonics (some other activity that depends on phonology) might be useful for some students who have access to the sound system via amplification. Some examples of activities can be found in well-known textbooks (Durkin, 1989; Johnson & Pearson, 1984; see Adams, 1990a, 1994 for a good explanation of why phonics is important for all students).

The focus here is on vocabulary knowledge or word meaning. The intent of repeating the highlights here is to make the point about developmental similarities in first- and second-language acquisition. It is necessary to begin with a lengthy (adapted) passage that addresses a question that was discussed in Chapter 2: What does it mean to *know* a word? This discussion is important for decisions with regard to the teaching of vocabulary to students learning English as a second language. The content of the passage is based on the work of Richards (1976) for hearing second-language students. However, the similarities are obvious and the examples are illuminating (Taylor, 1990, pp. 1–3).

1. *Knowledge of the* frequency *of the word in the language, i.e., knowing the degree of probability of encountering the word in speech or in print. Some lexical items in English are far more frequent in speech than in writing, such as 'indeed,' 'actually,' 'well.' Other items, like 'former,' 'latter,' may only occur in the written language.*

2. *Knowledge of the* register *of the word, i.e., knowing the limitations imposed on the use of the word according to variations of function and situation. For example, 'Would you like a cigarette?' is a neutral formula, appropriate in most contexts. 'Want a fag?' may be an acceptable utterance between friends, but if made to a stranger it would be perceived as rude or insubordinate.*

3. *Knowledge of* collocation, *both semantic and syntactic . . . i.e., knowing the syntactic behaviour associated with the word and also knowing the network of associations between that word and other words in the language.*

4. *Knowledge of* morphology, *i.e., knowing the underlying form of a word and the derivations that can be made from it.*

5. *Knowledge of* semantics, *i.e., knowing firstly what the word means or 'denotes.' It is relatively easy to teach denotation of concrete items like 'plate,' 'ruler,' or 'banana' by simply bringing these objects or pictures of these objects into the classroom. For more abstract concepts,* synonyms, paraphrases

or definitions *may be useful.* Antonymns *are also important, since it is necessary to know what a word does* not *mean as well as what it does mean. Semantic knowledge involves knowing secondly what the word 'connotes.' For example, in Western culture the word 'slim' is positively evaluated, whilst we have many euphemisms for the negatively evaluated term 'fat,' such as 'plump,' 'portly,' or 'well-built.' However, 'You've put on weight' may be perceived as a compliment in some cultures.*

6. *Knowledge of* polysemy, *i.e., knowing many of the different meanings associated with a word.*

7. *Knowledge of the equivalent of the word in the* mother tongue.

Vocabulary Activity: One Example

In one sense, there are aspects of this activity that are similar to those discussed in Chapter 7, particularly with respect to multimeaning words. There are, at least, two important differences or, rather, additions. It might be necessary for teachers to expend more time and energy on words so that both connotative and denotative features can be discussed (see previous section). The teacher might also need to relate these examples to their usage in the mother tongue, or the first language of the student.

From Chapter 7, recall that one of the most important ways to elicit and build background knowledge is to teach relevant vocabulary directly. However, direct vocabulary instruction does not necessarily mean step-by-step, precision-teaching techniques. It does mean that more than just a single meaning or usage of the word is covered. Traditional definition-and-sentence-approaches (e.g., see Nagy, 1988; Paul & O'Rourke, 1988) are too limiting for poor readers/writers and even more so for the students attempting to learn English as a second language. The use of a semantic elaboration approach, accompanied by class discussions, is probably a very effective approach (e.g., see discussion in Heimlich & Pittelman, 1986; Johnson & Pearson, 1984).

In Chapter 2 of this text, the reader was introduced to the concept of a word map (or web). That idea is expanded here within the framework of what is often called a semantic map (or web) (e.g., Heimlich & Pittelman, 1986). The word that serves as our example is *bank*. It is possible to start out with a word map by listing and discussing the three questions: What is it? What is it like? and What are some examples? (e.g., Mason & Au, 1986; see Figure 2-1). However, we are going to do more with this word than those three questions seem to suggest.

Let's suppose that the word bank is used in the story in a sentence such as: Julie sat on the bank of the river under a big tree. The recommended initial task is to elicit a meaning or description from the students (as a whole class activity) that fits the intention of the usage in this sentence. Nevertheless, we would be remiss if we ended on this note, that is, only to relate the meaning or nuance of *bank* as it is used in this story. This word, similar to many other multimeaning words, lends itself to more in-depth examples and discussion.

As it is used in the story, students might relate or describe this word as land, place, dirt, and so on, beside or near water. This can be refined to include the phrase: land beside a body of water. By now, the creative teacher can pop some very good questions in a discussion format.

A bank is land besides a body of water. The body of water in this picture is a river. What do we call the land beside a body of water such as an ocean? a lake? a sea?

These questions might have obvious answers; if not, the teacher might need to provide this background knowledge in this lesson or in another lesson.

Let's suppose we accomplished our purpose with answers such as shore, coast, or beach. Now, the teacher can proceed to another line of thinking. Where else can we find a bank? A river is one place. Let's think about this. What are the characteristics of a river? Do these features do something to the land near it? The focus of this approach is on the notion of *running water* that erodes (washes away) the land, creating a hump, pile, or mound. This focus should lead to the idea that land beside bodies of running water are likely to be called banks. Examples include canal, stream, and brook.

The question raised earlier, *Do these features do something to the land near it?,* can lead to yet another meaning or nuance associated with bank: a mound or pile. Examples for this emphasis include dirt, rocks, clouds, and snow (as in snowbank or a bank of clouds). Some students might be able to provide a creative response such as a bank of hay or hay stacks for racing tracks (i.e., a pile or bank of hay near the corner of a speedway to help stop runaway vehicles and protect car, driver, and spectators).

Because bank is a common multimeaning word, the teacher can and should elicit further discussion from the class. For example, the teacher might focus on prompting or probing the students with questions such as, Does anyone know another meaning or use for this word? If no response, the teacher can remark: Where do you save or keep your money? Where can you save or keep your money? Where do your parents or guardians save or keep their money? Where do some people save or keep their money? This should lead to a discussion of a *money* bank, including related concepts such as teller, automatic teller, drive-through, savings account, checking account, names of banks, and so on. Later on, the notion of *a place to save or store* can be elaborated upon. Here, a discussion can be started on what is or can be saved: money, clothes, food, and sperm (obviously, this depends upon the age of the students!).

It should come as no surprise that there is more to this word bank. If a teacher focuses on morphology or grammatical use (e.g., noun or verb or some other descriptors), the students might come up with examples such as a billiards table or the curve of a tilted road (i.e., the category is *inside the edge of something*). The use of the example, billiards table, might lead to a nice discussion of a bank shot. That there is still more to the word, bank, perhaps, the appropriate response is You can bank on that. Another fascinating, related lesson is how banks obtain their names or the significance of bank names such as First National, Fifth Third Bank, Banc Ohio, and so on. (*Note:* Even the spelling of the word, banc, in Banc Ohio is an interesting sidebar.)

The above can be covered in several lessons. More important, the teacher and class can create an evolving, creative word/semantic map as shown in Figure 8-1 After each group of words within a heading, such as Inside the Edge of Something or Things You Save or Store, the teacher should translate the above examples in the mother tongue of the students. In this case, this would be American Sign Language because our focus is on ASL/English bilingual/bicultural programs. This activity is related to the metacognitive ones discussed previously in the literature on deafness.

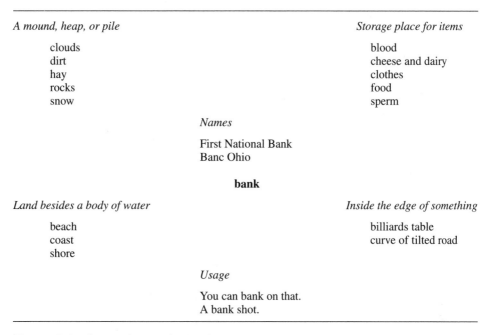

A mound, heap, or pile

    clouds
    dirt
    hay
    rocks
    snow

Storage place for items

    blood
    cheese and dairy
    clothes
    food
    sperm

Names

First National Bank
Banc Ohio

bank

Land besides a body of water

    beach
    coast
    shore

Inside the edge of something

    billiards table
    curve of tilted road

Usage

You can bank on that.
A bank shot.

Figure 8-1   Semantic map for bank.

More Vocabulary Activities

As expected, a number of activities described in literacy texts for first-language learners are also applicable to second-language learners (e.g., Clark, 1982; Durkin, 1989; Mason & Au, 1986; McCormick, 1987). For example, in one source (Clark, 1982), the activities seem to focus on grammatical and vocabulary features, which are also problematic for students who are deaf and learning English as a first or second language—multimeaning words, verb-particles (two-word verbs), and idiomatic and figurative language. These activities can be presented as games (concentration, hang-man or hang-person, twenty questions) or as exercises (matching, analogies, multiple-choice) or combinations of the two formats. In addition, similar to the activity on *bank* presented previously, it is critical to engage the students in a discussion of these features. If these features can be discussed relative to a storytelling, reading, or writing exercise, this would be more meaningful to the students (see Chapter 7 for some examples of writing activities).

The following examples are adapted from Clark, and the idea is that all of these can be used with index cards (see also, Bowen, Madsen, & Hilferty, 1985; Cook, 1991). The extent of the activities is limited by the imagination of the teacher. Although the level of the activity is indicated, it should be highlighted that these are guidelines. The actual level is dependent on the individual capabilities of the students within a particular teacher's classroom.

Prior to using an item such as synonym (or any other major concept), the teacher should discuss this entity with students. As argued by Johnson and Pearson (1984), synonyms are not two or more words that have exactly the same meanings. Rather, this concept should be presented as two or more words that are nearly similar in meaning. If two words were exactly the same, there would probably not be the need to have two words. For example, *big* and *large* are synonyms with nearly similar meanings. They can be used interchangeably for a number of situations and have basically the same meaning as in *big car, large car*. However, they do not completely overlap as indicated by the following examples: *big idea, large idea; big money, large money*. Thus, not only can the teacher have a discussion on words with similar meanings but also should present cases in which the words are not really synonymous.

Examples of synonym pairs follows:

Adjective Synonyms for the Elementary Level

big	large
near	close
simple	easy
certain	sure
angry	mad

Adjective Synonyms for the Intermediate Level

next	following
shy	timid
afraid	scared
enough	sufficient
terrible	awful

Adjective Synonyms for the Advanced Level

skeptical	doubtful
eccentric	strange
selfish	egotistical
uneasy	apprehensive
careful	cautious (Clark, 1982, pp. 7–9)

Additional ideas for words and their synonyms from fourth grade to the high school level and beyond can be obtained from a source that focused entirely on words and their meanings (e.g., Dale & O'Rourke, 1981). Using a thesaurus in conjunction with this word source book should result in numerous pairs of synonyms that might be appropriate for students at the specified grade level (e.g., see Dale & O'Rourke, 1981 for a description of the manner in which word meaning difficulty was determined).

One of the fastest growing idiomatic element in the English language is the two-word verb (or verb-particles). The work of Payne (1982; Payne & Quigley, 1987) has illustrated students' difficulty in this area. Similar to multimeaning words, many of these two-word verbs also have multiple usages and meanings. Again, from Clark, the following examples might be useful in creative activities (see also, the activities in Bowen et al., 1985; Cook, 1991):

Two-Word Verbs for the Elementary Level: Separable
(i.e., the two words of the verb can be separated)

call up	telephone
pick out	choose
talk over	discuss
do over	repeat
put back	replace

Two-Word Verbs for the Intermediate Level: Inseparable
(i.e., the two words of the verb cannot be separated)

come back	return
look after	take care of
run into	meet by chance
run out of	consume completely
look for	search

Two-Word Verbs for the Advanced Level: All Types

take up	begin to study
pass out	distribute
figure out	solve
put out	extinguish
throw away	discard (Clark, 1982, pp. 14–16)

There is no limit (except the teacher's imagination) for constructing activities with two-word verbs. In addition to the traditional *concentration game,* the teacher might ask the student: What does *put out* mean in the sentence: The firewoman put out the fire. The teacher will accept answers such as *make the fire disappear* or *go away, stop the fire,* or *extinguish the fire,* or even *throw water* or whatever on the fire. Later, the teacher might inquire whether it is possible to say, The firewoman *put* the fire *out.* As indicated in the examples above, some two-word verbs are separable and some are not. For example, one can *run into a friend,* but not *run a friend into.*

The teacher should also be on the look out (pun intended) for additional nuances or meanings associated with two-word verbs. For example, *put out* can refer to the retiring of a runner in baseball or a feeling of irritation or annoyance as in being put out by what someone said. In our view, when it comes to vocabulary instruction, it is a miscarriage of justice to only focus on one common meaning or nuance of a word. Each word represents an evolving universe that expands with usage and the experience of the individual during lifelong activities.

It is important to ensure that students understand these words. Feedback, however, can and should be conducted in the conversational mode (speech and/or signs) of English initially. When this does not yield satisfactory results, the teacher might need to conduct the explanation in ASL. With respect to feedback, there are several techniques, but only one will be discussed here. This involves the use of questions, either *wh -, yes–no,* or *tag,* and the use of additional, probing statements (*Note:* Tag questions, however, might be a little difficult for deaf students). For example, to obtain feedback on the use of the two-word verbs, teachers might ask the following questions and continue the interactions/conversations with the students with follow-up statements or probes:

1. Did you run into your friend yesterday or the day before? Tell me about it.
2. What happened when you ran into your friend yesterday? I want to know more about it.
3. You ran into your friend yesterday, didn't you? Tell me about it.

Grammatical Features of English

Additional activities for vocabulary and other grammatical features can be used and can be found in a number of sources (e.g., Clark, 1982; Dale & O'Rourke, 1971, 1981; Taylor, 1990; Verghese, 1989). Again, as indicated in Chapter 3, students who are deaf or hearing impaired might have difficulty with a variety of vocabulary and language features, for example, relative clauses, verb processes, question formation, figurative language, and so on. These grammatical features also cause problems for second-language learners (e.g., see discussion in Cook, 1991; McLaughlin, 1984, 1985; Taylor, 1990). For example, at the *word* level, students might need assistance with specific phrases that are associated with certain words. You go to the store and *buy a loaf of bread, a carton of milk, a head of lettuce, five pounds of sugar, two sticks of butter*, and so on.

Examples of other grammatical aspects follow (Clark, 1982, pp. 40, 41, & 44; see also the activities in Taylor, 1990).

Conditionals: Advanced Level (Adapted)

- I would not have been so angry yesterday if you had told me the truth.
- If I were President of the United States, I would live on Pennsylvania Avenue in Washington, DC.
- If I had invited you to my house yesterday, would you have come?

Clauses with When and While: Intermediate/Advanced Level (Adapted)

- What were you doing yesterday, when I called?
- We got married while she was living in Massachusetts.
- Someone stole her purse while she was shopping downtown.

Story: Scrambled Paragraphs, Intermediate Level (Adapted)

(Numbers reflect the actual order; this activity is similar to putting sentences in the correct order or sequence.)

(1) One day a large truck filled with one hundred penguins broke down on the highway outside of a large city. (2) The driver of the truck was trying to decide what to do when a man driving a big, empty bus stopped and offered to help. (3) The truck driver said, "I have to take these penguins to the zoo right away. If you will take them in your bus, I will give you two hundred dollars. (4) The bus driver agreed to take them. (5) Later that afternoon, after he had repaired the truck, the truck driver was driving

through the city when he saw the bus driver with the hundred penguins. (6) He was walking along the sidewalk followed by the penguins walking two by two in a line. (7) The truck driver got out of his truck and said to the bus driver, "I told you to take these penguins to the zoo!" (8) "I did, " replied the bus driver, "but I had some money left over, so now I'm taking them to the movies."

These lessons can be presented explicitly (i.e., structured) or implicitly (i.e., natural) or some combination of the two broad forms. For example, Clark (1982) has provided activities with conditionals, clauses with *when* and *where*, and one called *story* in which the students need to organize the sentences or paragraphs so that they make sense in a *story* (see example above). Each of the aforementioned exercises lends itself to a good discussion as a whole-class activity.

One of the most difficult grammatical elements of English is the use of figurative and idiomatic expressions (see also the discussion and examples in Chapter 7). This is problematic for both learners who are deaf and for second-language learners (e.g., Giorcelli, 1982). Regardless of the activities planned, students are going to need numerous exposures and experiences with these metaphorical, arbitrary expressions. In one sense, there is no real logic, only acceptance of the manner in which they are used in English. Some expressions need to be taught as whole phrases or sentences such as:

1. It's raining cats and dogs.
2. (He/she) is climbing the walls or going out of (his/her) mind.
3. (He/she) is running around like a chicken without a head.

Students are bound to be challenged by expressions such as a *pride of lions* and *a school of fish*. English is strange, indeed, if lions can be proud and fish can go to school, perhaps obtaining an advanced degree!

It might be helpful to teach related idioms or idiomatic expressions, that is, related in a particular sense. For example, people often use the phrase *as pretty as a picture* to describe another person. This is assuming, of course, that both the picture and the person are pretty! In any case, there are phrases that can be taught together in a variety of situations such as role playing, descriptions of the comparisons, and so on.

The following phrases are taken from Taylor (1990, p. 48) and are part of a matching activity. This activity should be conducted after the students have had various experiences and exposures to the phrases.

We often used these idioms to describe people.
Can you match them up? [Note: This author obviously used a separable two-word verb: *match up*].

As pretty as	an ox
As obstinate as	gold
As white as	a picture
As strong as	a mouse
As good as	a sheet
As quiet as	a mule

Equally as challenging are phrases that one cannot say even though the word seems to be acceptable in a different context. For example, it is acceptable to say or write, the *head of the class* and the *foot of the mountain*. However, the *foot of the class* and the *head of the mountain* are not acceptable. As noted by several researchers (e.g., Moores, 1987, 1996; Paul & Quigley, 1994a; Wilbur, 1987), difficulty with these so-called colorful expressions and word usage probably contributes to the stilted usage of words so often found in the written language of students who are deaf and hearing impaired.

Many students who are deaf are not likely to encounter these expressions in typical, everyday situations, including reading materials, especially if they have difficulty reading. Therefore, it is up to the teacher to create numerous opportunities for the students to interact with and use the various aspects of figurative and idiomatic language. Again, it might be necessary for teachers to teach or emphasize these structures directly (i.e., structured lessons). The teacher can also find printed materials that contain these structures or create their own stories with them.

Advanced Language/Literacy Skills in English

The reader is referred to Chapter 7 for additional information regarding the development of emerging and advanced literacy skills in English. Relevant exercises include the examples in both bottom-up and top-down skills for reading and both lower-level and higher-level skills for writing. The last point to discuss here is the use of materials that are either specially designed or modified for students who are deaf versus the use of unmodified materials typically used with hearing students.

Syntheses of the debates on this issue have been presented elsewhere (e.g., King & Quigley, 1985; McAnally et al., 1994; Paul & Quigley, 1994a). This debate has been fueled by the dichotomy on language-teaching and literacy-teaching approaches: naturalism versus structuralism. As discussed in this text and elsewhere (e.g., McAnally et al., 1994), this should not be construed as an either/or situation because research does not offer a clear-cut pattern on which approach is *superior*. Many teachers of children who are deaf use some combination of these two broad approaches.

The same applies to the use of materials, however, there are some additional issues to consider. Firstly, the research on the effectiveness of types of materials is typically based on comparisons of groups of students, that is, quantitative research. As discussed previously, this assumes that there is a separation between method and method user, material and material user, and so on, that undermines the complexity of the student-material interactions or the teacher-student interactions. Secondly, this *best material approach* violates one of the major strategies of effective instruction—the need to cater to the individual needs of the students. The crux is to find the level and type of material that best suits the needs of the individual student in the classroom. Finally, although a variety of materials should be used—children's literature, regular or special materials, and the child's or teacher's language in language experience approaches—there might be a need to modify the language and content of such materials. There is also evidence that this approach is effective for some hearing students in bilingual or second-language learning programs (e.g., Cummins, 1988; McLaughlin, 1985, 1987).

In essence, for some ASL-using students who are deaf, it might be of benefit to present information in what is called a spiraling or cyclical pattern. That is, the language structures and content of the stories are sequenced according to determined levels of student difficulty with these items. These features are typically arranged from simple to increasing levels of difficulty and appear frequently throughout the printed materials.

A Final Word

The main purpose of this chapter was to discuss issues relative to instruction and second-language literacy. The focus was on literacy instruction within an ASL/English bilingual program, although many of the principles and exercises are also applicable to other types of bilingual programs involving English and some other minority language. In addition, there was a focus on the importance of the visual modality and how this related to using ASL to teach some grammatical features of English.

The driving force behind the discussion and selection of instructional activities was the present authors' persuasion that development in L2 is essentially similar to development in L1. In fact, it was argued that an individual's position regarding this issue pervasively influences the type of research studies, the use of instructional approaches and curricular materials, and even the establishment of a particular bilingual education model. Specifically, it was averred that a position on this issue has led to the use of English literacy instructional models that are not strongly supported by theories and research with hearing children.

As discussed previously in this text, it is important to develop deafness theories of literacy development. However, at present, the theories and research on hearing children can be presented as guidelines. That was the intention of the few instructional examples illustrated in this chapter. Because of the complexity of the teaching-learning situation, it is also important for teachers to modify the activities (and materials) so that there is a best fit between these aspects and individual children's abilities and interests.

Further Readings

KRESS, J. (1993). *The ESL teacher's book of lists.* West Nyack, NY: The Center for Applied Research in Education.

MARTON, W. (1988). *Methods in English language teaching:* Frameworks and options. New York: Prentice Hall.

McCORMICK, K. (1994). *The culture of reading and the teaching of English.* New York: Manchester University Press.

OMARK, D., & ERICKSON, J. (1983). *The bilingual exceptional child.* San Diego, CA: College-Hill Press.

WALLACE, C. (1986). *Learning to read in a multicultural society: The social context of second language literacy.* New York: Pergamon.

Chapter 9

Literacy Assessment: Selected Issues

Tests on reading and writing are usually related to theoretical views of the nature of reading and/or writing. There is a growing body of evidence, however, that assessment has not kept pace with the emerging views of reading and writing.... (Paul & Quigley, 1990, p. 200).

The purposes of assessment are to evaluate the existing match and identify the optimal match between the reader and the reading context . . . However, the long-range goal of the entire assessment and instruction process is to produce strategic, motivated readers, and to develop mature readers who can and will apply their skills and strategies independently and in a flexible manner. The process of assessment and instruction requires that we find ways to break down reading into component parts that can be examined with the larger context of the reading process.... an interactive view of reading suggests that the components must include factors in the reading context.... because reading problems in school arise most frequently from interactions between the reader and the reading context (Lipson & Wixson, 1991, p. 45).

Standardized testing maintains its prominent position in the nation's schools because of both economic and political reasons. For example, as Americans we want our children to receive the best education possible, but we also want to get the most from the education dollars we spend. As a result, we have developed an "accountability mentality" for evaluating the education system, and opinion polls indicate consistently that the general public believes that standardized test scores are the best indicators of the quality of education that children are receiving . . . The economic force exerted by these scores is evident by the uses made of them. In some areas, for example, newspapers publish schools' test scores. Realtors then may quote the scores to prospective property buyers as part of their sales pitch, and, as a result, property values rise and fall according to the quality of the schools—as indexed by test scores . . . (Pearson & Stallman, 1994, p. 240).

The three passages above characterize the tone of much of the information in this chapter. It should be underscored that the metatheoretical and theoretical underpinnings of literacy measurements should be articulated by test developers. This is important for several reasons. One, it makes it easier to describe and follow through on the interrelations among theory, research, curriculum, instruction, and assessment. Two, it provides the rationale for how and why literacy skills should be measured. And three, it clarifies the nature of the assessment tools that should be employed or even if literacy should be assessed at all.

This chapter provides some basic information on selected issues in the assessment of English literacy. It is not a comprehensive treatment of the major issues; rather, it is a brief synthesis. There are brief discussions of some traditional assessment issues such as reliability, validity, and practicality. Also covered are the types and purposes of literacy assessment and how test results should be used.

There is no discussion of specific test instruments that are or should be used with students with severe to profound hearing impairment. However, some points are made relative to advantages or disadvantages with using certain types of tests. Readers who desire specific information on particular tests, including in-depth descriptions of types of tests, are advised to peruse other sources (e.g., a good discussion can be found in Bradley-Johnson & Evans, 1991; Salvia & Ysseldyke, 1991). A good discussion of reading assessment and deafness can be found in King and Quigley (1985) and of both reading and writing assessment in Luetke-Stahlman and Luckner (1991).

Relative to second-language assessment, the focus of this chapter is on the assessment of English. There is no discussion of assessment on the first language of second-language students, including ASL-using students who are deaf (the main bilingual/bicultural situation discussed in Chapter 6). In the field of second-language learning, much of the research and debate has been on assessing language proficiency, rather than reading and writing skills, and relevant points can be obtained in the following sources (e.g., see discussions in Cummins, 1984; Davies, 1990; McLaughlin, 1985; Verhoeven, 1992). However, there is some debate on the assessment of reading and writing (e.g., see discussions in Bernhardt, 1991; Hamp-Lyons, 1990; Heaton, 1990; Larsen-Freeman, 1991). The assessment issues discussed in this chapter are somewhat similar to those that have been discussed relative to second-language learners (e.g., see examples in Madsen, 1983). The development of assessment in ASL is also in its young stages (e.g., see Bellugi, 1991; Lucas, 1990; Wilcox & Wilcox, 1991).

It is critical for educators to consider their approaches to assessment. It is common to view assessment as administering a series of tests either at the end of instructional sessions or the school year in the form of achievement tests. These summative evaluations provide some information; however, they do not assist the teacher in evaluating particular teaching procedures or in developing programs that suit the individual needs of the students. To be sure, the latter is a time-consuming process—however, it is critical.

Another point to address is the amount of information that can be obtained by the use of assessments. It needs to be emphasized that no matter how comprehensive the tools or procedures, the results of an assessment (i.e., selected tests) can only provide a snapshot of the student's performance. It is not possible for teachers/evaluators to observe all instances of a student's use of language and literacy for a particular assessment period. Consider the following passage (Wray & Medwell, 1991):

This would involve making judgment about each particular language and literacy task—for example, how well the child performed; which aspects of the task were found difficult and which easy; what special strengths and weaknesses there appeared to be; and what the child's attitude was towards the task. Assuming the teacher knew how to assess these things accurately and reliably, this would give a reasonably comprehensive picture of a child's capabilities. There are, however, some problems with this approach, to say the least! It is simply not possible for a teacher to observe and assess every instance of a child's use of language and literacy. These are so integral a part of life that such an attempt would involve careful observation of almost everything the child did. (pp. 201–202)

One of the most important topics discussed in this chapter is the need for reform in assessment (e.g., Garcia & Pearson, 1991; Pearson & Stallman, 1994; Tierney, Carter, & Desai, 1991; Wiggins, 1991). As such, there should be a greater consideration of what can be called alternative measures, which are generally performance-based tools, that is, which seem to be closely related to classroom instruction or the curriculum. The call for the use of alternative measures does not mean the elimination of traditional formal tests, such as standardized tests, nor should we discontinue instruction in the use and interpretation of these measures. Nevertheless, there need to be improvements in current standardized literacy tests, particularly those that have not incorporated emerging views of the literacy process. As is seen in this chapter, assessment is a complex issue and any type of reform is influenced by political, economic, and philosophical pressures (e.g., Pearson & Stallman, 1994).

General Issues of Assessment

Regardless of the type of test used, there is growing evidence that assessment affects instruction, either directly or indirectly. In one sense, this seems to support the view that there should be a strong relationship between assessment and instruction (e.g., Dixon-Krauss, 1996; Lipson & Wixson, 1991). On the other hand, there are explicit dangers. For example, administrators and other educators might make decisions solely for the purpose of improving test scores. This leads to a discussion of direct and indirect effects, and the rendition here is based on the work of Pearson and Stallman (1994).

There are several ways in which assessment can directly affect instruction. The direct effects of assessment is most noticeable in school districts that place an inordinate amount of emphasis on test scores. The author of this text has observed and has heard from others, including specific teachers themselves, that chunks of classroom time are often set aside for the sole purpose of *getting students ready for the achievement test*. In other words, teachers are attempting to teach the test by focusing on similar prototypical test items.

Why is this happening? There are advantages for a school and the community to possess a large number of students with higher test scores. One of the most obvious advantages is the promise of increased financial support and a strong endorsement by prominent members of the community. As indicated in the quote at the beginning of this chapter, even businesses might use the results of high test scores to their advantage. There is also the assumption, mostly accurate, that high scores of students lead to acceptance into highly prestigious universities, and this, in turn, increases the likelihood of a high-paying job or career.

What is often forgotten, however, is that high test scores do not mean that students are well educated. For example, *teaching the test* might lead to the focus on only a narrow portion of the curriculum for developing literacy. This narrow focus might also make it difficult for students to acquire skills that can be generalized to non-test-taking situations. Finally, teaching the test seems to foster the idea that only certain types of information are worthwhile and prestigious; that is, only information that is going to be on the test is really worth knowing. In essence, this condition undermines educators' attempts to help students develop into creative, reflective, and critical thinkers.

Pearson and Stallman (1994) also provided examples of how assessment can affect instruction in an indirect manner. Because of the prestige associated with the results of tests, educators and administrators might make decisions for the purpose of improving students' scores on the test. For example, if there is a perception that a particular basal or other reading series contains items or information that are similar to what will appear on standardized tests, the series will be adopted by the school district. The same principle applies to any other decision regarding curricular and instructional activities, even research activities. That is, the use of certain instructional methods or the permission to do research on certain topics might take place only if school officials are convinced that these activities will result in improved test scores. The foregoing discussion suggests that it is not difficult to imagine that the bulk of educational decisions can evolve around the contents of standardized tests.

The last general issue to discuss here is the need for evaluation and what can be called evaluation research (e.g., see discussions in Hannon, 1995; McLaughlin, 1985). There are a number of views on the notion of evaluation; a few are discussed in the ensuing paragraphs. Much of this discussion is based on the work of Hannon (1995). One view of evaluation is that it is related to the values of education as perceived by educators, parents, and interested others. It is possible to state that literacy is a highly valued goal; that is, most individuals believe that students should learn to read and write well (see related discussion in Chapter 5 of this text). Controversy surrounds the manner in which this goal can be met, for example, the use of bottom-up (or phonics) skills predominantly or the use of top-down (or comprehension) skills. Regardless of the controversy, there needs to be some consensus on how the overall goal of literacy is to be measured.

Probably one of the most important functions of evaluations is to enable educators and parents to make informed decisions. These decisions might be in the areas of the use of instructional materials, the establishment of curricular models, or the selection of certain standardized tests. Parents might need information on whether or not to utilize a specific tutoring program for their children. Related also to this issue is the notion of practicality (see later discussion in this chapter). That is, evaluative procedures are necessary to provide data on costs and benefits of educational innovations or other educational projects. In essence, evaluative research aims for providing information that would be most helpful to practitioners, in our case, literacy practitioners.

Hannon (1995) emphasized that evaluative research is not the same as theoretical research. This confusion is often caused by the use of similar designs and methodologies in both types of research. Theoretical research is driven by the need for developing and refining theories (and models). This type of research might help us to better understand the process of literacy; however, it does not necessarily have immediate practical implications. Hannon (1995) remarked that, "In the long term, good practice does need sound theoretical underpinning but, in the short term, research to advance theory may not be all that helpful practically" (p. 110).

Assessment: Purpose and Use

There are numerous reasons why educators use assessment tools. Relative to literacy, they might want to use scores to place students in a *reading* program or discover the strengths and weaknesses of the student in a particular literacy program. It might be of interest to compare students' achievement levels with those of their age or grade peers. Perhaps, the best reason for conducting an assessment is to use the results to develop a literacy program that meets the individual needs of the student. Within this vein, administering tests, particularly formal and informal tests, is only one part of this plan.

Suffice it to say that the articulation of the purpose of assessment should provide guidelines on what types of tests to use and how to use the results to develop a literacy program for students. The selection of a particular test or even the use of a formal test is influenced by the philosophy (actually metatheory) of the individuals responsible for making these choices (e.g., see discussions in Ritzer, 1991, 1992). For example, individuals who favor a cognitive information-processing framework, specifically interactive theories, are more likely to utilize tests that account for reader-based skills such as prior knowledge and metacognition. Individuals who favor a naturalistic approach, particularly one based on a whole-language philosophy, might argue that formal tests are not reflective of the literacy process. In essence, the best way to measure progress is to use performance-based measures (actually unobtrusive measures) within a classroom setting. Regardless of one's metatheoretical bent, the use of one test or one approach to understanding literacy development might not be sufficient. At the least, the evaluator should consider the use of both formal and informal tests as well as alternative assessment measures.

Another perspective on assessment can be seen in the following points that were stated relative to classroom-based assessment, a form of alternative measure. Although some points seem to be directly related to classroom-based assessment, others can be generalized to different categories such as formal and informal assessment (see discussion in the ensuing sections).

1. *Assessment should reflect the philosophy and content of the curriculum;*
2. *Assessment should be based on a thorough understanding of the task a child is asked to complete;*
3. *Assessment should be varied in both its forms and contexts;*
4. *Assessment should be both reliable and valid;*
5. *Assessment should aim to put the child at ease and hence elicit a 'best' performance;*
6. *Assessment should show strengths as well as weaknesses;*

7. *Assessment should inform the next stage of the teaching process;*
8. *Assessment techniques should relate to the use to which the results are going to be put;*
9. *Record-keeping should reflect both the curriculum and the assessment philosophy of the school. (Brinton, 1986, p. 178)*

A Few Assessment Issues Related to Deafness

It is necessary to consider a few specific assessment issues related to children and adolescents with severe to profound hearing impairment. A number of these issues affect the selection, administering, and scoring of the tests. There are general issues that should be taken into account for any test; for example, it is critical to ascertain whether the test is appropriate for individuals who are deaf. That is, do the characteristics of the students match those of individuals who were part of the norming sample? A good discussion of these issues can be found elsewhere (Anastasi, 1982; Borg & Gall, 1983; Salvia & Ysseldyke, 1991).

Relative to individuals who are deaf, there are certain text-based, task-based, and reader-based issues to consider and be aware of. For example, the performance of these students might be affected by the format of the test, that is, the use of multiple-choice, yes/no, or even cloze procedures (e.g., for a detailed discussion of these problems, see King & Quigley, 1985; Moores, 1987, 1996; Paul & Quigley, 1990). The use of a cloze procedure (omitting every nth word) is particularly problematic. One reason for this is that it requires a knowledge of the English language, particularly syntax and grammar, in order to complete the sentences. This specific knowledge might prevent investigators from obtaining an accurate measure of reading comprehension or writing proficiency. This is not a novel idea; it has been reported previously by Babbini and Quigley (1970), who argued that most achievement tests, including reading achievement tests, were essentially general indices of English language proficiency.

Some of the reader-based (or person-based) variables that are of concern are the strategies that students who are deaf might use during the literacy tasks. For example, it has been observed that students use association strategies or visual matching strategies that are prompted by the wording of the items on the tests (e.g., see discussions in LaSasso, 1985; Wolk & Schildroth, 1984). Examples of visual matching strategies are illustrated in Table 9-1.

Awareness of these strategies might lead to the development of test items that are more appropriate for students with severe to profound impairment. More specifically, students can be shown that their incorrect answers are due to the use of inappropriate or inefficient strategies. A good discussion of the problems of literacy assessment relative to text-based, reader-based, and task-based variables can be found elsewhere (e.g., King and Quigley, 1985; Luetke-Stahlman & Luckner, 1991). In my view, Chapter 7 in the King and Quigley text is still one of the most accurate and comprehensive treatments of these issues in reading assessment and deafness.

The last point to address here is the danger of a predominant or total reliance on paper-and-pencil measures for a complete understanding of the literacy achievement of students

TABLE 9-1   Examples of visual matching strategies used by students who are deaf

Type of Strategy: Response (a) does not contain key words, (b) is within the sentence that contains key words, and (c) is vertically aligned with key words.

Text (sample)

Nature has a similar method for cooling off the body. When little particles of water, called perspiration, are evaporated from the skin, the body is cooled to 98.6 degrees.

Question: What is perspiration composed of?

Answer from student: 98.6 degrees

Type of Strategy: Response (a) does not contain key words, (b) is within the sentence that contains key words, (c) is neither vertically or horizontally aligned with key words, and (d) is within two lines above or below line containing key words.

Text (sample)

Question: How is the eel used by the Indians?

Answer from student: attacks of enemies

Source: Adapted from LaSasso (1985). See also the discussion in King & Quigley (1985).

who are deaf. These types of measures are purported to focus on text-based literacy skills, that is, the students' ability to understand information presented in the printed mode. As discussed in Chapter 5, this can be considered a narrow view of literacy, which might not be appropriate or feasible for a number of students with severe to profound hearing impairment.

What are some problems with this text-based approach? In general, literacy achievement tests require students to read and write their responses. These types of tests demand, at least, proficiency in the language in which the students are supposed to read and write. This is in addition to knowledge of the topics that are used in the literacy passages. In fact, it is possible that students have prior knowledge about a literacy topic, which they are unable to retrieve because of their struggles with the English language on the paper-and-pencil test. In other words, some students may know the answers to questions that are presented to them through speech and/or signs, but this knowledge is evident only if they are permitted to answer the questions in the same expressive, conversational mode (i.e., speech or signs). Students might not be able to demonstrate their knowledge through reading and/or writing as required by literacy standardized tests and other similar assessments. Obviously, this situation is most critical for educational achievement tests with subtests on content areas such as science or social studies. However, a strong case can also be made for tests on literacy, especially on reading tests (see discussions of literate thought and related issues in Chapter 5 of this text).

In essence, it could be argued that the ability of the students to do well on literacy achievement tests is strongly related to their knowledge and use of the English language rather than to their knowledge of the content on the tests. This issue is related also to the ongoing debate on whether students who are deaf should be required to take the same high-school proficiency exams as do typical hearing students or to take special tests designed for them (e.g., see discussion in Bloomquist, 1986). On the other hand, some educators maintain that "it can be argued that achievement tests measure the ability of students to understand information presented at a certain literate level in the majority language of mainstream society" (e.g., see discussion in Paul & Quigley, 1990, p. 16).

Characteristics of Good Assessment Tools

The terms selected here for a brief discussion are norm-referenced, criterion-referenced, reliability, validity, and practicality (for in-depth discussions, see Anastasi, 1982; Salvia & Ysseldyke, 1991). Some issues are important for all assessments, for example, reliability, and some pertain to specific tests, for example, the establishment of norms. These items, including the standardization process, should be discussed in any test-based evaluation report to teachers and parents. Specifically, this evaluation report should also contain the advantages and disadvantages of using objective tests and why a particular test was administered. Finally, there should be sufficient information on the manner in which the score can be interpreted and how the content of the test relates to the curriculum of the school.

Examples of questions for teachers and test administrators to ask in the selection and use of a test are presented in Table 9-2.

TABLE 9-2   Points to consider in the selection and use of a test

Step 1: Background Information

Name of test:
Type (e.g., norm-referenced, criterion-referenced, etc.):
Purpose of test:
Date of publication:
Author(s):
Directions for administration:
Interpretation of results:
Relation to instruction and curriculum:

Step 2: Technical Soundness

Reliability information:
Validity information:
Notes on practicality:
Plan for using the results:

Step 3: Evaluation of Use with Students

Amount of time required:
Attitude of students:
Observation of test-taking situation:
Other notes:

Norm-Referenced and Criterion-Referenced Issues

In discussing formal, and sometimes informal, tests, it is important to understand the nature of the terms, norm-referenced and criterion-referenced. The purpose of norm-referenced tests is to compare a student's score with other similar students at the same grade or age level (Anastasi, 1982; Salvia & Yesseldyke, 1991). These tests are administered to large numbers of representative students across several grade levels. A sufficient number of students are tested so that a table of norms (i.e., standards) can be developed. The average score is a representation of overall achievement, not a particular ability.

The use of grade equivalent scores is not recommended for comparing the performances of students or making decisions about instructional program or placement. Discussing the grade equivalent scores or grade means of students with hearing impairment in the present text was only used to provide readers with a rough idea of the literacy levels of these students. Additional information on grade equivalent scores and other related issues can be found elsewhere (Anastasi, 1982; Salvia & Ysseldyke, 1991).

If a test has been standardized, then there should be a uniform set of procedures used for administering and scoring a test (Anastasi, 1982; Salvia & Ysseldyke, 1991). This is necessary so that scores of different individuals can be compared. In addition to clear directions, it must be ensured that the content of the test is assessing a representative sample of literacy skills in school curricula.

Some remarks should be made relative to the use of norms. Norms indicate that a student's score can be compared to a representative group or sample of students who have taken the same test. As such, the characteristics of the student must be included or similar to the characteristics of the norming sample. Any test norm is restricted to the particular population from which it was derived. It should be underscored that norms should not be considered as absolute or permanent. The characteristics of the student population vary, and this needs to be reflected in the norming sample for the test. At the least, this requires updated editions of the achievement test on a periodic basis.

Criterion-referenced tests focus on the performance of students in a particular area or domain, for example, reading or writing or both. Informal reading inventories represent a good example of a criterion-referenced test (e.g., see discussions in Farr & Carey, 1986; Lipson & Wixson, 1991). The test score reflects the extent to which the student has mastered a particular skill or area of information. The student's score is compared to some arbitrarily defined absolute standard. The student's score is not compared with those of other students. Thus, criterion-referenced tests can be used to illustrate strengths and weaknesses in a particular domain (e.g., Berk, 1980).

It should be highlighted that criterion-referenced tests are constructed according to a set of concepts or skills that relate to a particular theory on the nature of the subject. For example, the Test of Syntactic Abilities (TSA; Quigley, Steinkamp, Power, & Jones, 1978) is considered to be representative of some major syntactic structures of English. The developers of the TSA were influenced by a linguistic theory labeled (at that time) transformational generative grammar (Chomsky, 1957, 1965). The students' mastery scores on a particular syntactic structure indicate their proficiency of that structure, at least at the sentential level.

Reliability, Validity, and Practicality

From one perspective, all types of tests should satisfy the notions of reliability, validity, and practicality. If a test is reliable, then the performances of the students should be consistent (Anastasi, 1982; Borg & Gall, 1983; Salvia & Ysseldyke, 1991). That is, reliability refers to the degree to which a test provides consistent measures of a student's performance. Again, this should be interpreted to apply to any type of measurement, whether formal, informal, or alternative. It might be somewhat difficult to assess the reliability of alternative measures (e.g., portfolios, instruction as assessment, curriculum-based, etc.) because of their qualitative nature. However, there have been attempts to do this so that comparisons can be made (e.g., see discussion in Pearson & Stallman, 1994).

Validity refers to the notion of whether a test measures what it was designed to measure. Differences among the tasks on literacy tests are most likely due to the test developer's views of validity. For example, it might be argued that free recall is a better measure of achievement than the use of multiple choice questions that requires students to select an answer from a list of alternatives (i.e., distractors). Other differences are dependent on the various views of the nature of reading and writing and how test items should be constructed. For example, an individual who ascribes to a bottom-up view of reading would construct a test that would be quite different from one who ascribes to an interactive view of reading. Finally, relative to validity, it is highly recommended that the findings of a test be compared to the findings from other types of situations such as those from classroom or home observations or clinical situations.

The common rendition of reliability and validity is that associated with a discussion of formal and some informal tests. Consider the following examples as a synopsis of some major tenets.

Reliability

- For formal (norm-referenced) tests, the most common procedures are alternate (or parallel) form, test-retest, and internal consistency. The alternate form requires the calculation of a correlation coefficient between the two forms of the same test (see Borg & Gall, 1983; Salvia & Ysseldyke, 1991). Test-retest means that the individuals take the same test again. Internal consistency requires the use of various computation procedures, for example, the use of Cronbach's coefficient alpha.
- For informal and alternative procedures, the commonly used procedures are intrarater and interrater procedures. With intrarater procedures, the evaluator judges two sets of highly similar data after a period of time has elapsed. Interrater procedures refer to the degree of agreement between two or more raters on the same data.

Validity

- Validity should be assessed by comparing the findings of a test with those from clinical and observational settings.
- There are several types of validity—face, content, construct, concurrent, and predictive.
- Face validity refers to the appropriateness of a specific test. For example, using a vocabulary picture test with adolescents is considered inappropriate because the students might have an adverse reaction to this format.

- To determine content validity, the content of one test can be compared with those of other similar tests.
- Construct validity is influenced by an individual's theoretical persuasion. A test is considered to have construct validity if it adheres to a specific theoretical construct.
- Concurrent validity requires the evaluation of one measure against another measure that purports to measure the same variable. This type of validity is often used for the adoption of new assessments. For example, the scores on the new test are compared to those on the older tests, which contain different items but are said to measure the same test behavior.
- Predictive validity reflects the degree to which a measure can predict an individual's performance in a future situation. This type of validity is important for classification purposes, for example, college entrance or selection of a special-education program.

Practicality

One of the most underrated issues in assessment is that of practicality. One of the concerns of practicality is the amount of time required for administering and scoring the test. Admittedly, it is nice to aim for cost-effectiveness and efficiency, but not at the expense of obtaining incomplete information. For example, multiple-choice questions require less time than retellings of stories, or the use of controlled measures can be completed much more quickly than free measures. Nevertheless, free measures, particularly retellings, might provide additional, in-depth information that is not possible with multiple-choice or other objective measures.

Another area of practicality is the need for special arrangements. For example, some individuals test better in quiet settings with no one else present, other than the test monitor. Other individuals might need special adaptations, for example, longer testing period (e.g., students with learning disabilities), alternative response modes (e.g., students with physical disabilities), a room free from visual distractions, or the use of certified interpreters for relating test instructions and directions (e.g., students with hearing impairment). These special arrangements should not impinge on the reliability and validity of the assessment.

Practicality also influences the marketability or usefulness of a test. This needs to be evaluated in relation to the overall purposes and uses of the assessment tools. The use of alternative tools such as classroom observations and curriculum-based procedures should be seriously considered in addition to formal and informal assessments, even though they are labor-intensive and time-consuming to administer, score, and interpret. Nevertheless, the issue of marketability cannot be ignored (e.g., Harrison (1983).

Categories of Literacy Assessment

Reading Assessments

There can be several approaches to take in presenting categories of literacy assessments, particularly reading assessments. The approach developed by King and Quigley (1985) provides a good starting point. They asserted that there are three broad categories: formal, informal, and *unobtrusive measures* (i.e., measures that do not interrupt typical classroom instructional or clinical activities). Instead of unobtrusive measures, the phrase adopted here is alternative measures, which includes unobtrusive measures and combinations of other measures such as curriculum-based and instructional-based assessments. It is also possible to talk about the use of free testing formats (e.g., free recall) and controlled testing formats (e.g., the use of objective tasks involving multiple-choice or forced-choice alternatives). As mentioned previously, the selection of the task or format is dependent upon the metatheoretical views of the test developers. A good discussion of the advantages and disadvantages of free and controlled formats of reading can be found in King and Quigley (1985).

In general, formal tests refer to the group of tests that can be labeled as survey, diagnostic, or achievement. Examples of this type of test used with students with severe to profound hearing impairment include the achievement batteries such as the California Achievement Test (CAT), the Metropolitan Achievement Test (MAT), and the Stanford Achievement Test (SAT). These tests might include subtests of literacy (mostly reading), mathematics, science, and social studies.

The SAT is probably the most widely used achievement test with students with hearing impairment (Allen, 1986; CADs, 1991). An adapted version of this test has been developed by the Center for Assessment and Demographic Studies (CADS). This adapted version has been standardized on students with hearing impairment, considering their special needs, for example, and eliminating inappropriate test items that depend on the use of hearing. Despite a few changes in test administration of some items, the performance of students with hearing impairment can be compared with the norms established for their hearing counterparts on the unadapted version of the SAT (Allen, 1986; Allen, White, & Karchmer, 1983; CADS, 1991).

Some common literacy standardized tools used with hearing students with potential for use with students with hearing impairment can be found in several sources (e.g., Bradley-Johnson & Evans, 1991; Farr & Carey, 1986; King & Quigley, 1985; Lipson & Wixson, 1991; McCormick, 1987; Schirmer, 1994). The above sources also contain a good discussion of the advantages and disadvantages of using these tests.

Informal assessments refer to the use of tests such as the cloze procedures, informal reading inventories (e.g., Informal Reading Inventory [IRI]), Reading Miscue Inventory (RMI), and placement and end of level tests associated with reading series (see King & Quigley, 1985, for a discussion of advantages and disadvantages). Informal reading inventories might be a useful tool for providing some information on the strengths and weaknesses of students with hearing impairment. That is, they can provide some information similar to the more formal diagnostic or criterion-referenced tests (for a detailed discussion of common IRIs and diagnostic assessments, see Farr & Carey, 1986; McCormick, 1987).

Two examples of informal reading inventories are discussed here. The first example can be thought of as a generic example in which the goal is to obtain a level of word recognition (typically from a spoken reading task) and a level of comprehension (e.g., the use of a modified Betts procedure; see discussion in Farr & Carey, 1986). This level can be considered to be the independent reading level. For the word recognition (identification) aspect, a score of 95% or better is needed. For the comprehension aspect, a score of 80% (can be higher) or better is needed. The steps for this procedure follow:

1. Select stories that are about one or two grades below and above the reading level that would be typically associated with the student's chronological age. Additional stories (or short books) can be used as needed.
   a. Select 50- to 100-word passages from the stories.
   b. Ask the student to read one passage silently. Ask about five to six comprehension questions on both literal and inferential levels (see Chapter 7). If the comprehension criterion is met, go to the next step. If the comprehension criterion is not met, go to a lower reading level.
   c. Have the student read the passage again orally (or via signing or both). Compute the word identification level. If the word identification level criterion is not met, go to a lower reading level. For deaf students, the use of a sign is considered acceptable. If the student fingerspells the word, it might be helpful to ask the student to tell you about or describe the word (not define it or use it in a sentence). For further information on this issue, see the discussions in King and Quigley (1985) and Moores (1987, 1996).
   d. The highest place where both criteria (word identification and comprehension) are met is the independent level. If the student does not meet both criteria, start at the level at which the comprehension criterion is met and at which the highest word identification score is obtained.

      The instructional level of the student is the level at which only one criterion has been met, in some cases, the instructional level may span two or three grade levels. The frustration level would be the place where neither criterion was met.

The second example described here is taken from *Silvaroli's Classroom Reading Inventory* (see discussions in Farr & Carey, 1986; McCormick, 1987). Table 9-3 illustrates some items of this inventory (reprinted with permission granted in the workbooks). The steps for this procedure are as follows:

1. Present the graded word lists, starting at the level that matches the child's chronological age or the level that represents the best estimate of the examiner.
2. Tell the child to pronounce (sign, etc.) each word. Encourage the child to try to tell you what the word is, even if she or he cannot pronounce or sign it.
3. Discontinue at the level at which the child mispronounces or indicates she or he does not know five of the 20 words at a particular grade level (75%). Each correct response is worth five points. The examiner is instructed to circle all mispronounced (missigned) words and is informed that corrected errors are acceptable.
4. When the cut-off level has been determined (75%), the oral (or signing) reading level should be started at the highest level in which the student successfully pronounced (or signed) all 20 words in the list.
5. The paragraphs are for estimating the child's independent, instructional, and frustration levels. In addition, the examiner can identify the types of word identification errors (e.g., via miscue analysis; see Chapter 7 and discussion in King & Quigley, 1985) and estimate the comprehension level. Ask the child to read the passage aloud the first time and silently the second time. Reading aloud permits the examiner to evaluate the word identification errors. Before the child reads silently, the examiner should explain that questions will be asked about the passage. The examiner will need to judge the

TABLE 9-3   Examples from Silvaroli's classroom reading inventory

Form A, Part I—Graded Word List (Teacher's Worksheet): A sample

(PP)	(P)	(1)	(2)
1. for	was	many	stood
2. blue	day	painted	climb
3. car	three	feet	isn't
4. to	farming	them	beautiful
5. and	bus	food	waiting

Form A, Part II—Level 1 (43 words)

PLANT SPIDERS

There are all kinds of spiders.
This black and green one is called a plant spider.
A plant spider has small feet.
All spiders have small feet.
Plant spiders live in nests.
They soon learn to hunt for food and build new nests.

Sample Comprehension Questions

1. _____ Is there more than one kind of spider? (Yes—many more)
2. _____ What two things do plant spiders quickly learn? (Hunt for food and build new nests).
3. _____ What color was the spider in this story? (Black and green)

Source: Adapted from discussion in Silvaroli (1990).

adequacy of the responses. Answers in the Teacher Edition are to be used as guidelines or probable answers.

6. The examiner should follow the procedures in the manual for determining the three levels of reading.

Referring to Table 9-3, consider the following example. Suppose the student obtains 100% at the *PP*, *P*, and *1* levels, but obtains 75% at the *2* level for the word recognition task. The student begins reading the paragraph (short story) at the *1* level. The name of the story at this level is Plant Spiders. There are five comprehension questions, and the scoring guide is as follows (see discussion in Silvaroli, 1990):

Scoring Guide: First
    WR Errors   COMP Errors
    IND   0   IND 0-1
    INST   2   INST 1 1/2-2
    FRUST   4+   FRUST 2 1//2 +

    Where WR = word recognition, COMP = comprehension, IND = independent, INST = instruction, and FRUST = frustration. (p. 23)

A description of other common informal tools for reading can be found in the following sources (e.g., Bradley-Johnson & Evans, 1991; Farr & Carey, 1986; King & Quigley, 1985; Lipson & Wixson, 1991; McCormick, 1987; Schirmer, 1994).

Assessments on Writing

Considerations

Prior to discussing the categories of writing assessments, it is important to present some considerations. As stated by Wray and Medwell (1991, p. 213):

1. *An assessment of writing must begin with a consideration of the aims which were originally formulated for this piece of work. The product cannot be judged unless these are taken into account.*
2. *The assessment must also take into consideration the capabilities of the children producing the work. A piece of writing may be good for one child, but well below another's capability.*
3. *The assessment should also focus on the intended audience for the writing, and whether it is appropriate for this audience. The only real way of judging this is for the writing to be given to the intended audience for assessment of whatever kind is feasible.*
4. *Finally the assessment should take into account the context in which the writing was produced, which includes such things as the resources which were available to the child, the kind of help he or she received, and the time which was taken to produce this outcome.*

Consider the following example, which incorporates all four points mentioned above. With respect to point number 1, the fifth-grade class project involved a trip to the zoo and the reading of books on animals in this particular zoo. The assignment was to write an account of the zoo visit and to include a discussion of the types of animals. The teacher encouraged students to brainstorm on what to include in their stories. Some students decided to inform their readers of the history, evolution, and classification of animals. Others focused on the notion of endangered species. Despite the variations, the intentions of the written reports were twofold: (1) to inform readers about certain types of animals, and (2) to encourage actions to be taken to save some animals. The readers of these reports will be students from an adjacent classroom.

With this blueprint in mind, the teacher can evaluate the productions of the students. The general comments of the teacher should focus on whether or not a particular piece of work adhered to the intent of the class project. With respect to point 2 above, the teacher can comment on the specific output of the student writers, and the evaluations might vary according to the capabilities of the students. A student, who rarely writes anything and who produces a one-page paper, which is somewhat stilted but pertinent to the intent of the project, should receive accolades from the teacher. A similar output by a good student and writer is not acceptable. The same evaluation procedure applies to the quality and amount of errors in mechanics. From the first student above, a certain number of errors is acceptable whereas the same quality and quantity of errors from the second student are not acceptable.

The writings of the students in one class are read by students in the adjacent class. The students in the adjacent class provide remarks on the quality of the papers. The focus here is on the papers of the two students in the previous paragraph. For example, it might be commented that neither paper was ready for publication or dissemination to a wider audience; that is, additional work needed to be done on both of them. Students might also comment on whether either paper adhered to the principles as developed by the class for the class project.

With respect to the fourth point, it can be stated that our two student writers had access to similar resources and were subject to the same time constraints. Relative to time constraints, the report had to be written in an 80-minute period on the day after the general class discussion. Both of our students only produced one draft of their reports; neither one wanted to revise their first drafts.

This four-point framework should allow teachers to approach the writing products of students in a differential, individualized manner, attempting to evaluate each student's output relative to the history, attitude, and previous productions of the respective student. This might appear to be a labor-intensive approach, especially when the class size is large. However, it is possible for the teacher to select only a few papers of students to focus on per day.

Types of Assessments

It should be clear here that the reference is to external evaluations of written language, not to students' evaluations of their writing as part of the writing process (also known as self-evaluations). For simplistic purposes, it is possible to divide written language assessments into two broad areas: (1) the focus on specific written language features such as vocabulary and grammar or (2) the use of holistic evaluation schemes based on the total output. The focus on specific features is an indirect measure of written language and is conducted primarily through the use of objective, norm-referenced tests (as discussed previously). Holistic evaluations are considered to be direct measures of writing because they involve a complete writing sample from the students (e.g., see discussions in Hillocks, 1986; Mosenthal, Tamor, & Walmsley, 1983). It is also possible, and desirable, to combine both types in one assessment or to use both types in evaluating students' written language productions.

Advantages and criticisms of indirect, norm-referenced tests are similar to those levied against reading assessments. One benefit is that these tests, particularly those that employ a multiple-choice format, can be administered and scored in an efficient, cost-saving manner. Purportedly, the biases, relating to topic or mode, can be kept to a minimum and, thus, have little influence on the output. For example, students in one school or district might be more familiar with a specific topic or mode and, because of this, are likely to perform better or achieve a higher score on the test. The strongest argument in favor of this type of test is that it can provide a fairly reliable prediction of a student's success with composition. In addition, it is argued that actual writing tests (i.e., use of writing samples) are highly unreliable (see previous discussion of the concept of reliability).

On the contrary, there are a number of criticisms that can be raised here. One of the most serious problems of norm-referenced tests can be labeled as validity (see previous discussion of validity). The passage below by Phelps-Gunn and Phelps-Terasaki (1982) is still applicable today:

. . . objective tests have a serious drawback: validity. They do not directly measure what they directly evaluate: writing. The examination results are used to infer competence, yet the test never elicits nor measures actual writing. Instead, they measure such factors as punctuation, capitalization, mechanics, grammar, or sentence structure. Moreover, objective tests cannot as yet measure the whole composition. Such compositional abilities as unity, coherence, organization, development, focus, support, logic, and clarity do not lend themselves to objective testing. In fact, tests do not tap the very act of writing—generating sentences that are formulated into paragraphs and essays by means of compositional abilities. (p. 245)

Literacy Assessment: Improvements for Formal Tests

A number of problems associated with present literacy assessments, both reading and writing, have been documented in several reviews (e.g., Nystrand & Knapp, 1987; Pearson & Stallman, 1994; Pearson & Valencia, 1986). For example, Pearson and Valencia (1986) argued that the assessments on reading do not match the new, emerging views of the reading process. It has been shown that prior knowledge is an important variable in reading comprehension; however, some of the current assessments continue to use short passages or numerous short topics, which preclude any relationship between prior knowledge and reading comprehension. Consider another example: Asking good questions about the reading selection, as well as answering them, is a good index of expert reading skill. Nevertheless, on assessments, students are rarely required to create or select questions about the selection after reading it. Finally, one more example: As argued by Adams (1990a), skilled readers are fluent, especially with respect to their word identification skills (see also the discussion in Chapter 2). Yet, fluency is rarely considered or measured as a factor in these assessments.

Similar criticisms can also be made on standardized writing assessments. Nevertheless, standardized writing tests can be useful, and it has been argued that this format again is becoming a predominant mode of testing in second-language writing (e.g., Hamp-Lyons, 1990). To improve the quality of standardized reading/writing tests, however, several recommendations need to be implemented:

1. *Test writers should provide adequate context for testing the skills which they seek to measure.*
2. *Tests and sections of tests should require students actually to do what they say they test.*
3. *Tests of genitive skills, such as writing, should reveal and identify the actual errors of the test taker.*
4. *Tests should use actual, not contrived texts, i.e., texts specially composed for the tests.*
5. *In reading, tests should use a range of prose and text types.*
6. *In writing, tests should elicit more than one type of writing sample, on different topics in different genres. (Nystrand & Knapp, 1987, pp. 5–6)*

Alternative Measures

For the purposes of this text, alternative measures refer to the use of unobtrusive measures and others that seem to focus mainly on the improvement of instruction, curriculum, and student's performance in the classroom setting, for example, curriculum-based measures to some extent, ecological assessments (e.g., portfolios), and mediated learning activities (i.e., instruction as assessment). Before discussing the major types of alternative measures in some detail, it should be underscored that one salient aspect of these assessments is (or should be) the gathering and interpretation of the experiences, activities, and perspectives of pertinent individuals in the literacy process: teachers, support personnel, parents, and the readers/writers themselves.

Obviously, collecting this type of information is often perceived as labor intensive, but it is necessary for what is often referred to as a collaborative process between parents and educators/specialists (e.g., see Bigner, 1994; Lambie & Daniels-Mohring, 1993; Turnbull & Turnbull, 1990). At the heart of this process is the gathering of information from parents on the issue of literacy activities and behaviors of their children and adolescents.

It has been argued that the best method for obtaining and interpreting parental views is through the use of structured interviews (e.g., see discussions in Hannon, 1995; Turnbull & Turnbull, 1990). A list of questions can be developed that relates to literacy skills and behaviors. It is probably best for parents to be interviewed by a third person (not teachers) so that both positive and negative comments can be solicited. Parents can be guaranteed anonymity; however, their views should be related to teachers and other professionals. This situation is different from obtaining specific information about their child that will be used for developing and improving literacy programs. Nevertheless, both types of evaluations are necessary.

The critical role of parents in the development of their children's literacy has been reported in several prominent sources (e.g., Adams, 1990a, 1990b; Anderson et al., 1985). As aptly stated by Hannon (1995) on literacy practices in England:

> Since the early 1980s there has been a very significant change in educators' thinking about literacy at home and in school, and of the role of parents in the teaching of literacy. It is now almost inconceivable that there could be a return to school-centered views of literacy as something children only learn as a result of being taught in school, of parents as marginal or even harmful in children's literacy development of direct parental involvement in the teaching process as impracticable and undesirable. We have learned that much literacy—perhaps most—is learned at home, that parents or other family members are central to children's development, that parental exclusion is unjustifiable, and that involvement is feasible, rewarding, and can help meet the goals of schools and families. (pp. 150–151)

Other specific unobtrusive aspects to be included in alternative assessments entail information from student-teacher conferences, lesson plans, instructional records, combination of instruction and assessment within the classroom setting, and, probably the most common measure, systematic observation of classroom situations and, it should be added, systematic observation of home literacy situations (e.g., for readable accounts, see Friend

& Bursuck, 1996, Chapter 8; King & Quigley, 1985, Chapter 7). Unobtrusive measures with a dynamic aspect include the evaluations of conditions under which students can improve their performance (e.g., mediated learning or instruction as assessment). In one sense, there is no limit to their potential; in another sense, one is attempting to help students reach their highest potential (e.g., related discussions in Brown & Campione, 1986; Feuerstein, Rand, & Hoffman, 1979; Feuerstein, Rand, Hoffman, & Miller, 1980; Vygotsky, 1978).

Curriculum-Based Assessment

Curriculum-Based Assessment (CBA) has been touted as one alternative to standardized testing (e.g., Brinton, 1986: Pearson & Stallman, 1994). This type of assessment typically includes informal tests and measures. It is also possible to use an ecological approach (see discussion in next section); in fact, depending on the description, CBA can be considered ecological in nature. In essence, CBA is a form of criterion-referenced assessment in which the curriculum of the school is the standard and the basis for the content of the assessments.

There have been some attempts to standardize CBAs so that comparisons can be made across groups of students within the same school (e.g., see discussions in Kane & Khattri, 1995; Pearson & Stallman, 1994). Nevertheless, the focus is on what students need to know in the classroom setting, and the CBA is defined as a method of assessing that level of achievement (e.g., Blankenship & Lilly, 1981; Tucker, 1985). In one sense, CBA can be related to the dynamic type of unobtrusive measures (i.e., mediated learning or instruction as assessment) because of the relation between instruction (i.e., what is taught) and assessment (i.e., what is tested); however, as mentioned previously, it can include a variety of testing situations within the classroom. In general, students are compared to other students within a class or school, rather than to students in other schools or national norms.

There are several disadvantages of using CBAs. One, test items are often difficult to construct. Two, because of its focus on instructional content, there is a tendency to neglect areas that might not be taught directly, due to lack of emphasis or even lack of time. That is, what's worth testing is what has been taught only. This situation is similar to the narrow focus associated with instruction that is used mainly to teach the content of standardized tests (e.g., see discussions in Kane & Khattri, 1995; Pearson & Stallman, 1994). CBAs focus on skills within an educational setting; thus, these tools might not be adequate for assessing skills needed in real-world contexts. However, it is possible to simulate some real-world activities in a classroom setting. The last disadvantage to mention is the problem of comparing students to other students at the state or national level or to established norms or standards. However, there have been attempts to address this situation (Kane & Khattri, 1995; Pearson & Stallman, 1994).

There are several purposes associated with the use of CBAs; these include identification, establishment of instructional groups, monitoring of student progress, and the planning and evaluation of programs (e.g., Hasbrouck & Tindal, 1992). Fuchs, Fuchs, and Hamlett (1990) have demonstrated how CBAs can be used to improve the quality of instructional programs. As an example, if students are performing better than expected, then there should be attempts to raise the standards or goals. In addition, instructional methods can be compared with the goal of selecting the most effective or best methods.

It should be clear that CBA can be heavily influenced by reductionistic models of teaching and learning (see Chapter 1). This can be seen in the tasks of systematic analyses of the curriculum and the construction of specific assessment formats such as the use of questions and cloze procedures. Finally, as stated by Smith, Polloway, Patton, and Dowdy (1995):

> Although manuals and other resources for developing curriculum-based instruments exist, they serve primarily as guides because instruments used in the classroom should reflect the curriculum being followed in that venue. (p. 47)

Ecological Models

Education and other professions have been influenced by a perspective called system theory. System theory involves the perception that an individual or entity is part of a system and that whatever affects the individual or entity affects the whole system. System theory has been based on the operations of natural, physical systems such as the solar system and the environment.

In referring to children in homes, the model that has been used is called the family system theory (e.g., Bigner, 1994; Lambie & Daniels-Mohring, 1993; Turnbull & Turnbull, 1990). Within the school environment, the concept has lent itself to a sociological (or sociocultural) description of the classroom and school, including the functions and purposes of instruction and assessment. In addition, this concept has influenced the use of more ecologically-valid materials in the assessment process (e.g., Pearson & Valencia, 1986; Pearson & Stallman, 1994).

Within family system theory, a family is not simply a collection of individuals who behave independently of each other. A family needs to be considered from a wholistic perspective, as an entity. Whatever affects one member of the family affects all members. In essence, the family is a social system that has complex rules and interactions. Family system theory provides a framework for understanding how families make decisions, establish and achieve goals, and establish rules for regulating behaviors.

The influence of system theory in literacy can be seen in the development of the whole-language approach (Chapters 1 and 2). Relative to assessment, there has been a tendency to view the students and their academic and social behaviors within the realm of the overall classroom environment. In essence, this means that the selection and use of assessments and the data collected should be undertaken for the purpose of improving and understanding a student's academic and social behaviors within a classroom setting. Thus, the use of ecological assessments emphasizes the classroom setting as one context of the evaluation process.

From another perspective, this should result in a broadening of the assessment process; that is, a move away from the total or predominant reliance on paper-and-pencil, standardized tasks. More importantly, as stated previously, the educator has opportunities for validating the results of the more formal tests. Several strategies have been suggested along these lines (Luckasson et al., 1992), some of which have been mentioned previously:

1. Conduct observations of the student in a variety of natural educational and home settings.
2. Obtain in-depth information from interviews of significant others in the student's life. If possible, interview and/or interact with the student in semi-structured and natural academic and social activities.
3. Collect and peruse case histories, individualized educational plans, teacher reports, and other paperwork on the student (obviously, this needs to be done with parental and/or student permission).
4. Use several types of assessments to collect information on the desired academic and social behavior. Involve other professionals in administering and participating in the assessment process so that findings can be compared.

The above information might be most presentable in a portfolio approach (e.g., Tierney et al., 1991). The portfolio documents literacy progress in an individualized manner. It contains descriptive data, which include samples of writings and recorded observations on reading performance. The portfolio can also include reports, narratives, and checklists, some of which focus on specific skills and strategies that readers and writers have utilized over the specified period of assessment. As with any labor-intensive project, the development of an adequate, useful portfolio requires the implementation of a systematic plan for gathering and recording information (e.g., for a detailed account, see Tierney et al., 1991).

Mediated Learning
To determine conditions for improving students' performance, it might be necessary to use what has been called a dynamic version of the unobtrusive measures. Because of the potentials of these types of tools, this section ends with a brief discussion of one dynamic tool—Vygotsky's zone of proximal development, operationalized as mediated learning and often referred to as instruction as assessment (e.g., Vygotsky, 1978). Vygotsky's model has also been operationalized in a procedure known as the DAP, the Dynamic Assessment Procedure (e.g., Dixon-Krauss, 1996).

The notions of zone of proximal development, mediated learning, learning enrichment, or other learning potential aspects have been motivated by the cognitive-processing movement in the field of intelligence testing (e.g., see Blennerhassett, 1990; Paul & Jackson, 1993). It has also been viewed as the test-teach-test philosophy for both assessment and instructional situations. For example, the instructor/examiner might question the individual about the nature of his or her given responses and provide immediate feedback. There is a retest/reevaluation to see if the feedback and other techniques are effective in improving the performance of the individual (e.g., see discussions in Kragler, 1996; Stanley, 1996).

The dynamic assessment model is heavily influenced by the content of the dialogue between student and teacher. The potential ability/growth of the student is typically assessed by these interactions. As indicated in the previous paragraph, teachers can determine which responses of students are conducive to further learning and which seem to impede learning. The goal is an improvement in the student's learning behaviors.

It should be emphasized that the social dialogues/mediations (i.e., guided social interactions) between teacher and student (and, perhaps, between student and student) are important and must occur often in meaningful classroom situations. This is an evolving process, as described by Kragler (1996):

> Within the zone are varying degrees of adult support. At first, adults may do most of the thinking, reading, or problem solving. As children begin to process and learn the strategies needed to complete the task, the adult support gradually fades. The children begin to be more self-directed and assume more responsibility for the task. Eventually, the transition from other-directed to self-directed behavior is complete, and the students can perform the task without mediation. For example, in reading a new story, at first the adult may need to read most of the text. However, as children start learning the words, they read more of the text until they can read it all without adult support or intervention. (p. 155)

In essence, some of the techniques associated with mediated learning are similar to those discussed in Chapters 7 and 8 on instruction in this text: demonstrations, modeling, scaffolding, and reciprocal teaching. Kragler (1996) has applied these techniques to the areas of vocabulary and comprehension. At present, there is limited literacy research dealing with Vygotsky's zone of proximal development in both children who are deaf and who are hearing. Nevertheless, there seems to be great potential for this type of research with benefits for both reading and writing instruction.

A Final Word

This chapter provided a snapshot of some of the major issues in literacy assessment. There is a great need to utilize alternative assessments in addition to the more formal norm-referenced and criterion-referenced instruments. It is important to reiterate two themes associated with assessment, particularly with assessment and deafness: (1) obtaining complete and useful results for students with hearing impairment is a labor-intensive, time-consuming task, and (2) there should be an interrelationship among theory, assessment, and practice. As argued by Bradley-Johnson and Evans (1991): "An assessment that does not result in improved academic performance by a student experiencing difficulty serves no useful purpose. The assessment process is a means to an end, not an end in itself" (p. 2).

It can be inferred from the statement above that there is a need for reform in assessment. This chapter provided some perceptions on this issue. In essence, much work still needs to be accomplished to convince the general public that there is more to education than obtaining high scores on standardized achievement tests.

In sum, the adoption of alternative measures should not be undertaken without extensive research and analysis. There are a number of questions that should be addressed about both these measures and the issue of assessment reform. For example:

> What knowledge and skills are students expected to demonstrate after a certain period of schooling? What other systemic reforms must be undertaken in order for assessment reforms to be effective? Which assessment formats are most useful for which specific purposes? (Kane & Khattri, 1995 p. 32).

Further Readings

BLOOM, B. (1968). *Learning for mastery. Evaluation comment.* Los Angeles, CA: University of California, Center for the Study of Evaluation.

BERK, R. (Ed.). (1982). *Handbook of methods for detecting test bias.* Baltimore, MD: Johns Hopkins University Press.

COHEN, L., & MANION, L. (1980). *Research methods in education.* London: Croom Helm.

COOPER, P. (1984). *The assessment of writing ability: A review of research.* Research Report 84-12. Princeton, NJ: Educational Testing Service.

RUTH, L., & MURPHY, S. (1988). *Designing writing tasks for the assessment of writing.* Norwood, NJ: Ablex.

SCHOLES, R., & COMLEY, N. (1989). *The practice of writing* (3rd ed.). New York: St. Martin's Press.

Literacy, Literate Thought, and Deafness: A Brief Synthesis

A liberal education . . . frees a man from the prison-house of his class, race, time, place, background, family, and even his nation.   Robert M. Hutchins (in Seldes, 1985, p. 196)

The pleasure and delight of knowledge and learning, it far surpasseth all other in nature . . . We see in all other pleasures there is satiety, and after they are used their verdure departeth; which showeth well they be but the deceits of pleasure, and not pleasure: and that it was the novelty that pleasured, not the quality.   Francis Bacon (in Seldes, 1985, p. 27)

The intent for including the above passages is not to debate the merits of a liberal education or the pursuit of knowledge. Rather, it is to suggest that these two entities can and should become by-products of literate thought. As discussed in this text, literate thought is the ability to think creatively, critically, and reflectively. This can be manifested through the use of the conversational forms of a language (e.g., speech, sign), the written forms (e.g., reading, writing), and other avenues (e.g., computers, mathematics).

The traditional assumption has been that literate thought is facilitated and enhanced by an individual's ability to read and write printed texts. That is, an individual cannot achieve a high level of complex, rational thought without a concomitant development in advanced text-based literacy skills. This assumption is also fueled by the importance of English text-based literacy skills for access to and participation in a scientific, technological society such as the United States.

It is argued here (and elsewhere in this text) that literate thought should be the major goal of the education of children and youth who are deaf. Furthermore, the development of literate thought is not predominantly dependent upon the acquisition of text-based literacy skills. This assertion does not denigrate the importance of English text-based literacy skills nor does it downplay the mainstream value of the development of receptive and expressive skills in the conversational form of the English language (i.e., speech and/or signs).

Nevertheless, educators and scholars have found it difficult to address the question of whether English literacy is a realistic goal or can become an oppressive situation for many students with severe to profound hearing impairment. Obviously, the more difficult challenge is to convince the larger society to broaden its values and standards; this requires, at least, a discussion of ethics from several different philosophical perspectives (e.g., see related discussions in Paul & Ward, 1996; Turnbull & Turnbull, 1990). It might be that educators need to consider this situation from a critical theoretical perspective (e.g., Gibson, 1986).

The aim of this brief final chapter is to provide some reflections and directions concerning the development of literacy and literate thought in children and youth who are deaf. If English text-based literacy is a major, realistic goal, it is argued that educators need to decide if the basic fundamentals of literacy can be developed by students with severe to profound hearing impairment, especially in light of what is known about literacy development and instruction. There is evidence that English text-based literacy seems to be dependent on certain fundamentals, regardless of the literacy framework used: cognitive information processing, naturalism, or social constructionism.

This chapter reemphasizes several issues relative to the development of literacy and literate thought: (1) the interrelations of metatheory, theory, research, and practice; (2) the reciprocal relations between word identification and comprehension and between the conversational and written forms of a phonetic language such as English; and (3) the contributions of a well- and early-developed language to the subsequent development of literate thought. For each issue, the intent is to present in capsule form some general conclusions and implications from the relevant chapters in this text in conjunction with the personal reflections of the present author.

Effects of Metatheory and Metatheorizing

As discussed in this text and elsewhere (e.g., Paul & Jackson, 1993; Paul & Quigley, 1994a; Ritzer, 1991, 1992), the importance and relevance of metatheory and metatheorizing cannot be overemphasized. A metatheory is a way of thinking about a particular discipline. It influences the types of theories developed, the research tools and analyses employed, and the practices followed. Of course, it is a metatheoretical assumption that there *ought to be* an interrelation among theory, research, and practice. Nevertheless, many practitioners and scholars might not often be cognizant of the underpinnings of their practices or research, and they might assume that it is not important to possess such knowledge.

Articulation of a Metatheory

The lack of a metatheoretical awareness makes it difficult for professionals to communicate effectively or to articulate their agreements and disagreements. More importantly, as suggested by the passage by Hutchins at the beginning of this chapter, this indifference to basic assumptions can create a prison or mind-set that precludes the acceptance or understanding of an alternative point of view (e.g., literate thought) as one effective route for some individuals in our society. In addition, most educators and other professionals might not have the resources or tools to reflect on the implications or resolutions of common *either–or* situations in the field of deafness and literacy (e.g., bottom-up or top-down models of reading; ASL or English; text-based literacy or literate thought). There is no intent here to place the blame solely on educators and teachers because there are numerous complex factors that have contributed to this state of affairs, for example, cultural experiences, educational background and training, societal views, and personality factors (e.g., self-esteem, perception of educational career, etc.).

There is little doubt that all professionals in every discipline adhere to certain philosophical views, whether they are aware of or articulate them to others. As aptly remarked by Bunge and Ardila:

> . . . every psychologist *(and educator),* no matter how indifferent or even hostile he or she may feel toward philosophy, cannot help holding some philosophy of mind or other. Whereas in exceptional cases this philosophy may be an outcome of reflections on scientific findings, in most cases it is learned from teachers, colleagues, or publications. (1987, p. 7; emphasis and words added)

In this text, the attempt was to provide information on the major metatheoretical and theoretical views in deafness and literacy. Among the views discussed were reductionism/constructionism, reading-comprehension/literary critical, and clinical/cultural perspectives. These views were related to research and practice. More importantly, it was shown that adherence to a particular view influences markedly the manner in which literacy is defined and whether or not English text-based literacy should be the major goal of schooling and society. For example, if text-based literacy (reading and writing) is the major aim, then scholars and educators will expend the greatest proportion of their time, energy, and resources on discovering and constructing effective methods (perhaps, best methods) for developing skills in reading and writing. That these skills can and should be developed is not always open to debate or question. The major stress is on *how*, not *why* or *what else is comparable.*

By employing metatheorizing as a tool of analysis, it can be inferred that the foregoing discussion has been influenced by a clinical, mainstream view of deafness. This view is not positive or negative; it is simply one view, which happens to be the majority view of most scholars and educators. Conflicts arise when proponents of this view come in contact with proponents of another, seemingly opposing, perspective, the cultural view. The cultural view has been influenced by many forces, for example, the views of DEAF-WORLD proponents (e.g., Lane, Hoffmeister, & Bahan, 1996), the tenets of literary critical theorists, and even the basic principles of social constructivism.

As discussed in Chapters 5 and 6, these *cultural critical* influences have led to the questioning of the feasibility of English literacy skills for all individuals with severe to profound hearing impairment, especially for those who have struggled with obtaining proficiency in this mode for the majority of their formal school years. With a focus on questions such as, Whose interests are being served? or Whose values are being promoted? buttressed by a deep discussion of terms such as oppression and empowerment, the establishment of absolute, often narrow, standards for all individuals has been and should continue to be debated. As a result of these debates, we have gained, at least, a better understanding of the importance and influence of the early development of a bona fide first language, particularly its conversational form (speaking or signing), on the subsequent development of other areas such as cognition, psychosocial development, and literacy.

In this text, several points were made on the importance of metatheorizing in literacy and deafness. The one that needs to be highlighted here is the dearth of research in the field of deafness. A number of scholars have commented on the little available research on deafness and issues in language and literacy development, particularly the assessment of methods and materials (e.g., King & Quigley, 1985; Moores, 1987, 1996; Paul & Quigley, 1994a). Admittedly, these remarks have been stated mostly within a particular framework, namely, cognitive information processing, which has dominated research on deafness. Research within the purviews of naturalism and social constructionism is in its infancy (e.g., see Lemley, 1993; Williams, 1994; Williams & McLean, 1996).

Emerging Literacy Research Thrusts

There seem to be two, emerging, literacy research thrusts. One is focused on the development of *deafness* models/theories of literacy, and the other is on showing that there are qualitative similarities between the literacy development of hearing children and children who are deaf, necessitating the prudent use of existing, mainstream theories. Both of these research thrusts are critical, although the latter one is more advanced and well-developed. The former thrust assumes either that the literacy development of students who are deaf is pervasively different from that of hearing students or needs to be approached differently. For example, there might be a need to either bypass or explicate phonology by placing a stronger emphasis on the development of morphology or on the development of top-down, comprehension processes (see discussions in Chapters 6 & 7).

It has become necessary to utilize the theoretical and research results from the literature on hearing children in conjunction with the little existing research on children who are deaf to obtain a better understanding of the problems of literacy and deafness. This approach can also be gleaned from the research on children with disabilities in other special-education programs, especially within the purview of cognitive information-processing theories of literacy (e.g., Lipson & Wixson, 1991). This does not mean that mainstream theories should be applied indiscriminately; however, these theories do provide a strong starting point for understanding the so-called literacy problems of children with disabilities, including children who are deaf (e.g., see discussion in Paul & Jackson, 1993; for another perspective see Gliedman & Roth, 1980).

Despite the predominance of the cognitive information-processing perspective, it is not sufficient for a complete understanding of literacy and deafness, or for understanding literacy with other children (e.g., McCarthey & Raphael, 1992; see also the discussion in Chapter 4 on written language in this text). The same, however, can be said for naturalism and socialconstructivism. Perhaps a worthy endeavor for theorists and researchers is to develop models that incorporate the overlapping tenets of these major frameworks.

There is another view, as stated aptly by McCarthey and Raphael:

The three theories can work together to build a picture of the converging processes of reading and writing. The information processing lens focuses on questions related to the components of writing and reading, relationships among the components, effects of one process on the other, expert/novice and good/poor reader differences, and the structure of knowledge. The lens of the naturalist theory focuses on questions related to the type of environment that facilitates and supports reading and writing, issues in creating child-centered curricula, and children's underlying cognitive structures. Finally, social-constructivist theories focus our attention on the issues of the social origins of reading and writing, emergent literacy (including connections between oral and written language), the developmental priorities of reading, writing, and oral language, how language and literacy tools have been used historically and across cultures, and how children learn to use literacy in unique and personal ways. (1992, pp. 25–26)

Teachability of Literacy

One of the most critical issues for educators and scholars to address is the teachability of literacy. This issue is not only related to one's metatheory, but, also, it seems to be affected by the principles of the Matthews effect: the rich (i.e., good readers/writers) get richer and the poor (i.e., poor readers/writers) become poorer or stay the same (e.g., see discussion in Stanovich, 1986). Despite our best instructional efforts, most children with severe to profound hearing impairment do not reach functional literacy levels (e.g., fourth-, fifth-, or sixth-grade levels). From one perspective, the response has been either to develop more effective instructional methods or to reframe the notion of instruction itself (see discussion in Chapter 1 on reductionism and constructionism). This has led to debates on what is teachable in literacy or what is the role of the *teacher* in a classroom setting.

As an example, Pearson and Johnson (1978) have articulated three views on the teachability of comprehension:

At the one extreme, there is a position that contends that in teaching reading, we can only teach word identification processes. After that it is up to native intelligence and experience to aid children in understanding what we have taught them to read. A middle position argues that while we may not be able to teach comprehension per se, we can arrange instructional and practice conditions in such a way as to increase the likelihood that children will understand what they read. Then there are those, ourselves included, who contend that comprehension can be taught directly—that we can model comprehension processes for students, provide cues to help them understand what they are reading, guide discussions to help children know what they know, ask pointed, penetrating, or directional questions, offer feedback (both informational and reinforcing) at the appropriate time, and generate useful independent practice activities. (p. 4)

If the notion of teachability is accepted as plausible, then instructional practices should adhere to the basic principles of salient theories and metatheories. Although atheoretical practices have some value, these practices cannot become the norm because of the difficulty in understanding or evaluating them. In addition, in order to have *effective practices*, there is a need to improve teacher-education programs with a focus on literacy, especially for teachers who want to work with children who are deaf. Many preservice teachers of children and adolescents who are deaf still take only one or two courses in literacy at the university level (e.g., see discussions in King & Quigley, 1985; Paul & Quigley, 1990; Moores, 1987, 1996). It is difficult for teachers to be creative and effective with their instruction and materials when they have had few educational courses in literacy.

More importantly, not only must our practices be evaluated periodically, but, also, our goals need to be assessed on an ongoing basis. The legitimacy of English text-based literacy for all students who are deaf needs to be evaluated in light of the persistent low achievement levels, which, according to some scholars, have not changed much since the inception of standardized testing (e.g., see historical review and synthesis in Quigley & Paul, 1986). To understand some possible reasons for this condition, any assessment should take into consideration the reciprocal relationship between the conversational and written forms of the English language, the topic of the ensuing section.

Reciprocal Relation Between Conversational and Written Forms

To address whether English literacy is a realistic goal for students with hearing impairment, it is important to focus on the reciprocal relations between (1) word identification and comprehension, and (2) the conversational and written forms of the same language. It seems that realistic expectations of literacy are dependent upon the extent to which these reciprocal relations can be established. It should be clear that both of these reciprocal relations are influenced pervasively by the conceptual framework of reading-comprehension models (see Chapters 1 and 2). Proponents are interested mostly in the manner in which children and adolescents acquire literacy skills and why some of them have difficulty. The goal is to improve the literacy levels; indeed, it is assumed that it is possible to develop the literacy skills of most individuals up to a reasonable level.

Assumptions and Implications of Reciprocity Across Models

Despite the differences within and across cognitive information-processing theories of literacy, it is reasonable to assume that a working knowledge of the language of print (i.e., conversational English) is critical during emerging and later development of text-based literacy skills. This working knowledge refers to, at least, an intuitive cognitive awareness of the components of a language, namely, phonology, morphology, syntax, semantics (i.e., meaning in language), and pragmatics (i.e., use of the language). Also important is an understanding of the culture (e.g., world knowledge, school knowledge) related to the language and knowledge of topics that individuals are required to address and read about in print. It is also possible to find proponents of naturalism and social constructionism in agreement with the gist of the foregoing discussion.

Whether these skills, particularly language skills, can and should be taught, especially in a reductionist manner, is open to debate. There seems to be little debate that they are present in proficient readers and writers. Can students with severe to profound hearing impairment access the conversational form of a spoken language? Can they develop a sufficient level of proficiency in this form so that it can be used in a reciprocal manner with text-based skills? Can deaf students develop this level of reciprocity at an early age?

From one perspective, it should be asked whether students with hearing impairment can develop adequate word identification skills. This seems to be a necessary step for the reciprocal relation between word identification and comprehension. More importantly, this relation is dependent on the overall reciprocal relation between the conversational and written forms of the language (discussed previously), which is activated by the association between phonology and orthography (e.g., Brady & Shankweiler, 1991; Templeton & Bear, 1992).

Regardless of the theoretical underpinnings, there seems to be sufficient evidence that students with hearing impairment, and other students, need to understand the connection between the phonemes of speech of a phonetic language and the graphemes of print, especially for a language such as English. There needs to be an awareness that English speech can be segmented into phonemes (e.g., vowels and consonants) and that these are represented by an alphabetic orthography. Again, whether this information needs to be taught directly or can be assimilated indirectly through interactions with print is a separate issue.

How critical is this situation for students who are deaf and other students? As concluded by Adams (1990b):

> Skillful reading depends uncompromisingly upon thorough familiarity with individual letters, words, and frequent spelling patterns. Only to the extent that we have developed such familiarity can the written word flow effortlessly from print to meaning. Moreover, insufficient familiarity with the spellings and spelling-to-sound correspondences of frequent words and syllables may be the single most common source of reading difficulties.
>
> What are the prerequisites to acquiring such knowledge? Children should embark on reading instruction with solid visual knowledge of the letters of the alphabet. They must also have a broad, general appreciation of the nature of print—how it is formatted; that its basic meaningful units are specific, speakable words; and that its words are comprised of letters. And they should have a sense of its various functions and its potential personal use. We know that familiarity with individual letters and familiarity with the nature of written text are strong predictors of the ease with which young children will learn to read. (p. 115)

Reciprocity and the Use of a Phonological Code

It was argued in Chapter 3 that fluent word reading is influenced by a reader-based factor, namely, the use of a phonological code in short-term memory. The use of this type of code allows the reader who is deaf (and other types of readers) to expend more time and energy on higher-level comprehension processes. Even more interesting is the fact that there is an interrelationship among reading comprehension, the use of a phonological code, and short-term memory. This interrelationship documents strongly the importance of a deep knowledge of the alphabetic principle, which is dependent upon the development of the phonological and morphological properties of English.

These assertions are mainly within the purview of cognitive information-processing theories of literacy. However, it is my opinion that these assertions are fundamental; the findings of research within the conceptual frameworks of naturalism and social constructionism will not alter them, only refine them. In addition, these assertions force us to inquire about the accessibility of phonology and morphology by many students with severe to profound hearing impairment. This, in turn, compels us either to develop better techniques to promote this accessibility or to question the legitimacy of developing high-level text-based English literacy skills in all of these students.

Reciprocity and Second-Language Learning

It is becoming clear that the link between the conversational and written forms of English is also critical for students learning English as a second language (see Chapter 6). This is, indeed, a surprising—perhaps unacceptable—finding, even for most proponents of ASL/English bilingual programs. Perhaps the best recourse is to develop *deafness* theories of literacy, as mentioned previously. However, it might be more productive in the short term to conduct further research that shows the deep reasoning and logical abilities of literate thinkers who are deaf, many of whom do not have the ability to read and write English well.

Although it is possible for second-language learners to learn about the English culture for the purposes of reading and writing through the use of their native language, there is no compelling evidence that these students can achieve a high level of literacy along this route. Exposure to the print of a phonetic language with explanations in another language (spoken or signed) is simply not sufficient or efficient (see discussion in Chapter 6). This process precludes a reciprocal relationship that can and should exist between the conversational and written forms of the same language. Thus, in most cases, individuals need to learn to manipulate the conversational form of the language of print, especially a phonetic language such as English. Perhaps, reading-comprehension proponents need to develop more effective instructional methods to assist students who are deaf, and other poor readers and writers, in learning the connections between the phonemes of speech and the graphemes of print.

Should there be a limit or restriction on the time line for applying the reading-comprehension models with the sole, dominant focus on developing English text-based literacy skills? For example, if a students has not developed adequate reading/writing skills by—say—13 years of age, should we proceed with an alternative route? Should we think about this issue earlier, perhaps during the early childhood years (e.g., from birth to 8 years old)? Perhaps, as implied by the discussion in this section and elsewhere, there is a need for a better understanding of how to develop a bridge from proficiency in ASL to proficiency in English (e.g., see discussions in Drasgow & Paul, 1995; Luetke-Stahlman & Luckner, 1991; Paul & Quigley, 1994a, 1994b). Perhaps, there should be additional research on the aspects of using a visual language with children and youth who are deaf (e.g., see discussion in Gaustad, 1986).

Literacy, Literate Thought, and Deafness: A Final Word

Most educators, indeed, most people in mainstream society, believe that the reading-comprehension framework is the only acceptable model of literacy and literate thought. That is, the focus should be on developing the ability to read and write English at a high literate level.

In this text, it has been demonstrated that many students who are deaf begin their formal education with little knowledge of any social-conventional language. With our predominant emphasis on English language and literacy, educators and scholars might encounter situations in which many students who are deaf have acquired low levels of proficiency in English by the time they graduate from high school. It might be wondered if professionals in the field of deafness have failed to understand the growing research on the advantages of possessing a bona fide first language system at as early an age as possible (see related discussions in Lane et al., 1996; Paul & Quigley, 1994a). In addition, as many teachers of students who are deaf have wondered, how is it possible to teach or interact on a deep, meaningful level with school subjects such as science and social studies if you are working with students who possess neither communicative proficiency nor academic proficiency in the language of instruction or the language of print?

These concerns provide support for considering another group of models: literary critical. In addition, it can be inferred that there should be periodic evaluations of strongly-articulated goals such as the development of English language and English text-based literacy skills. The periodic evaluations should include the progress of students attempting to answer complex, academic questions or performing complex tasks in both the conversational mode and/or the printed mode of *any* language.

As elaborated in Chapter 5, literate thought is dependent upon the acquisition of a first language (especially the conversational form) at as early an age as possible. This should be the major concern for establishing and implementing ASL/English bilingual programs. The goal of acquiring English as a second language is an important, albeit secondary goal, and one that might not be realized for a large number of students with severe to profound hearing impairment.

In essence, there is little question that English text-based literacy is a critical educational goal for success in school and society. Nevertheless, educators and parents might need to decide if and when this goal, by itself, becomes unrealistic for a particular child with hearing impairment. The development of a first language at as early an age as possible should be of paramount importance. This is essential for the subsequent development in all other areas, including the development of literate thought.

It should be underscored that this situation should not be construed as an *either–or* one, that is, text-based literacy or literate thought. Given what we know about paradigms, it is not the case of one being better than the other. It is a matter of choice and that choice is driven by a myriad of factors that are and should be considered, for example, society's values, parental and student values, student's interests and needs, and the length of time in school required to develop certain skills.

Educators need to deal with the implications of developing instructional practices that adhere to either the reading-comprehension or literary-critical framework or both. They need also to understand the underpinnings of their practices and views in order to resolve or manage conflicts that are certain to arise when two different paradigms clash. At the very least, of course, there needs to be a better understanding of effective practices in both literacy and literate thought. Some possible general, research questions include the following:

- Because of the importance of the relationship between the conversational and secondary modes of English, what needs to be done to improve understanding of conversational English for students who are deaf (i.e., speech and/or signs)?
- How can we improve the word identification skills of students who are deaf so that these can be used in a reciprocal relationship with existing comprehension skills?
- What can be suggested to develop better metacognitive and other higher-level comprehension skills?
- How can we enrich the literacy education training of both preservice and inservice teachers?
- What do we know about the relationship between motivation and skilled reading and writing in students who are deaf?
- Given the importance of early literacy development, how can we foster and enhance the emerging literacy skills of children who are deaf?
- What is the relationship between text-based literacy skills and literate thought in children and youth who are deaf?

The above questions do not represent an exhaustive, comprehensive list; however, they do address some of the major areas in literacy and deafness.

Finally, as most teachers and practitioners know, it is counterproductive to espouse one literacy philosophy or perspective for *all* of these children and youth. Perhaps the focus should be not on finding the best or most effective method for all children but on possible literacy techniques to use with each child in an interactive, custom-made manner. In light of the abundance of *either–or* paradigms that exist in literacy and deafness, I would hope that educators and other professionals see the need to create a deeper paradigm or a composite paradigm—one that focuses on the development of critical, logical, and reflective thinking, and this should be the ultimate educational goal for all students who are deaf, indeed for *all* students.

Further Readings

HEDLEY, C., ANTONACCI, P., & RABINOWITZ, M. (Eds.). (1995). *Thinking and literacy: The mind at work.* Hillsdale, NJ: Erlbaum.

KELLY, E. (1971). *Philosophical perspectives in special education.* Columbus, OH: Merrill.

POSTMAN, N. (1995). *The end of education: Redefining the value of school.* New York: Knopf.

RAWLS, J. (1971). *A theory of justice.* Cambridge, MA: Harvard University Press.

Comprehension Questions and Challenge Questions

Chapter 1: Introduction to Literacy and Deafness

Comprehension Questions

1. How is *metaanalysis* described in this chapter? Discuss the three major reasons, mentioned in the chapter, for conducting metaanalyses in the field of literacy or that of literacy and deafness.

2. One of the major literacy perspectives is labeled the reading-comprehension framework (or metatheory). What are the interests and foci of theorists and researchers within this framework?

3. It is possible to categorize reading-comprehension theories into three broad groups. Describe the salient characteristics of each group briefly and include some remarks about metatheoretical underpinnings. (*Note:* More detailed descriptions of the groups are provided in Chapter 2.)

4. Another major perspective (or metatheory) is called the literary critical framework. This perspective is based on critical theory. What are some salient tenets of critical theorists? How are the skills of reading and writing viewed within this framework?

5. What is literate thought? How is it related to the use of text-based reading and writing skills?

6. In this chapter, two broad aspects of writing are discussed: product and process. Describe the major characteristics of the two aspects. According to the author, which aspect has dominated the research on deafness and writing?

7. According to the chapter, what are some (five are listed) questions regarding the use of American Sign Language and English in a bilingual or second-language learning program?

8. Why is it important to address the question of whether similarities and/or differences exist between first- and second-language acquisition of English?

9. In this chapter, there is a brief description of two world-views for theorizing, research, and instruction: reductionism and constructivism. Describe the major characteristics of each view and relate each view to the two major literacy frameworks, reading-comprehension and literary criticism.

10. It is stated in the chapter that there are two broad dichotomous paradigms or perspectives in the field of deafness: clinical and cultural. Describe each paradigm briefly and show its relation to the development of literacy in individuals who are deaf.

11. What are some major points (e.g., general research findings, interpretations of general findings, etc.) in the section providing a brief overview of literacy achievement and deafness?

Challenge Questions

1. In the chapter, there is a brief discussion of types of metaanalyses, for example, meta-data-analysis and translative research. Select a prominent journal in the field of deafness (e.g., *American Annals of the Deaf, Journal of Deaf Studies and Deaf Education, Sign Language Studies,* and *Volta Review*), and peruse all the articles (i.e., research) for the most recent year (i.e., 1994, 1995, 1996). How many of the research studies are examples of metaanalyses? (*Note:* Most likely, the article might be an integrative review article.) Do the authors of these articles list specific research questions similar to the use of the scientific method as described briefly in the chapter? Is it clear how the authors selected their research studies for analysis?

2. This activity is similar to the first except that the focus should be on categorizing articles as being examples of either the reading-comprehension framework or the literary critical framework. Was it possible to categorize articles as examples of both frameworks? Was it possible to determine whether a research or instructional study within the reading-comprehension framework is an example of a specific model, that is, bottom-up, top-down, or interactive? Do some studies use aspects from more than one model? (You might want to read Chapter 2 of this text for an additional perspective; in addition, there are some references listed for each model in that chapter in the reference section of this text.)

3. In the chapter, there is a brief discussion of whether similarities and/or differences exist between first- and second-language acquisition of English. Is this discussion related to the issue of whether there is a psychology of deafness? Why or why not? (A perspective on this issue can be found in Paul & Jackson, 1993, listed in the reference section of this text.)

4. Metatheorizing is a form of metaanalysis. What is metatheorizing? What are some salient types and their characteristics? What is the relationship between metatheorizing and theorizing? (Additional information can be found in Ritzer, 1991, 1992, listed in the reference section of this text.)

5. How are the following terms similar or different to each other: Metatheory, theory, paradigm, conceptual framework, and philosophy? (Additional information can be found in Paul & Jackson, 1993 and Ritzer, 1991, 1992, listed in the reference section of this text.)

Chapter 2: Reading-Comprehension Perspective: Theories and Research on Hearing Students

Comprehension Questions
1. In this chapter, it is stated that the differences among reading-comprehension theories can be seen in the treatment of two concepts (or components). What are these two components? What is the purported relationship between the two components?
2. Describe briefly the concept of *model*. How is this concept related to the concept of theory?
3. Describe the major tenets of prototypical bottom-up theories of reading. Describe some implications for instruction. Be sure to provide some instructional examples *similar* to the ones illustrated in the chapter.
4. Describe the major tenets of prototypal top-down theories of reading. Describe some implications for instruction. Provide some instructional examples that are *similar* to the ones presented in the chapter.
5. Describe the major principles of interactive theories of reading. What are some implications for instruction? Be sure to provide some instructional examples.
6. What are some major criticisms of each group (bottom-up, top-down, and interactive) of reading-comprehension models?
7. In the section on *Word Identification,* three questions were posed: (1) What is word identification? (2) What process is involved for accessing a word (i.e., lexical access)? and (3) What does research offer relative to instruction (i.e., focus on word identification strategies such as phonics, structural analysis, etc.)? What information does the section offer relative to these three broad questions? (*Note:* Discuss briefly the author's perspectives on these questions in this section. For example, for the first question, you should discuss the various interpretations of the term word identification and also, the meaning of word-identification *skills*.)
8. Describe briefly the two responses to the question, What does it mean to know a word? (*Note:* See quote by Beck and McKeown (1991).) Which response seems to hold the most promise for improving vocabulary instruction? Why?
9. Describe briefly the three major hypotheses that have been proffered to explain the relationship between vocabulary knowledge and reading comprehension. What are some instructional implications, if any, of each hypothesis?
10. Describe briefly the two general kinds of learning from context: deliberate and incidental.
11. Describe briefly the major findings from studies on the learning of words during reading (i.e., context) either via deliberate learning or via incidental learning. What are the effects of vocabulary instruction on the learning of words? (*Note:* Focus on one general finding at a time and discuss qualifications if necessary. For example, learning

words from context does occur, and it occurs in small increments. If learning from context does occur . . .). How does the author feel about the either–or situation of vocabulary versus the use of context? According to the chapter what should the goals of vocabulary research studies be?

12. Describe the following terms:
    a. Prior knowledge
    b. Passage-specific prior knowledge
    c. Topic-specific prior knowledge
    d. Metacognition

13. Why is prior knowledge important for reading comprehension? Why is metacognition important for reading comprehension? (*Note:* You can summarize the research on these two major aspects.) Which of these two aspects refers to students' comprehension of the text (i.e., text comprehension)? Which refers to improving students' ability to comprehend the text (i.e., comprehension ability)? (*Note:* It is difficult to separate these two aspects of comprehension. One refers to attempts to help children comprehend more of the text, e.g., use of summarizing, pre-story questions and discussion, use of semantic elaboration techniques, and the other refers to the development and improvement of specific strategies to improve comprehension ability, for example, self-monitoring activities such as asking comprehension questions, rereading sections, use of strategies to answer specific types of questions, etc.)

Challenge Questions

1. Assuming that both word identification and comprehension are important, do you think that it is possible to *teach* these skills? Do these skills need to be taught or can they be acquired during actual reading situations with no intervention by the teacher? Why or why not? What does the word *teach* mean to you? Should literacy be taught? Why or why not?

2. The development, assessment, and even understanding of a particular model need to be undertaken within a scientific framework, which is typically a metatheoretical framework. Why is a metatheoretical framework important? (For additional information, see Ritzer, 1991, 1992, listed in the reference section of this text.)

3. Consider the following statement: ". . . deep and thorough knowledge of letters, spelling patterns, and words, and of the phonological translations of all three, are of inescapable importance to both skillful reading and its acquisition" (Adams, 1990a, p. 416; listed in the reference section of this text). What does it mean to have a deep and thorough knowledge of these entities? Provide some examples. (A good source is Adams, 1990a.)

4. In general, it can be inferred from the chapter that research syntheses do not support an either/or dichotomy relative to the teaching of reading and/or writing. Select examples in the field of deafness concerning the teaching of language, particularly conversational English skills, for example, spoken and/or signed language. Do you think the natural versus structural language-teaching approaches dichotomy is justified? Why or why not?

5. Should the use of literacy instructional practices be based on theory and research? Why or why not? Select several common literacy practices in your area and see if you can describe the metatheoretical and theoretical underpinnings.

Chapter 3: Reading-Comprehension Perspective: Research on Students Who Are Deaf

Comprehension Questions

1. The answer to the question posed by Hanson (1989), "Is reading different for deaf individuals?" has pervasive implications for the instruction and assessment of reading (and writing) for students with severe to profound hearing impairment. Discuss the dual nature of her answer: *yes* and *no*. (*Note:* That is, what are the implications if the answer is *yes* or if the answer is *no*.)

2. In the chapter, it was stated that prior to the 1970s, at least three observations (general statements) can be made about the nature of reading research and deafness. List the three observations.

3. The major findings of the research of Pintner have not changed dramatically since the inception of the studies (early 1900s). List the four findings delineated in the chapter.

4. Pintner attributed his findings to two salient variables. Discuss the variables and include the qualifications from later research studies and analyses.

5. In addition to documenting the low achievement levels of students who are deaf, Babbini and Quigley observed that there were high intercorrelations among all subtests of the *Stanford Achievement Test*. What were the significance and the effects of this finding?

6. The findings of national surveys should be interpreted with caution because they tend to obscure the performances of select subgroups within the population of students with hearing impairment. According to the chapter, what contributes to the superior performance of these students? How can this superior performance be interpreted? That is, how can it be interpreted within a particular theoretical framework?

7. What are text-based variables?

8. There have been several studies on deaf students' knowledge of words and word meanings. At least three major thrusts of this research can be identified. Describe the three thrusts and provide some research findings in each area by discussing one or two studies and their results. (*Note:* This information can be located in the section entitled *Word Knowledge.*)

9. The research on syntax has provided insights and debates on a number of issues; only a few major issues were examined in this chapter. Describe briefly the two major issues. Discuss one study (i.e., results and implications) for each issue. (*Note:* For example, the work of Quigley [see review in Paul & Quigley, 1994], Ewoldt [1981], McGill-Franzen & Gormley [1980], and Nolen & Wilbur [1985] are associated with one of the two issues.)

10. What are reader-based variables, including those often associated with students with hearing impairment?

11. Relative to prior knowledge and metacognition, describe the major findings of the studies conducted by Strassman (1992) and Yamashita (1992).

12. A review of the literature reveals three major generalizations, at least, with regard to the effects of the English-based signed systems on the development of literacy. What are these generalizations, according to the chapter?

13. In the section on *Internal Mediating Systems,* the purpose was fourfold: to describe briefly (1) the nature of the coding strategies used by individuals who are deaf; (2) the

reason why the use of a phonological-based code is important for reading; (3) the case for the qualitative similarity of literacy; and (4) the relation of the development of a phonological-based code to literacy instruction. Discuss the salient conclusions for each area as presented in this section of the chapter.

Challenge Questions

1. Accept the assertion that knowledge of the sound system is important for developing good literacy skills. If the use of phonics is unrealistic for most students with severe to profound hearing impairment, what are some comparable, alternative strategies that might be used to develop morphophonological awareness in students who are deaf? Provide some specific examples of these strategies. (*Note:* Some ideas can be gleaned from texts such as Adams (1990a, 1990b) and Johnson & Pearson (1984), listed in the reference section of this text.)

2. Observe several classrooms in your district and describe the theoretical underpinnings (i.e., reading-comprehension or literary critical) of the literacy instructional approaches used. If the school adheres to a reading-comprehension model, is it solely or completely bottom-up, top-down, or interactive, or is it some combination of these approaches? Do combinations of approaches require a refinement of the typical model? Why or why not?

3. In the chapter, it is mentioned that many students with severe to profound hearing impairment could be labeled as functionally illiterate. What is functional illiteracy? Does it refer to a specific reading grade level of text-based materials? Is this a fixed, unchanging level? Is this level relative to the culture in which one resides? Was functional illiteracy in the early 1900s the same level as it is now? (*Note:* For another perspective on this issue, see the discussion in Chapter 5.)

4. What is morphology? Derivational morphology? Inflectional morphology? Be sure to provide some examples. What is the relationship of morphology to phonology? To syntax? Is knowledge of morphology important for developing high-level literacy skills? Why or why not?

5. Assume that a working knowledge of the alphabetic code is necessary for beginning reading and for reaching a high-level of literacy. What does this knowledge entail? Does it mean an understanding of phonics generalizations? Does it mean simply the knowledge of letter-sound relationships? (For some information, see Adams [1990a, 1990b] and Shankweiler & Liberman [1989], listed in the reference section of this text.)

Chapter 4: The Development of Writing

Comprehension Questions

1. In this chapter, it is stated that there is a marked influence of the knowledge level of the individual on the development of literacy skills. Hillocks (1986) differentiated four major types of knowledge. Describe these four types:
   a. declarative knowledge of substance
   b. procedural knowledge of substance

      c. declarative knowledge of form

      d. procedural knowledge of form

2. How are reading and writing viewed within the following frameworks: cognitive information-processing theories, naturalistic theories, and social-constructionist theories?

3. Cognitive information-processing theorists are interested in delineating and studying subprocesses of writing. Describe the following subprocesses: planning, composing (also translating), and revising (also reviewing).

4. List three major concerns with both cognitive information-processing and naturalistic theories. What is the major concern with social-constructionist theories?

5. List some of the major findings of research studies with hearing individuals conducted within the purviews of cognitive information-processing, naturalistic, and social constructionist theories.

6. According to the chapter, at least two major themes can be inferred from the research synthesis on the written language of students who are deaf, particularly a synthesis of the most recent research. What are these two themes?

7. Relative to students who are deaf, the chapter delineated four major problems associated with the use of their written language samples. Describe these problems.

8. The research on deafness and writing was presented relative to three broad areas: traditional/structural, transformational generative grammar, and the process approach. Provide a brief description of the major findings within each area, using the following information as guidelines:

    A. traditional/structural

      1. Discuss the focus on products rather than process.

      2. Discuss results relative to productivity, sentence complexity, and types of errors reported.

    B. transformational generative grammar

      1. Describe results relative to the use of morphological rules.

      2. Discuss results relative to the use of transformational rules.

    C. Process approach

      1. Describe results of the focus on the intersentential level (e.g., the works of Gormley & Sarachan-Deily and Wilbur).

      2. Discuss the focus on revision (e.g., the work of Livingston).

      3. Describe some results of children's response to literature (i.e., reader-response focus as in the work of Williams).

9. Describe free-response and controlled-response measures.

10. Ruddell and Haggard (1985) have proposed research needs with respect to hearing students. These areas are also deemed important for students who are deaf. Discuss the six major areas for further research needs.

Challenge Questions

1. Research on writing (and reading) can be categorized within one or more of the three major frameworks: cognitive information processing, naturalism, and social constructionism. Peruse research studies in one of the major journals in the field of deafness (See Challenge Questions in Chapter 1 of Appendix A.) and see if you can place the studies within one or more of the three major frameworks. If a study does not fit into any specified framework, try to provide some reasons for this lack of fit.

2. According to the chapter, naturalistic theorists emphasize the reciprocal relationship between oral and written language, and the oral aspect has referred to the spoken component of a language. What is the nature of this reciprocal relationship? Is it described in a similar manner by cognitive information-processing theorists? Why or why not? Is this oral-literacy (reading-writing) reciprocity the same as the sign-literacy one? Why or why not? (*Note:* For information on the two groups of theories and the reciprocity principle see references cited in this chapter. For some information on the comparison of the oral-literacy and sign-literacy reciprocity, see Chapter 6 of this text.)

3. Solicit impromptu written language samples of students in your district who are deaf (i.e., students with severe to profound hearing impairment). Compare the samples with those illustrated in the chapter. Can you describe similarities or differences? (*Note:* You might want to use some of the techniques described in the chapter for soliciting the samples or you can ask the classroom teacher to assist you.)

4. One of the prominent process theories of writing is reader-response theory. Describe the major tenets of this theory and its metatheoretical underpinnings. Are these theorists concerned with the improvement of reading and writing? Why or why not?

5. Research needs for hearing individuals have been proposed by Ruddell & Haggard (1985). The author of the text has argued that these are also important areas for individuals who are deaf. Peruse research studies in one of the major journals in the field of deafness (See Challenge Questions in Chapter 1 of Appendix A.), and see if you can place that research within one of the six areas delineated by Ruddell & Haggard.

Chapter 5: Literary Critical Perspectives

Comprehension Questions

1. There are three modes of inquiry—empirical, interpretative, and critical. Which of these three modes is considered "scientific"? Which of the three modes is concerned with issues such as empowerment, enlightenment, and emancipation?

2. What is critical theory? Why is it a reaction against the positivistic and objective assumptions of the scientific method?

3. Describe the following terms: enlightenment, emancipation, and instrumental rationality. What examples did the author provide on enlightenment issues in the field of deafness? (*Note:* This refers to the uncovering of the interests of certain individuals or groups.)

4. In dealing with the question, What does it mean to read?, the author preferred "One possible interpretation (a traditional one) is to argue that there are levels of literacy . . . Given the fact that a high-level of literacy is difficult, a plausible goal for most students with severe to profound hearing impairment is functional literacy, and reading the newspaper is one manifestation of this goal." Discuss the problems associated with this interpretation. Include also in your discussion the description and implication of illiteracy from the chapter.

5. According to critical theories, is literature, especially great literature, important for high thought? Why or why not? (*Note:* Discuss the common-sense view and critical theorists' reactions to this view. Be sure to include the notion of having knowledge of these texts, that is, knowledge of the contents of great literature.)

6. What does the author mean by the assertion that there is a significant, reciprocal relationship between the conversational (i.e., speech) and written forms of the same language?

7. Provide a summary of the discussion on the relationship between literate thought and text-based materials. Are literacy skills essential for the development of the ability to engage in critical and reflective thought? Give examples from the chapter to support or refute this assertion. (*Note:* Be sure to include the discussion on the complexity of oral or conversational forms as compared to the written forms.)

8. The last section of the chapter attempted to relate the two macro paradigms of deafness, clinical and cultural, to the two broad perspectives on literacy and deafness: reading comprehension and literary critical.

Describe the major points of this section. (*Note:* Discuss how the tenets of each literacy perspective, reading comprehension and literary critical, are similar to or different from the tenets of the two macro paradigms, clinical and cultural. Also include a discussion of instructional practices.)

Challenge Questions

1. How do you think critical theorists would address issues such as the establishment and use of educational standards (e.g., proficiency exams for high-school students, statewide certification testing for teachers, etc.) and the adoption of curricula (e.g., who decides the content of subjects such as science, history, etc.)?

2. In this chapter, the author provided a few examples of the concept of enlightenment in the field of deafness. Can you think of other examples? Discuss the relevance of emancipation and instrumental rationality in the field of deafness and areas such as English language development and English literacy development.

3. The chapter briefly addressed the following questions: (1) Is it cost efficient to duplicate everything that is already available in print; that is, to present all information in several forms—print, video and/or audio recordings, Braille, and sign? If there are bilingual programs, does that mean all information has to be duplicated via translation into the home language of the students? (2) Is literate thought, without text-based literacy skills, sufficient for participation in a scientific, technological society such as the United States?

What are your opinions/feelings on the above questions? (*Note:* You might want to do a literature review or conduct interviews with professionals to obtain additional information.)

4. The last section of the chapter attempted to relate the two macro paradigms of deafness, clinical and cultural, to the two broad perspectives on literacy and deafness: reading comprehension and literary critical.

Can you relate the two macro paradigms to other areas of deaf education, for example, language development and psychosocial development? (Some discussion of this issue can be found in Paul & Jackson 1993, listed in the reference section of the text.)

Chapter 6: Second-Language Literacy

Comprehension Questions

1. Based on the discussion of the quote at the beginning of the chapter, what are the three major issues in the development of English as a second language in students who are deaf?

2. For the purposes of this chapter, how is bilingualism described or defined? Why is bilingualism difficult to define?

3. Describe briefly the following terms:
    a. communicative proficiency
    b. academic proficiency
    c. simultaneous acquisition of two languages
    d. successive acquisition of two languages

4. Describe the major tenets of the:
    a. balance theory
    b. threshold model
    c. developmental interdependence model
    d. interlanguage
    e. vernacular advantage model
    f. direct approach

5. Grabe (1988) discussed five major standard constraints associated with typical second-language learners. What are they?

6. Discuss and synthesize the research on both students who are deaf and those who are hearing relative to the following question, Is the development of English as a first language (i.e., L1) similar to the development of English as a second language (i.e., L2)? That is, do hearing or deaf second-language learners of English proceed through stages, make errors, or use strategies that are similar to those of native first-language learners of English?

7. According to the chapter, what are the major points to be made about the "effects of ASL on the subsequent development of English?"

8. Describe the following terms:
    a. majority-language and minority-language student
    b. language shift, maintenance, and enrichment
    c. L2 submersion; L2 monolingual immersion; L2 bilingual immersion; L1 bilingual immersion: Which of the above programs are supported by research as being effective for minority-language students?
    d. the notion of transfer

9. The author remarked that many ASL/English bilingual proponents have misinterpreted the notion of transfer, particularly because of their predominant focus on the works of Cummins and Vygotsky. What are the author's criticisms relative to this focus?

Challenge Questions

1. This chapter presented evidence that, in general, L1 is similar to L2. Some theorists/researchers believe that this is a gross oversimplification of the issue. Conduct a literature review and compile a list of the arguments against this generalization. (*Note:*

You might want to focus on the notions of individual differences and interference in your review.)

2. In the chapter, there is a brief discussion of the differences between ASL and the English-based signed systems. Provide a more detailed discussion of the differences between these two entities. (*Note:* Some information can be obtained in Paul & Quigley, 1990, 1994a; Wilbur, 1987, listed in the reference section of this text.) Why is this issue important for the development and implementation of ASL/English bilingual programs?

3. Obtain a complete description of Cummins' models (threshold and interdependence models described in 1984). Do you agree with the author on the feasibility of these models for understanding second-language literacy and deafness? (*Note:* Another good discussion of Cummins' models can be found in Meyer & Wells, 1996.)

4. What do you think are the literacy instructional implications for the following theories/models:
   a. balance theory
   b. developmental interdependence model
      (*Note:* As indicated in the chapter, these models are not necessarily literacy models; however, it is still possible to derive instructional practices. In fact, many ASL/English bilingual programs have been influenced by Cummins' developmental interdependence model.)

5. Conduct a review of the literature and interview relevant professionals to gather information on this question posed near the end of the chapter, Is it possible to determine if and when a child should be encouraged to learn a spoken or signed language based on his or her processing abilities?

Chapter 7: Instruction and First-Language Literacy

Comprehension Questions

1. The intent of the chapter was to provide instructional examples that could be related to one of the three broad literacy conceptual frameworks; cognitive information processing, naturalism, and social constructionism. However, the authors made four points relative to this issue. Discuss the four points.

2. What are the authors' major points with regard to the teachability/learnability issue?

3. What are some general instructional issues for teachers of students with hearing impairment?

4. Describe the major points in the section on letter-sound association.

5. What are the authors' major arguments for the use of a morphographic approach with students who are deaf?

6. List at least three guidelines for teachers in making decisions on the selection of vocabulary words for a particular story.

7. What do the authors mean by "higher-level comprehension skills"? Describe the various skills that were discussed in the chapter.

8. List at least five guidelines for teachers to consider in the development of comprehension activities.

9. List and describe the five stages of writing.

Challenge Questions

1. Should practice be grounded in theory? Why or why not? Review the literature and select about 10 to 15 instructional studies on literacy and deafness. Is it possible to state the theoretical persuasion of the authors of the articles? Why or why not?

2. The teachability/learnability issue has also been debated relative to language acquisition. Perform a review of the literature and summarize the major points of the debate.

3. The authors argued that morphology is a reasonable substitute for phonics in the decoding process. Conduct a review of the literature and summarize the major points regarding the interchangeability of phonics and morphology or structural analysis. Do the authors of the chapter have widespread support on this issue? Why or why not?

4. Select three stories and develop activities that focus on the following features:
   a. question-answer relationships
   b. metacognitive skills
   c. figurative language

Chapter 8: Instruction and Second-Language Literacy

Comprehension Questions

1. This chapter reiterates two major points from Chapter 6. These are second-language students are dependent on their first-language skills, particularly their first-language literacy skills, and there needs to be a reciprocal relationship between the conversational and written forms of the same language. Elaborate on these two points; that is, provide some additional information that was also discussed in the chapter. (*Note:* The additional information can be found in the same section that contains these two broad points.)

2. According to the authors, some researchers/program developers might have failed to consider the two points in question 1. What might have been the effects of overlooking these issues?

3. What are some major points that were emphasized relative to the selection of the students and teachers for an ASL/English bilingual program?

4. It was argued that the language-teaching approach of individuals is pervasively influenced by their position with regard to the similarity/difference hypothesis. What does this mean?

5. According to the chapter, individualized instruction can be conceptualized in several ways. Describe the three ways that were presented.

6. In the section on ASL and the Visual Modality, the authors attempted to provide an understanding of how modality can influence linguistic expression and how aspects of the visual mode are and can be used to heighten clarity in the communication of people who are deaf. Discuss the authors' main points in:

   The use of space
   Modulation of signs
   Nonverbal aspects of sign
   Simultaneity

7. Why do the authors think that multiple readings are very important?
8. In the section on Visual Techniques for Teaching English Structures, select a construction (e.g., direct and indirect object, passive voice, progressive and indicative verbs) and state the authors' main points.
9. If ASL is to be developed as a first language, then all instructional activities and materials need to be presented and conducted via the use of American Sign Language. What does this mean? Why did the authors feel that "it is important to emphasize (this) visual component" of American Sign Language?
10. Developing the conversational form of English via the use of signed systems is considered to be problematic. Discuss briefly some of the problems mentioned in the chapter.

Challenge Questions

1. The notion of transfer skills has traditionally been an intense area of debate. Peruse the literature and report examples of specific transfer skills for hearing second-language learners of English literacy. Do you agree with the authors that the notion of transfer does not specifically apply to the learning of English literacy skills by ASL students? Why or why not? Can you support your points with information from your literature review? (*Note:* This question is concerned with the beneficial effects of transfer skills, not the interference effects.)
2. Consider the following scenario as true. Suppose there is a shortage of ASL/English teachers who are Deaf (i.e., culturally Deaf) because of difficulty in passing the national teacher examinations. This situation is due mostly to the Deaf participants' difficulty with the use of English on the exam, not to the knowledge of concepts. These Deaf participants are, however, proficient in the use of ASL. How can or should this situation be remedied? Is this an oppressive situation for these Deaf participants (e.g., see Chapter 5)? Why or why not?
3. Many of the instructional techniques in this chapter are influenced by the authors' position with regard to the similarity/difference hypothesis, that is, L2 is developmentally similar to L1. Review the literature and provide examples of instructional strategies that seem to follow the principle that L2 is not the same as L1. Do the authors of the strategies provide theoretical or research support for their instructional techniques?
4. The chapter illustrated a lengthy lesson dealing with a multimeaning vocabulary word—bank. Develop similar lessons, including a class discussion protocol, for the following multimeaning words: *bat*, *check*, and *run*. Share your lessons with your classmates and your teacher.

Chapter 9: Literacy Assessment: Selected Issues

Comprehension Questions

1. According to the passage by Wray and Medwell (1991, pp. 201–202), what can teachers/practitioners expect with regard to the results of an assessment on language and literacy?

2. Describe the direct and indirect results of assessment (particularly the use of standardized assessments) on instructional and curricular issues. Use the work of Pearson and Stallman (1994) as a guide.
3. Discuss the author's point(s) with regard to "the danger of a predominant or total reliance on paper-and-pencil measures" for students who are deaf.
4. Discuss the characteristics of norm-referenced and criterion-referenced tests.
5. Describe the following terms and provide some major characteristics of each one:
    a. reliability
    b. validity
    c. practicality
6. According to the author, what are the three categories of assessments? Describe and provide examples of each category.
7. Written language assessments can be divided into two areas. Describe and list some advantages and disadvantages of each area.
8. What are some recommendations for improving both reading and writing tests?
9. Describe the following terms:
    a. classroom-based assessment
    b. ecological model
    c. mediated learning assessment

Challenge Questions

1. Pearson and Stallman (1994) argue that high scores on standardized tests do not result in a highly-educated student. Conduct interviews with school personnel in your area. What are their opinions on this issue? How do they think this situation can be remedied?
2. Do you think that the minimum proficiency tests for high-school students need to include additional formats? For example, in addition to a literacy format (reading and writing), should students be able to provide responses orally (or via the use of signs)? Why or why not? Conduct a review of the literature and summarize the research on this issue.
3. The science and social studies subtests of the SAT for hearing-impaired students might not be appropriate because of reliability and validity problems. Conduct a review of the literature and summarize the discussion on this issue. What are some solutions?
4. In one sense, the dynamic mediated learning assessment is a reaction against the use of *static* paper-and-pencil assessment of, for example, reading and writing. Why is this the case? Does this have to be set up as an either–or situation? Why or why not? (Some information can be obtained in Dixon-Krauss (1996), located in the reference section of the text.)

Chapter 10: Literacy, Literate Thought, and Deafness: A Brief Synthesis

Comprehension Questions

1. According to the author, what are two problems associated with a lack of metatheoretical perspectives on the part of educators and scholars?
2. Describe the two emerging literacy research thrusts.

3. According to the passage by McCarthey and Raphael (1992, pp. 25–26), how can the three literacy theories (cognitive information processing, naturalism, and social constructionism) "work together to build a picture of the converging processes of reading and writing?"

4. Discuss the three views of Pearson and Johnson (1978) with regard to the teachability of reading comprehension.

5. Describe what is meant by the reciprocity between (a) word identification and comprehension and (b) the conversational and written forms of the same language.

6. List at least three critical points in the passage by Adams (1990b, p. 115)?

7. According to the chapter, is the link between the conversational and written forms of English critical for students learning English as a second language? Why or why not?

8. What are some of the author's arguments in support of the idea that educators should also wear literary critical glasses?

9. What are some of the author's arguments in support of literate thought being the ultimate goal for students who are deaf?

Challenge Questions

1. In this chapter, two emerging literacy research thrusts were discussed briefly. Conduct a review of the literature and provide examples of research that can be placed into one or both thrusts. Are there other research thrusts that can be identified from your review?

2. The passage by McCarthey and Raphael (1992, pp. 25–26) seems to suggest that the three literacy theories (cognitive information processing, naturalism, and social constructionism) can work together to provide a better understanding of literacy. Based on your understanding of these three theories, what are some general implications for instruction and assessment that would be common across all three theories? (*Note:* The chapter by McCarthey and Raphael, 1992, is a good starting point for answering this question. See complete citation in the reference of this text.)

3. What does the phrase, the teachability of literacy, mean to you? (*Note:* Reread the three views on the teachability of reading comprehension by Pearson and Johnson (1978) for some additional information.) What is your position on this issue? Can your position be related to a particular theory of literacy as discussed in the text? (Some additional points with regard to teachability and learnability can be found in Paul & Quigley, 1994a and Quigley & Paul, 1994; complete citations in the references of this text.)

4. Do you think it is possible to read phonetic languages such as English and French without having a reciprocity between the conversational and written forms? That is, can students learn to read and write at high literate levels in English without manipulating the conversational form (either via speaking or signing). Support your answer with both theoretical and research evidence. (For some insights, good references are Adams, 1990a and Bernhardt, 1991.)

5. What are your opinions with regard to the following questions raised in this chapter: (a) Should there be a limit or restriction on the time line for wearing reading-comprehension glasses with the sole, dominant focus on developing English text-based literacy skills? (b) Will this heavy emphasis on English text-based literacy preclude or impede the development of high-level cognitive skills? (c) What happens if we are unsuccessful after 12 to 15 years of literacy instruction for students who are deaf?

Suggested Books and Materials for Children and Adolescents

In addition to the books and materials listed below, other recommended books are those that have won the Caldecott Medal, the John Newbery Medal, the Coretta Scott King Award, and the Jane Addams Children's Book Award. Suggested materials and methods for deaf children and adolescents can also be found in Appendix B of King and Quigley (1985; citation in the reference of this text). This is a comprehensive list.

Wordless Books and Almost Wordless Books: A Selection

Carle, E. (1973). *I see a song.* New York: Crowell.

DePaola, T. (1981). *The hunter and the animals.* New York: Holiday House.

Goodall, J. (1988). *Little Red Riding Hood.* New York: McElderry.

Krahn, F. (1974). *The self-made snowman.* New York: Lippincott.

Krahn, F. (1977). *The mystery of the giant footprints.* New York: Dutton.

Mayer, M. (1969). *Frog goes to dinner.* New York: Dial.

McCully, E. (1988). *New baby.* New York: Harper & Row.

Ormerod, J. (1982). *Moonlight.* New York: Lothrop, Lee, & Shepard.

Prater, J. (1986). *Gift.* New York: Viking.

Spier, P. (1988). *Rain.* New York: Doubleday.

Turk, H. (1987). *Bon appetit.* Natick, MA: Picture Book Studio.

Turke, H. (1987). *Chocolate Max.* Natick, MA: Picture Book Studio.

Winter, P. (1976). *The bear and the fly.* New York: Crown.

A Few Books Involving the Alphabet

Arnosky, J. *Mouse writing.* New York: Harcourt Brace Jovanovich.

Base, G. (1986). *Animalia.* New York: Viking/Kestrel.

Bayer, J. (1984). *A my name is Alice.* New York: Dial.

Bridwell, N. (1983). *Clifford's ABC.* New York: Scholastic.

Chess, V. (1969). *Alfred's alphabet walk.* New York: Greenwillow.

Domanska, J. (1973). *Little red hen.* New York: Macmillan.

Duke, K. (1983). *The guinea pig ABC.* New York: Dutton.

Eichenberg, F. (1952). *Ape in a cage: An alphabet of odd animals.* San Diego, CA: Harcourt, Brace, & World.

Elting, M., & Folsom, M. (1980). *Q is for duck.* New York: Clarion.

Farber, N. (1975). *As I was crossing Boston Common.* New York: Dutton.

Feelings, M., & Feelings, T. (1974). *Jambo means hello: A Swahili alphabet book.* New York: Dial.

Fisher, L. (1978). *Alphabet art: Thirteen ABC's from around the world.* New York: Scholastic.

Fujikawa, G. (1974). *A to Z picture book.* New York: Grosset & Dunlap.

Garten, J. (1964). *The alphabet tale.* New York: Random House.

Harrison, T. (1982). *A northern alphabet.* Plattsburg, NY: Tundra.

Hawkins, C., & Hawkins, J. (1983). *Pat the cat.* New York: Putnam.

Hawkins, C., & Hawkins, J. (1988). *Zug the bug.* New York: Putnam.

Hoban, T. (1982). *A, B, see!* New York: Greenwillow.

Hoguet, S. (1983). *I unpacked my grandmother's trunk.* New York: Dutton.

Kellogg, S. (1987). *Aster aardvark's alphabet adventures.* New York: Morrow.

Kitchen, B. (1984). *Animal alphabet.* New York: Dial.

Isadora, R. (1983). *City seen from A to Z.* New York: Greenwillow.

Langoulant, A. (1989). *A prize for Percival.* Milwaukee, WI: Gareth Stevens's Children's Books.

Larcher, J. (1976). *Fantastic alphabet: 24 original alphabet.* New York: Dover.

Lobel, A. (1977). *Mouse soup.* New York: Harper.

Obligado, L. (1983). *Faint frogs feeling feverish: And other terrifically tantalizing tongue twisters.* New York: Viking.

Pearson, T. (1986). *A apple pie.* New York: Dial.

Pigeen, S. (1985). *Eat your peas, Louise.* Chicago, IL: Children's Press.

Rosenblaum, R. (1986). *The airplane ABC.* New York: Atheneum.

Ruben, P. (1976). *Apples to zippers.* New York: Doubleday.

Schermer, J. (1979). *Mouse in house.* Boston: Houghton Mifflin.

Schwartz, A. (1980). *Ten copycats in a boat and other riddles.* New York: Harper.

Seuss, Dr. (1958). *Cat in the hat comes back.* New York: Beginner.

Seuss, Dr. (1965). *Fox in socks.* New York: Beginner.

Sloane, E. (1963). *The ABC book of early Americana.* New York: Doubleday.

Stove, R. (1975). *Because a little bug went ka-choo!* New York: Beginner.

Van Allsburg, C. (1987). *The Z was zapped.* New York: Houghton Mifflin.

Winder, J. (1979). *Who's new at the zoo?* New York: Aro.

Yolen, J. (1979). *All in the woodland early.* New York: Collins.

Zion, G. (1960). *Harry and the lady next door.* New York: Harper.

Some Predictable Books

Ahlberg, J. (1979). *Each peach pear plum.* New York: Viking.

Barrett, J. (1980). *Animals should definitely not act like people.* New York: Atheneum.

Barrett, J. (1983). *A snake is totally tail.* New York: Atheneum.

Becker, J. (1985). *Seven little rabbits.* New York: Scholastic.

Berenstain, S., & Berenstain, J. (1970). *Old hat new hat.* New York: Random House.

Bishop, C. (1938). *Five Chinese brothers.* New York: G. P. Putnam's Sons.

Brown, M. (1947). *Goodnight moon.* New York: Harper & Row.

Brown, M. (1949). *The important book.* New York: Harper & Row.

Brown, M. (1957). *The three billy goats gruff.* New York: Harcourt Brace Jovanovich.

Carle, E. (1975). *The mixed up chameleon.* New York: Crowell.

Carle, E. (1977). *The grouchy ladybug.* New York: Crowell.

Carle, E. (1987). *Have you seen my cat?* New York: Picture Book Studio.

Carle, E. (1989). *The very busy spider.* New York: G. P. Putnam's Sons.

Child, L. (1975). *Over the river and through the woods.* New York: Scholastic.

Christelow, E. (1989). *Five little monkeys jumping on the bed.* New York: Clarion.

De Regniers, B. (1990). *Jack and the beanstalk.* New York: Aladdin/Macmillan.

Elting, M. (1980). *Q is for duck.* New York: Clarion.

Emberley, E. (1974). *Klippity klop.* Boston: Little, Brown.

Galdone, P. (1968). *Henny Penny.* New York: Scholastic.

Galdone, P. (1970). *The three little pigs.* New York: Seabury Press.

Galdone, P. (1972). *The three bears.* New York: Scholastic.

Galdone, P. (1984). *The teeny tiny woman.* New York: Clarion.

Ginsburg, M. (1981). *Where does the sun go at night?* New York: Greenwillow.

Hutchins, P. (1968). *Rosie's walk.* New York: Macmillan.

Hutchins, P. (1972). *Good-night owl.* New York: Macmillan.

Kellogg, S. (1985). *Chicken little.* New York: Morrow.

Krauss, R. (1952). *A hole is to dig.* New York: Harper & Row.

Langstaff, J. (1955). *Frog went a-courtin'.* New York: Harcourt Brace Jovanovich.

Lobel, A. (1979). *A treeful of pigs.* New York: Greenwillow.

Martin, B., Jr. (1986). *Barn dance.* New York: Holt.

Martin, B., Jr. (1989). *Chicka chicka boom boom.* New York: Simon & Schuster.

Nodset, J. (1963). *Who took the farmer's hat?* New York: Scholastic.

Peppe, R. (1970). *The house that Jack built.* New York: Delacorte.

Quackenbush, R. (1973). *She'll be comin' round the mountain.* Philadelphia: Lippincott.

Raffi. (1988). *The wheels on the bus.* New York: Random House.

Sendak, M. (1963). *Where the wild things are.* New York: Scholastic.

Seuss, Dr. (1960). *Green eggs and ham.* New York: Random House.

Seuss, Dr. (1968). *The foot book.* New York: Random House.

Silverstein, S. (1983). *Who wants a cheap rhinoceros?* New York: Macmillan.

Wildsmith, B. (1987). *All fall down.* Toronto, Canada: Oxford University Press.

Williams, B. (1977). *Never hit a porcupine.* New York: Dutton.

Zolotow, C. (1958). *Do you know what I'll do?* New York: Harper & Row.

Emerging and Beginning Literacy Books: A Sample

Ackerman, K. (1988). *Song and dance man.* New York: Knopf.

Alexander, M. (1969). *Blackboard bear.* New York: Dial.

Andersen, H. C. (1979). *The emperor's new clothes.* Boston: Houghton Mifflin.

Baylor, B. (1974). *Everybody needs a rock.* New York: Scribner's.

Bonsall, C. (1980). *Who's afraid of the dark?* New York: Harper & Row.

Brown, M. (1976). *Once a mouse.* New York: Scribner's.

Browne, A. (1983). *Willy the wimp.* New York: Knopf.

Cherry, L. (1990). *The great kapok tree.* New York: Harcourt Brace Jovanovich.

Cohen, B. (1983). *Molly's pilgrim.* New York: Lothrop, Lee & Shepard.

Cohen, M. (1985). *Liar, liar, pants on fire!* New York: Greenwillow.

Coie, J. (1986). *The magic school bus at the waterworks.* New York: Scholastic.

Cole, J. (1989). *The magic school bus: Inside the human body.* New York: Scholastic.

Crews, D. (1978). *Freight train.* New York: Greenwillow.

DePaola, T. (1980). *Now one foot, now the other.* New York: G. P. Putnam's Sons.

Fatio, L. (1986). *The happy lion.* New York: Scholastic.

Fox, M. (1989). *Koala Lou.* New York: Harcourt Brace Jovanovich.

Gag, W. (1928). *Millions of cats.* New York: Coward, McCann & Geoghegan.

Greenfield, E. (1979). *Grandma's joy.* New York: Collins.

Hawthorne, N. (1959). *The golden touch.* New York: McGraw-Hill.

Hoban, L. (1981). *Arthur's funny money.* New York: Harper & Row.

Kessler, L. (1966). *Kick, pass, and run.* New York: Harper & Row.

Lee, D. (1974). *Alligator pie.* New York: Macmillan.

Lindgren, A. (1950). *Pippi Longstocking.* New York: Viking.

Shulevitz, U. (1967). *One Monday morning.* New York: Scribner's.

Surat, M. (1983). *Angel child, dragon child.* New York: Raintree.

Westcott, N. (1989). *Skip to my Lou.* New York: Little, Brown.

White, E. B. (1952). *Charlotte's web.* New York: Harper & Row.

Williams, M. *The velveteen rabbit.* New York: Holt.

Yolen, J. (1987). *Owl moon.* New York: Philomel.

Zemach, H. (1990). *It could always be worse.* New York: Farrar, Straus & Giroux.

A Selection of Additional Reading Books

Aardema, V. (1975). *Why mosquitoes buzz in people's ears: A west African folk tale.* New York: Dial.

Arthur, R. (1964). *The secret of Terror Castle.* New York: Random House.

Baker, O. (1981). *Where the buffaloes begin.* New York: Warne.

Blume, J. (1971). *Freckle juice.* New York: Dell.

Blume, J. (1972). *Tales of a fourth grade nothing.* New York: Dutton.

Brown, D. (1979). *Teepee tales of the American Indians.* New York: Holt.

Bunting, E. (1991). *The wall.* New York: Clarion.

Cameron, E. (1980). *Beyond silence.* New York: Dutton.

Carroll, L. (1985). *Jabberwocky.* Niles, IL: Whitman.

Cleaver, V., & Cleaver, B. (1969). *Where the lilies bloom.* Philadelaphia: J. B. Lippincott.

Collier, J. (1974). *My brother Sam is dead.* New York: Four Winds Press.

Cooney, B. (1983). *Miss Rumphius.* New York: Viking.

Corcoran, B. (1986). *I am the universe.* New York: Atheneum.

Coville, B. (1989). *My teacher is an alien.* New York: Minstel Books.

Douglass, B. (1982). *Good as new.* New York: Lothrop.

Esbensen, B. (1984). *Cold stars and fireflies.* New York: Crowell.

Fisher, A. (1960). *Going barefoot.* New York: Crowell.

Gag, W. (1928). *Millions of cats.* New York: Coward.

George, J. C. (1959). *My side of the mountain.* New York: Dutton.

Gwynne, F. (1970). *The king who rained.* New York: Windmill Books.

Hautzig, E. (1968). *Endless steppe: A girl in exile.* New York: Crowell.

Hill, E. (1967). *Evan's corner.* New York: Holt, Rinehart, & Winston.

Hoban, J. (1989). *Quick chick.* New York: Dutton.

Hoban, R. (1960). *Bedtime for Frances.* New York: Harper & Row.

Howe, J. (1983). *The celery stalks at midnight.* New York: Atheneum.

Hunt, I. (1966). *Up a road slowly.* New York: Follett.

Ivimey, J. (1987). *The complete story of the three blind mice.* New York: Clarion.

Keats, E. (1965). *In a spring garden.* New York: Dial.

Kipling, R. (1912). *Just so stories.* New York: Doubleday.

Larrick, N. (1988). *Cats are cats.* New York: Philomel.

Lear, E. (1983). *The owl and the pussycat.* New York: Holiday House.

Lee, D. (1983). *Jelly belly.* New York: Bedrick.

Lord, B. (1984). *In the year of the boar and Jackie Robinson.* New York: Harper & Row.

MacLachlan, P. (1982). *Mama one and Mama two.* New York: Harper & Row.

MacLachlan, P. (1985). *Sarah plain and tall.* New York: Harper & Row.

McCloskey, R. (1976). *Homer Price.* New York: Viking.

Morey, W. (1965). *Gentle Ben.* New York: Dutton.

Myers, W. (1988). *Scorpions.* New York: Harper & Row.

Neufield, J. (1968). *Edgar Allen.* New York: New American Library.

O'Dell, S. (1978). *Island of the blue dolphins.* New York: Houghton Mifflin.

Peck, R. (1975). *The ghost belonged to me.* New York: Viking.

Perl, L. (1979). *Me and fat Glenda.* New York: Clarion.

Potter, B. (1908). *The tale of Peter Rabbit.* London: Warne.

Prelutsky, J. (1984). *The new kid on the block.* New York: Greenwillow.

Reigot, B. (1988). *A book about planets and stars.* New York: Scholastic.

Rockwell, T. (1973). *How to eat fried worms.* New York: Dell.

Ryder, J. (1988). *Step into the night.* New York: Four Winds Press.

Silverstein, S. (1974). *Where the sidewalk ends.* New York: Harper & Row.

Silverstein, S. (1981). *A light in the attic.* New York: Harper & Row.

Smith, D. (1973). *Taste of blackberries.* New York: Crowell.

Sobol, D. (1961). *The Wright brothers at Kitty Hawk.* New York: Dutton.

Speare, E. (1958). *The witch of Blackbird Pond.* Boston: Houghton Mifflin.

Taylor, M. (1976). *Roll of thunder, hear my cry.* New York: Dial.

Thayer, E. (1988). *Casey at the bat.* New York: G. P. Putnam's Sons.

Tolkein, J. R. R. (1938). *The hobbit.* Boston: Houghton Mifflin.
Webster, J. (1988). *Daddy-long-legs.* New York: New American Library.
Whitehouse, J. (1984). *I have a sister, my sister is deaf.* New York: Harper & Row.
Wilder, L. (1941). *Little house on the prairie.* New York: Harper & Row.
Wildsmith, B. (1988). *Squirrels.* New York: Oxford University Press.

High-Interest/Easy Reading: Books for Selected Content Areas

Recommended for instruction with upper elementary to high school students. The reading grade levels are estimates.

Topic: Teaching of English—a sample

Title and Publisher	Reading Level (Grades)
The world of vocabulary series (Globe)	2–7
Writing a research paper (Globe)	5–6
The business of basic English (Holcombs)	4–6
English for everyday living (Holcombs)	3–4
Writing to other programs (Holcombs)	3–4
Webster's alphabetical thesaurus (Holcombs)	5–7
Spinning grammar game set (Holcombs)	3–4
Spotlight on sentences (Holcombs)	2–4
Sentence writing learning lab (Holcombs)	3–4
Paragraph writing learning lab (Holcombs)	3–5
Activities for writing and rewriting (Holcombs)	3–5
Fundamental English review (Steck-Vaugh)	8–12

Topic: Geography—a sample

The Earth: Regions and peoples (Globe)	3
Exploring the western world (Globe)	5
Exploring the urban world (Globe)	5–6
The Nile: Lifeline of Egypt (Garrard)	5
The Rhone: River of contrasts (Garrard)	5
The Seine: River of parts (Garrard)	5
The Thames: London's river (Garrard)	5
The Mississippi: Giant at work (Garrard)	5
A world explorer: Roald Amundsen (Garrard)	4

Topic: History—a sample

Cultures in conflict (Globe)	5–6
Inquiry: Western civilization (Globe)	5–7
The Afro-American in United States history (Globe)	5–6
The war between the states (Educational Insights)	4

The new exploring American history (Globe)	5–6
Civilizations of the past: Peoples and cultures (Globe)	6
The American Revolution (Educational Insights)	4
Exploring civilizations: A discovery approach (Globe)	5–6
The United States in the making (Globe)	5–6
Insights about America (Educational Insights)	4
Martin Luther King (New Readers Press)	4–5
The men who won the west (Scholastic)	4–7
Explorers in a new world (Children's Press)	4

Topic: Mathematics—a sample

Real-life math program (Holcombs)	4–6
Survival math skills program (Holcombs)	4–5
Basic skills in using money (Holcombs)	4–5
Payroll deductions activity unit (Holcombs)	5–7
Math marathon (Holcombs)	2–4
Metric puzzles duplicating module (Holcombs)	5–6
Money makes sense activity book (Holcombs)	2–3
Figure it out (Xerox)	2–4
The learning skills series arithmetic, 2/e (McGraw-Hill)	2–3
Basic math operations (Holcombs)	2–4
Whole number operations (Holcombs)	3–5

Topic: Science—a sample

Spaceship Earth/Earth science (Houghton Mifflin)	7–8
Curie/Einstein (Pendulum)	4–6
Physics workshop 1: Understanding energy (Globe)	4–5
What is an atom? (Benefic)	4
What is gravity? (Benefic)	4
What is matter? (Benefic)	4
What is sound? (Benefic)	4
What makes a light go on? (Little, Brown)	3
Experiments for young scientists (Little, Brown)	3

References

Adams, M. (1990a). *Beginning to read: Thinking and learning about print.* Cambridge, MA: The MIT Press.

Adams, M. (1990b). *Beginning to read: Thinking and learning about print. A summary.* Prepared by S. Stahl, J. Osborn, & F. Lehr. Urbana-Champaign, IL: University of Illinois, Center for the Study of Reading, The Reading Research and Education Center.

Adams, M. (1994). Phonics and beginning reading instruction. In F. Lehr & J. Osborn (Eds.), *Reading, language, and literacy: Instruction for the twenty-first century* (pp. 3–23). Hillsdale, NJ: Erlbaum.

Aitchison, J. (1994). *Words in the mind: An introduction to the mental lexicon* (2nd ed.). Cambridge, MA: Blackwell.

Akamatsu, C. T. (1988). Instruction in text structure: Metacognitive strategy instruction for literacy development in deaf students. *ACEHI/ACEDA, 14,* 13–32.

Akamatsu, C. T., & Armour, V. (1987). Developing written literacy in deaf children through analyzing sign language. *American Annals of the Deaf, 132,* 46–51.

Albertini, J., & Shannon, N. (1996). Kitchen notes, "the grapevine," and other writing in childhood. *Journal of Deaf Studies and Deaf Education, 1:1,* 64–74.

Alexander, J., & Colomy, P. (1992). Traditions and competition: Preface to a postpositivist approach to knowledge cumulation. In G. Ritzer (Ed.), *Metatheorizing* (pp. 27–52). Newbury Park: Sage.

Allen, T. (1986). Patterns of academic achievement among hearing impaired students: 1974 and 1983.

In A. Schildroth & M. Karchmer (Eds.), *Deaf children in America* (pp. 161–206). San Diego, CA: Little, Brown.

Allen, T., White, C., & Karchmer, M. (1983). Issues in the development of a special edition for hearing-impaired students of the seventh edition of the Stanford Achievement Test. *American Annals of the Deaf, 128,* 34–39.

Altenberg, E., & Vago, R. (1983). Theoretical implications of an error analysis of second language phonology production. *Language Learning, 33,* 427–447.

Anastasi, A. (1982). *Psychological testing* (5th ed.). New York: Macmillan.

Anderson, R. (1985). Role of reader's schema in comprehension, learning, and memory. In H. Singer & R. Ruddell (Eds.), *Theoretical models and processes of reading* (3rd ed.) (pp. 372–384). Newark, DE: International Reading Association.

Anderson, R., & Freebody, P. (1979). *Vocabulary knowledge* (Tech. Rep. No. 136). Urbana, IL: University of Illinois, Center for the Study of Reading. (ERIC Document Reproduction Service, No. ED 177 480).

Anderson, R., & Freebody, P. (1985). Vocabulary knowledge. In H. Singer & R. Ruddell (Eds.), *Theoretical models and processes of reading* (3rd ed.) (pp. 343–371). Newark, DE: International Reading Association.

Anderson, R., Hiebert, E., Scott, J., & Wilkinson, I. (1985). *Becoming a nation of readers: The report of the commission on reading.* Washington, DC: The National Institute of Education and The Center for the Study of Reading.

Anderson, R., & Nagy, W. (1991). Word meanings. In R. Barr, M. Kamil, P. Mosenthal, & P. D. Pearson (Eds.), *Handbook of reading research* (2nd ed.) (pp. 690–724). New York: Longman.

Anderson, R., & Pearson, P. D. (1984). A schema-theoretic view of basic processes in reading comprehension. In P. D. Pearson, R. Barr, M. Kamil, & P. Mosenthal (Eds.), *Handbook of reading research* (pp. 255–291). New York: Longman.

Anderson, T., & Armbruster, B. (1984). Studying. In P. D. Pearson, R. Barr, M. Kamil, & P. Mosenthal (Eds.), *Handbook of reading research* (pp. 657–679). New York: Longman.

Andrews, J., & Gonzales, K. (1991). Free writing of deaf children in kindergarten. *Sign Language Studies, 74,* 63–78.

Andrews, J., & Mason, J. (1991). Strategy usage among deaf and hearing readers. *Exceptional Children, 57,* 536–545.

Andrews, J., & Taylor, N. (1987). From sign to print: A case study of picture book "reading" between mother and child. *Sign Language Studies, 56,* 261–274.

Antonacci, P., & Hedley, C. (Eds.). (1994). *Natural approaches to reading and writing.* Norwood, NJ: Ablex.

Argyris, C., Putnam, R., & Smith, D. (1985). *Action science: Concepts, methods, and skills for research and intervention.* San Francisco: Jossey-Bass.

Baars, B. (1986). *The cognitive revolution in psychology.* New York: The Guilford Press.

Babb, R. (1979). *A study of the academic achievement and language acquisition levels of deaf children of hearing parents in an educational environment using signing exact English as the primary mode of manual communication.* Unpublished doctoral dissertation, University of Illinois, Urbana-Champaign.

Babbini, B., & Quigley, S. (1970). *A study of the growth patterns in language, communication, and educational achievement in six residential schools for deaf students.* Urbana, IL: University of Illinois, Institute for Research on Exceptional Children. (ERIC Document Reproduction Service No. ED 046 208).

Bailey, K. (1983). Competitiveness and anxiety in adult second language learning: Looking AT and THROUGH the diary studies. In H. Seliger & M. Long (Eds.), *Classroom-oriented research in second language acquisition* (pp. 67–103). Rowley, MA: Newbury House.

Bailey, N., Madden, C., & Krashen, S. (1974). Is there a "natural sequence" in adult second language learning? *Language Learning, 24,* 235–243.

Baker, C., & Cokely, D. (1980). *American Sign Language: A teacher's resource text on grammar and culture.* Silver Spring, MD: T. J. Publishers.

Baker, L., & Brown, A. (1984). Metacognitive skills and reading. In P. D. Pearson, R. Barr, M. Kamil, & P. Mosenthal (Eds.), *Handbook of reading research* (pp. 353–394). New York: Longman.

Balota, D., Flores d'Arcais, G., & Rayner, K. (Eds.). (1990). *Comprehension processes in reading.* Hillsdale, NJ: Erlbaum.

Balow, B., Fulton, H., & Peploe, E. (1971). Reading comprehension skills among hearing-impaired adolescents. *Volta Review, 73,* 113–119.

Balow, I., & Brill, R. (1975). An evaluation of reading and academic achievement levels of 16 graduating classes of the California School for the Deaf, Riverside. *Volta Review, 77,* 255–266.

Barr, R., Kamil, M., Mosenthal, P., & Pearson, P. D. (Eds.). (1991). *Handbook of reading research* (2nd ed.). New York: Longman.

Bartine, D. (1989). *Early English reading theory: Origins of current debates.* Columbia, SC: University of South Carolina Press.

Bartine, D. (1992). *Reading, criticism, and culture: Theory and teaching in the United States and England, 1820–1950.* Columbia, SC: University of South Carolina Press.

Bates, E. (1976). *Language and context: The acquisition of pragmatics.* New York: Academic Press.

Beardsmore, H. (1986). *Bilingualism: Basic principles* (2nd ed.). Clevedon, Avon (England): Multilingual Matters Ltd.

Beck, E. (Ed.). (1980). *John Bartlett's familiar quotations: A collection of passages, phrases, and proverbs traced to their sources in ancient and modern literature.* Boston: Little, Brown.

Beck, I., & McKeown, M. (1991). Conditions of vocabulary acquisition. In R. Barr, M. Kamil, P. Mosenthal, & P. D. Pearson (Eds.), *Handbook of reading research* (2nd ed.) (pp. 789–814). New York: Longman.

Beck, I., McKeown, M., & McCaslin, E. (1983). Vocabulary development: All contexts are not created equal. *Elementary School Journal, 83,* 177–181.

Becker, W. (1977). Teaching reading and language to the disadvantaged—What we have learned from field research. *Harvard Educational Review, 47,* 518–543.

Bellugi, U. (1991). The link between hand and brain: Implications from a visual language. In D. Martin (Ed.), *Advances in cognition, education, and deafness* (pp. 11–35). Washington, DC: Gallaudet University Press.

Bereiter, C., & Scardamalia, M. (1983). Levels of inquiry in writing research. In P. Mosenthal, L. Tamor, & S. Walmsley (Eds.), *Research on writing: Principles and methods* (pp. 3–25). New York: Longman.

Bereiter, C., & Scardamalia, M. (1987). *The psychology of written composition.* Hillsdale, NJ: Erlbaum.

Berk, R. (Ed.). (1980). *Criterion-referenced measurement: The state of the art.* Baltimore: Johns Hopkins University Press.

Berko, J. (1958). The child's learning of English morphology. *Word, 14,* 150–177.

Bernhardt, E. (1991). *Reading development in a second language.* Norwood, NJ: Ablex.

Besner, D. (1990). Does the reading system need a lexicon? In D. Balota, G. Flores d'Arcais, & K. Rayner, K. (Eds.), *Comprehension processes in reading* (pp. 73–99). Hillsdale, NJ: Erlbaum.

Bigner, J. (1994). *Parent-child relations: An introduction to parenting* (4th ed.). New York: Macmillan.

Blankenship, C., & Lilly, M. S. (1981). *Mainstreaming students with learning and behavior problems.* New York: Holt, Rinehart, & Winston.

Blanton, R., Nunnally, J., & Odom, P. (1967). Graphemic, phonetic, and associative factors in the verbal behavior of deaf and hearing subjects. *Journal of Speech and Hearing Research, 10,* 225–231.

Blennerhassett, L. (1990). Intellectual assessment. In D. Moores & K. Meadow-Orlans (Eds.), *Educational and developmental aspects of deafness* (pp. 255–280). Washington, DC: Gallaudet University Press.

Bloom, L., & Lahey, M. (1978). *Language development and language disorders.* New York: Wiley.

Bloome, D. (Ed.). (1989). *Classrooms and literacy.* Norwood, NJ: Ablex.

Bloomquist, C. (1986). Minimum competency testing programs and hearing-impaired students. In A. Schildroth & M. Karchmer (Eds.), *Deaf children in America* (pp. 207–229). San Diego, CA: College-Hill.

Bohannon, J., & Warren-Leubecker, A. (1985). Theoretical approaches to language acquisition. In J. Berko-Gleason (Ed.), *The development of language* (pp. 173–226). Columbus, OH: Merrill.

Bongaerts, T. (1983). The comprehension of three complex English structures by Dutch learners. *Language Learning, 33,* 159–182.

Borg, W., & Gall, M. (1983). *Educational research* (4th ed.). White Plains, NY: Longman.

Bornstein, H., Saulnier, K., & Hamilton, L. (1980). Signed English: A first evaluation. *American Annals of the Deaf, 125,* 467–481.

Bornstein, H., Saulnier, K., & Hamilton, L. (1983). *The comprehensive signed English dictionary.* Washington, DC: Gallaudet College Press.

Bowen, J., Madsen, H., & Hilferty, A. (1985). *TESOL: Techniques and procedures.* Rowley, MA: Newbury House.

Bradley-Johnson, S., & Evans, L. (1991). *Psychoeducational assessment of hearing-impaired students.* Austin, TX: Pro-Ed.

Brady, S., & Shankweiler, D. (Eds.). (1991). *Phonological processes in literacy: A tribute to Isabelle Y. Liberman.* Hillsdale, NJ: Erlbaum.

Brasel, K., & Quigley, S. (1977). The influence of certain language and communication environments in early childhood on the development of language in deaf individuals. *Journal of Speech and Hearing Research, 20,* 95–107.

Bridwell, L. (1980). Revising strategies in twelfth grade students' transactional writing. *Research in the Teaching of English, 14,* 197–222.

Brinton, P. (1986). Classroom-based assessment. In A. Cashdan (Ed.), *Literacy: Teaching and learning language skills* (pp. 162–179). New York: Basil Blackwell.

Bronowski, J. (1977). *A sense of the future.* Cambridge, MA: MIT Press.

Brown, A. (1975). The development of memory: Knowing, knowing about knowing and knowing how to know. *Advances in Child Development and Behavior, 10,* 103–151.

Brown, A., Armbruster, B., & Baker. L. (1986). The role of metacognition in reading and studying. In J. Orasanu (Ed.), *Reading comprehension: From research to practice* (pp. 49–75). Hillsdale, NJ: Erlbaum.

Brown, A., & Campione, J. (1986). Academic intelligence and learning potential. In R. Sternberg & D. Detterman (Eds.), *What is intelligence? Contemporary viewpoints on its nature and definition* (pp. 39–43). Norwood, NJ: Ablex.

Brown, P., & Long, G. (1992). The use of scripted interaction in a cooperative learning context to probe planning and evaluating during writing. *Volta Review, 95,* 411–424.

Brown, R. (1973). *A first language: The early stages.* Cambridge, MA: Harvard University Press.

Brynes, J., & Gelman, S. (1991). Perspectives on thought and language: Traditional and contemporary views. In S. Gelman & J. Byrnes (Eds.), *Perspectives on language and thought: Interrelations in development* (pp. 3–27). New York: Cambridge University Press.

Bunge, M., & Ardila, R. (1987). *Philosophy of psychology.* New York: Springer-Verlag.

CADS. (1991). Center for Assessment and Demographic Studies. *Stanford Achievement Test, eighth edition: Hearing-impaired norms booklet.* Washington, DC: Gallaudet University, Gallaudet Research Institute, Center for Assessment and Demographic Studies.

Calfee, R (1994). Critical literacy: Reading and writing for a new millennium. In N. Ellsworth, C. Hedley, & A. Baratta (Eds.), *Literacy: A redefinition.* Hillsdale, NJ: Erlbaum.

Calkins, L. (1983). *Lessons from a child.* Exeter, NH: Heinemann.

Calkins, L. (1986). *The art of teaching.* Portsmouth, NH: Heinemann.

Carnine, D., Silbert, J., & Kameenui, E. (1990). *Direct instruction reading* (2nd ed.). Columbus, OH: Merrill.

Carroll, J., Davies, P., & Richman, B. (1971). *The American heritage word frequency book.* New York: American Heritage.

Cazden, C. (1965). *Environmental assistance to the child's acquisition of grammar.* Unpublished doctoral dissertation. Boston: Harvard University.

Chall, J. (1967). *Learning to read: The great debate.* New York: McGraw-Hill.

Chall, J. (1983). *Learning to read: The great debate* (Updated ed.). New York: McGraw-Hill.

Chamot, A. (1983). Toward a functional ESL curriculum in the elementary school. *TESOL Quarterly, 17,* 459–472.

Chaplin, J. (1975). *Dictionary of psychology* (Rev. ed.). New York: Dell.

Charrow, V. (1975). A psycholinguistic analysis of deaf English. *Sign Language Studies, 7,* 139–150.

Charrow, V., & Fletcher, J. (1974). English as the second language of deaf children. *Developmental Psychology, 10,* 463–470.

Chomsky, C. (1969). *The acquisition of syntax in children from 5 to 10.* Cambridge, MA: MIT Press.

Chomsky, N. (1957). *Syntactic structures.* The Hague: Mouton.

Chomsky, N. (1965). *Aspects of the theory of syntax.* Cambridge, MA: The MIT Press.

Chomsky, N. (1975). *Reflections on language.* New York: Pantheon Books.

Chomsky, N. (1988). *Language and problems of knowledge: The Managua lectures.* Cambridge, MA: The MIT Press.

Chun, J. (1980). A survey of research in second language acquisition. *The Modern Language Journal, 64,* 287–296.

Cicourel, A., & Boese, R. (1972a). Sign language acquisition and the teaching of deaf children: Part I. *American Annals of the Deaf, 117,* 27–33.

Cicourel, A., & Boese, R. (1972b). Sign language acquisition: Conclusion. *American Annals of the Deaf, 117,* 403–411.

Clark, R. (1982). *Index card games for ESL: Supplementary materials handbook one.* Brattleboro, VT: The Experiment Press/Pro Lingua Associates.

Clay, M. M. (1979). Reading: *The pattening of complex behavior* (2nd ed.). Auckland, New Zealand: Heinemann.

Cole, E., & Gregory, H. (Eds.). (1986). Auditory learning. *Volta Review, 88*(5), September. [Special Issue].

Coltheart, M. (1977). Critical notice on E. Gibson & H. Levin (Eds.), *The psychology of reading. Quarterly Journal of Experimental Psychology, 29,* 157–167.

Conley, J. (1976). Role of idiomatic expressions in the reading of deaf children. *American Annals of the Deaf, 121,* 381–385.

Conrad, R. (1979). *The deaf school child.* London: Harper & Row.

Cook, V. (1991). *Second language learning and language teaching.* New York: Edward Arnold.

Cooper, H. (1982). Scientific guidelines for conducting integrative reviews. *Review of Educational Research, 52,* 291–302.

Cooper, J., Heron, T., & Heward, B. (1987). *Applied behavior analysis.* Columbus, OH: Merrill.

Cooper, R. (1967). The ability of deaf and hearing children to apply morphological rules. *Journal of Speech and Hearing Research, 10,* 77–86.

Cooper, R., Olshtain, E., Tucker, G., & Waterbury, M. (1979). The acquisition of complex English structures by adult native speakers of Arabic and Hebrew. *Language Learning, 29,* 255–275.

Copeland, K., Winsor, P., & Osborn, J. (1994). Phonemic awareness: A consideration of research and practice. In F. Lehr & J. Osborn (Eds.), *Reading, language, and literacy: Instruction for the twenty-first century* (pp. 25–44). Hillsdale, NJ: Erlbaum.

Copleston, F., S. J. (1985). *A history of philosophy, Book Two, Vol. IV, V, & VI.* Garden, NY: Image.

Corson, H. (1973). *Comparing deaf children of oral deaf parents and deaf parents using manual communication with deaf children of hearing parents on academic, social, and communication functioning.* Unpublished doctoral dissertation, University of Cincinnati, Ohio.

Crandall, K. (1978). Inflectional morphemes in the manual English of young hearing impaired children and their mothers. *Journal of Speech and Hearing Research, 21,* 372–386.

Crittenden, J. (1993). The culture and identity of deafness. In P. Paul & D. Jackson, *Toward a psychology of deafness: Theoretical and empirical perspectives* (pp. 215–235). Boston: Allyn & Bacon.

Cromer, R. (1988a). Differentiating language and cognition. In R. Schiefelbusch & L. Lloyd (Eds.), *Language perspectives: Acquisition, retardation, and intervention* (2nd ed., pp. 91–124). Austin, TX: Pro-Ed.

Cromer, R. (1988b). The cognition hypothesis revisited. In F. Kessel (Ed.), *The development of language and language researchers: Essays in honor of Roger Bown* (pp. 223–248). Hillsdale, NJ: Erlbaum.

Cross, D., & Paris, S. (1988). Developmental and instructional analyses of children's metacognition and reading comprehension. *Journal of Educational Psychology, 80,* 131–142.

Crutchfield, P. (1972). Prospects for teaching English Det + N structures to deaf students. *Sign Language Studies, 1,* 8–14.

Cummins, J. (1977). Cognitive factors associated with the attainment of intermediate levels of bilingual skill. *The Modern Language Journal, 61,* 3–12.

Cummins, J. (1978). Educational implications of mother tongue maintenance in minority-language groups. *Canadian Modern Language Review, 34,* 395–416.

Cummins, J. (1979). Linguistic interdependence and the educational development of bilingual children. *Review of Educational Research, 49,* 222–251.

Cummins, J. (1984). *Bilingualism and special education: Issues in assessment and pedagogy.* San Diego, CA: College-Hill Press.

Cummins, J. (1988). Second language acquisition within bilingual education programs. In L. Beebe (Ed.), *Issues in second language acquisition: Multiple perspectives* (pp. 145–166). New York: Newbury House.

Cummins, J. (1989). A theoretical framework for bilingual special education. *Exceptional Children, 56,* 111–119.

Czerniewska, P. (1992). *Learning about writing: The early years.* Cambridge, MA: Basil Blackwell.

Cziko, G. (1992). The evaluation of bilingual education: From necessity and probability to possibility. *Educational Researcher, 21*(2), 10–15.

Dale, E., & Chall, J. (1948). A formula for predicting readability. *Educational Research Bulletin, 27,* 11–20, 37–54.

Dale, E., & Eicholtz, G. (1960). *Children's knowledge of words.* Columbus, OH: Ohio State University, Bureau of Educational Resources.

Dale, E., & O'Rourke, J. (1971). *Techniques of teaching vocabulary.* Menlo Park, CA: Benjamin/Cummings.

Dale, E., & O'Rourke, J. (1981). *The living word vocabulary: A national vocabulary inventory.* Chicago: World Book.

Dale, E., & O'Rourke, J. (1986). *Vocabulary building: A process approach.* Columbus, OH: Zaner-Bloser.

Daneman, M., Nemeth, S., Stainton, M., & Huelsmann, K. (in press). Working memory as a predictor of reading achievement in orally educated hearing-impaired children. *Volta Review.*

d'Anglejan, A., & Tucker, G. (1975). The acquisition of complex English structures by adult learners. *Language Learning, 25,* 281–296.

Davey, B., & King, S. (1990). Acquisition of word meanings from context by deaf readers. *American Annals of the Deaf, 135,* 227–234.

Davey, B., LaSasso, C., & Macready, G. (1983). Comparison of reading comprehension task performance for deaf and hearing readers. *Journal of Speech and Hearing Research, 26,* 622–628.

Davies, A. (1990). *Principles of language testing.* Cambridge, MA: Basil Blackwell.

Davies, A., Criper, C., & Howatt, A. (1984). *Interlanguage.* Edinburgh, Scotland: Edinburgh University Press.

Davis, H. (1978). Anatomy and physiology of the auditory system. In H. Davis & S. R. Silverman, *Hearing and deafness* (4th ed.) (pp. 46–83). New York: Holt, Rinehart, & Winston.

Delaney, M., Stuckless, E. R., & Walter G. (1984). Total communication effects—A longitudinal study of a school for the deaf in transition. *American Annals of the Deaf, 129,* 481–486.

deVilliers, J., & deVilliers, P. (1973). A cross-sectional study of the acquisition of grammatical morphemes in child speech. *Journal of Psycholinguistic Research, 2,* 267–278.

deVilliers, J., & deVilliers, P. (1978). *Language acquisition.* Cambridge, MA: Harvard University Press.

deVilliers, P., & Pomerantz, S. (1992). Hearing-impaired students learning new words from written context. *Applied Psycholinguistics, 13,* 409–431.

Devine, T. (1986). *Teaching reading comprehension: From theory to practice.* Boston: Allyn & Bacon.

Dewey, J. (1938). *Experience and education.* New York: Macmillan.

DiFrancesca, S. (1972). *Academic achievement test results of a national testing program for hearing-impaired students—United States, Spring* (Series D, No. 9). Washington, DC: Gallaudet College, Office of Demographic Studies.

Dixon-Krauss, L. (Ed.). (1996). *Vygotsky in the classroom: Mediated literacy instruction and assessment.* White Plains, NY: Longman.

Dolman, D. (1992). Some concerns about using whole language approaches with deaf children. *American Annals of the Deaf, 137,* 278–282.

Douglas, M. (1989). *Learning to read: The quest for meaning.* New York: Teachers College, Columbia University.

Drasgow, E., & Paul, P. (1995). A critical analysis of the use of MCE systems with deaf students: A review of the literature. *ACEHI/ACEDA, 21* (2/3), 80–93.

Dulay, H., & Burt, M. (1973). Should we teach children syntax? *Language Learning, 23,* 245–258.

Dulay, H., & Burt, M. (1974a). Natural sequences in child second language acquisition. *Language Learning, 24,* 37–53.

Dulay, H., & Burt, M. (1974b). Errors and strategies in child second language acquisition. *TESOL Quarterly, 8,* 129–136.

Durkin, D. (1966). *Children who read early.* New York: Columbia University, Teachers College Press.

Durkin, D. (1981). Reading comprehension instruction in five basal reader series. *Reading Research Quarterly, 16,* 515–544.

Durkin, D. (1989). *Teaching them to read* (5th ed.). Boston: Allyn & Bacon.

Eacker, J. (1975). *Problems of philosophy and psychology.* Chicago: Nelson-Hall.

Eacker, J. (1983). *Problems of metaphysics and psychology.* Chicago: Nelson-Hall.

Ehri, L. (1991). Development of the ability to read words. In R. Barr, M. Kamil, P. Mosenthal, & P. D. Pearson (Eds.), *Handbook of reading research* (2nd ed.) (pp. 383–417). White Plains, NY: Longman.

Ehri, L., & Wilce, L. (1985). Movement into reading: Is the first stage of printed word learning visual or phonetic? *Reading Research Quarterly, 20,* 163–179.

Ellsworth, N. (1994). Critical thinking and literacy. In N. Ellsworth, C. Hedley, & A. Baratta (Eds.), *Literacy: A redefinition* (pp. 91–108). Hillsdale, NJ: Erlbaum.

Ellsworth, N., Hedley, C., & Baratta, A. (Eds.). (1994). *Literacy: A redefinition.* Hillsdale, NJ: Erlbaum.

Erickson, M. (1987). Deaf readers reading beyond the literal. *American Annals of the Deaf, 132,* 291–294.

Everhart, V., & Marschark, M. (1988). Linguistic flexibility in signed and written language productions of deaf children. *Journal of Experimental Child Psychology, 46,* 174–193.

Ewoldt, C. (1981). A psycholinguistic description of selected deaf children reading in sign language. *Reading Research Quarterly, 17,* 58–89.

Ewoldt, C. (1994). Booksharing: Teachers and parents reading to deaf children. In A. Flurkey & R. Meyer (Eds.), *Under the whole language umbrella* (pp. 331–342). Urbana, IL: National Council of Teachers of English.

Ewoldt, C., Israelite, N., & Dodds, R. (1992). The ability of deaf students to understand text: A comparison of the perceptions of teachers and students. *American Annals of the Deaf, 137,* 351–361.

Farr, R., & Carey, R. (1986). *Reading: What can be measured?* (2nd ed.). Newark, DE: International Reading Association.

Felix, S. (1981). The effect of formal instruction on second language acquisition. *Language Learning, 31,* 87–112.

Feuerstein, R., Rand, Y., & Hoffman, M. (1979). *The dynamic assessment of retarded performers.* Baltimore: University Park Press.

Feuerstein, R., Rand, Y., Hoffman, M., & Miller, R. (1980). *Instrumental enrichment.* Baltimore: University Park Press.

Fillmore, L. (1979). Individual differences in second language acquisition. In C. Fillmore, D. Kempler, & W. Wang (Eds.), *Individual differences in language ability and language behavior* (pp. 203–228). New York: Academic Press.

Fitzgerald, J. (1992). Variant views about good thinking during composing: Focus on revision. In M. Pressley, K. Harris, & J. Guthrie (Eds.), *Promoting academic competence and literacy in school* (pp. 337–358). New York: Academic Press.

Flavell, D. (1985). *Cognitive development* (2nd ed.). Englewood Cliffs, NJ: Prentice-Hall.

Flower, L., & Hayes, J. (1980). The dynamics of composing: Making plans and juggling constraints. In L. W. Gregg & E. R. Steinberg (Eds.), *Cognitive processes in writing* (pp. 31–50). Hillsdale, NJ: Erlbaum.

Fodor, J. (1983). *The modularity of mind: An essay on faculty psychology.* Cambridge, MA: The MIT Press.

Foucault, M. (1973). *The order of things: Archaeology of the human sciences.* London: Tavistock.

Friedlander, A. (1990). Composing in English: Effects of a first language on writing in English as a second language. In B. Kroll (Ed.), *Second language writing: Research insights for the classroom* (pp. 109–125). New York: Cambridge University Press.

Friend, M., & Bursuck, W. (1996). *Including students with special needs: A practical guide for classroom teachers.* Boston: Allyn & Bacon.

Fruchter, A., Wilbur, R., & Fraser, B. (1984). Comprehension of idioms by hearing-impaired students. *Volta Review, 86,* 7–18.

Fuchs, L., Fuchs, D., & Hamlett, C. (1990). Curriculum-based measurement: A standardized, long-term goal approach to monitoring student progress. *Academic Therapy, 25,* 615–632.

Furth, H. (1966). A comparison of reading test norms of deaf and hearing children. *American Annals of the Deaf, 111,* 461–462.

Furth, H. (1973). *Deafness and learning: A psychosocial approach.* Belmont, CA: Wadsworth.

Gamez, G. (1979). Reading in a second language: Native language approach vs. direct method. *The Reading Teacher, 32,* 665–670.

Gannon, J. (1981). *Deaf heritage: A narrative history of deaf America.* Silver Spring, MD: National Association of the Deaf.

Garcia, G., & Pearson, P. D. (1991). The role of assessment in a diverse society. In E. Hiebert (Ed.), *Literacy in a diverse society: Perspectives, practices, and policies* (pp. 253–278). New York: Teachers College Press.

Garton, A., & Pratt, C. (1989). *Learning to be literate: The development of spoken and written language.* New York: Basil Blackwell.

Gaustad, M. (1984). *Phonological evolution of American manual English: A decade of development.* Paper presented to the Center for Studies in Education and Human Development, Gallaudet University, Washington, DC, December.

Gaustad, M. (1986). Longitudinal effects of manual English instruction on deaf children's morphological skills. *Applied Psycholinguistics, 7,* 101–128.

Gaustad, M., & Messinheimer-Young, T. (1991). Dialogue journals for students with learning disabilities. *Teaching Exceptional Children, 23*(3), 28–32.

Geers, A., & Moog, J. (1989). Factors predictive of the development of literacy in profoundly hearing-impaired adolescents. *Volta Review, 91,* 69–86.

Genesee, F. (1987). *Learning through two languages: Studies of immersion and bilingual education.* Cambridge, MA: Newbury House.

Gentile, A., & DiFrancesca, S. (1969). *Academic achievement test performance of hearing-impaired students—United States, Spring* (Series D, No. 1). Washington, DC: Gallaudet College, Office of Demographic Studies.

Gibbs, K. (1989). Individual differences in cognitive skills related to reading ability in the deaf. *American Annals of the Deaf, 134,* 214–218.

Gibson, E., & Levin, H. (1975). *The psychology of reading.* Cambridge, MA: The MIT Press.

Gibson, R. (1986). *Critical theory and education.* London, England: Hodder & Stoughton.

Gillis, M., & Weber, R. (1976). The emergence of sentence modalities in the English of Japanese-speaking children. *Language Learning, 26,* 77–94.

Gilman, L., Davis, J., & Raffin, M. (1980). Use of common morphemes by hearing impaired children exposed to a system of manual English. *Journal of Auditory Research, 20,* 57–69.

Giorcelli, L. (1982). *The comprehension of some aspects of figurative language by deaf and hearing subjects.* Unpublished doctoral dissertation, University of Illinois, Urbana-Champaign.

Glass, G., McGaw, B., & Smith, M. (1981). *Meta-analysis in social research.* Beverly Hills, CA: Sage.

Gleidman, J., & Roth, W. (1980). *The unexpected minority: Handicapped children in America.* New York: Harcourt Brace Jovanovich.

Godzich, W. (1994). *The culture of literacy.* Cambridge, MA: Harvard University Press.

Goetzinger, C., & Rousey, C. (1959). Educational achievement of deaf children. *American Annals of the Deaf, 104,* 221–231.

Goldberg, J., & Bordman, P. (1975). The ESL approach to teaching English to hearing impaired students. *American Annals of the Deaf, 120,* 22–27.

Goldin-Meadow, S., & Feldman, H. (1975). The creation of a communication system: A study of deaf children of hearing parents. *Sign Language Studies, 8,* 225–236.

Goodman, K. (1976). Reading: A psycholinguistic guessing game. In H. Singer & R. Ruddell (Eds.), *Theoretical models and processes of reading* (2nd ed.) (pp. 497–508). Newark, DE: International Reading Association.

Goodman, K. (1985). Unity in reading. In H. Singer & R. Ruddell (Eds.), *Theoretical models and processes of reading* (3rd ed.) (pp. 813–840). Newark, DE: International Reading Association.

Gormley, K., & Sarachan-Deily, A. (1987). Evaluating hearing-impaired students' writing: A practical approach. *Volta Review, 89,* 157–170.

Gough, P. (1972). One second of reading. *Visible Language, 6,* 291–320.

Gough, P. (1984). Word recognition. In P. D. Pearson, R. Barr, M. Kamil, & P. Mosenthal (Eds.), *Handbook of reading research* (pp. 225–253). White Plains, NY: Longman.

Gough, P. (1985). One second of reading: Postscript. In H. Singer & R. Ruddell (Eds.), *Theoretical models and processes of reading* (3rd ed.) (pp. 687–688). Newark, DE: International Reading Association.

Gough, P., Ehri, L., & Treiman, R. (Eds.). (1992). *Reading acquisition.* Hillsdale, NJ: Erlbaum.

Gough, P., & Hillinger, M. (1980). Learning to read: An unnatural act. *Bulletin of the Orton Society, 30,* 179–196.

Grabe, W. (1988). Reassessing the term "interactive." In P. Carrell, J. Devine, & D. Eskey (Eds.), *Interactive approaches to second language reading* (pp. 56–70). New York: Cambridge University Press.

Grabe, W. (1991). Current developments in second-language reading research. *TESOL Quarterly, 25,* 375–406.

Graves, D. (1983). *Writing: Teachers and children at work.* Portsmouth, NH: Heinemann.

Graves, M. (1986). Vocabulary learning and instruction. *Review of Research in Education, 13,* 91–128.

Gunning, T. (1992). *Creating reading instruction for all children.* Boston: Allyn & Bacon.

Gustason, G., & Zawolkow, E. (1993). *Signing exact English.* Los Alamitos, CA: Modern Signs Press.

Habermas, J. (1984). *The theory of communicative action. Volume One: Reason and the rationalization of society.* London: Heinemann.

Hakuta, K., & Cancino, H. (1977). Trends in second-language acquisition research. *Harvard Educational Review, 47,* 294–316.

Halliday, M. (1984). Three aspects of children's language development: Learning language, learning through language, and learning about language. In Y. Goodman, M. Haussler, & D. Strickland (Eds.), *Oral and written language development research: Impact on the schools* (pp. 165–192). Urbana, IL: National Council of Teachers of English.

Hamp-Lyons, L. (1990). Second language writing: Assessment issues. In B. Kroll (Ed.), *Second language writing: Research insights for the classroom.* New York: Cambridge University Press.

Hannon, P. (1995). *Literacy, home and school: Research and practice in teaching literacy with parents.* Washington, DC: The Falmer Press.

Hanson, V. (1989). Phonology and reading: Evidence from profoundly deaf readers. In D. Shankweiler & I. Liberman (Eds.), *Phonology and reading disability: Solving the reading puzzle* (pp.

69–89). Ann Arbor, MI: University of Michigan Press.

Hanson, V. (1991). Phonological processing without sound. In S. Brady & D. Shankweiler (Eds.), *Phonological processes in literacy: A tribute to Isabelle Y. Liberman* (pp. 153–161). Hillsdale, NJ: Erlbaum.

Harris, T., & Hodges, R. (Eds.). (1981). *A dictionary of reading and related terms.* Newark, DE: International Reading Association.

Harrison, A. (1983). *A language testing handbook.* London: Macmillan.

Harste, J., Burke, C., & Woodward, V. (1982). Children's language and world: Initial encounters with print. In J. Langer & M. T. Smith-Burke (Eds.), *Reader meets author: Bridging the gap* (pp. 105–131). Newark, DE: International Reading Association.

Hasbrouck, J., & Tindal, G. (1992). Curriculum-based oral reading fluency norms for students in grades 2 through 5. *Teaching Exceptional Children, 24*(3), 41–44.

Hatch, E. (1978). *Second language acquisition.* Rowley, MA: Newbury House.

Hatfield, N., Caccamise, F., & Siple, P. (1978). Deaf students' language competency: A bilingual perspective. *American Annals of the Deaf, 123,* 847–851.

Hayes, P., & Arnold, P. (1992). Is hearing-impaired children's reading delayed or different? *Journal of Research in Reading, 15,* 104–116.

Heath, S. (1982). What no bedtime story means: Narrative skills at home and school. *Language and Society, 2,* 49–76.

Heaton, J. (1990). *Classroom testing.* New York: Longman.

Hedley, C. (1994). Theories of natural language. In P. Antonacci & C. Hedley, *Natural approaches to reading and writing* (pp. 3–18). Norwood, NJ: Ablex.

Heider, F., & Heider, G. (1940). A comparison of sentence structure of deaf and hearing children. *Psychological Monographs, 52,* 42–103.

Heimlich, J., & Pittelman, S. (1986). *Semantic mapping: Classroom applications.* Newark, DE: International Reading Association.

Herman, P., Anderson, R., Pearson, P. D., & Nagy, W. (1987). Incidental acquisition of word meaning from expositions with varied text features. *Reading Research Quarterly, 22* (3), 263–284.

Heward, W., & Orlansky, M. (1992). *Exceptional children* (4th ed.). Columbus, OH: Merrill.

Hickman, J. (1979). *Response to literature in a school environment, Grades K-5.* Unpublished doctoral dissertation, The Ohio State University, Columbus.

Hillocks, G. (1986). *Research on written composition: New directions for teaching.* Urbana, IL: National Conference on Research in English.

Holmes, J. (1953). *The substrata-factor theory of reading.* Berkeley, CA: California Book.

Houck, J. (1982). *The effects of idioms on reading comprehension of hearing impaired students.* Unpublished doctoral dissertation, University of Northern Colorado (Abstract).

Hunt, K. (1965). *Grammatical structures written at three grade levels.* Champaign, IL: National Council of Teachers of English.

Hunt, K. (1970). Syntactic maturity in school children and adults. *Monographs of the Society for Research in Child Development, 35*(134).

Hunter, C., & Harman, D. (1979). *Adult illiteracy in the United States: A report to the Ford Foundation.* New York: McGraw-Hill.

Iran-Nejad, A., Ortony, A., & Rittenhouse, R. (1981). The comprehension of metaphorical uses of English by deaf children. *Journal of Speech and Hearing Research, 24,* 551–556.

Irwin, J., & Doyle, M. (Eds.). (1992). *Reading/writing connections: Learning from research.* Newark, DE: International Reading Association.

Israelite, N. (1981). *Direct antecedent context and comprehension of reversible passive voice sentences by deaf readers.* Unpublished doctoral dissertation, University of Pittsburgh.

Jenkins, J., Stein, M., & Wysocki, K. (1984). Learning vocabulary through reading. *American Educational Research Journal, 21,* 767–787.

Johnson, D., & Baumann, J. (1984). Word identification. In P. D. Pearson, R. Barr, M. Kamil, & P. Mosenthal (Eds.), *Handbook of reading research* (pp. 583–608). White Plains, NY: Longman.

Johnson, D., Moe, A., & Baumann, J. (1983). *The Ginn word book for teachers: A basic lexicon.* Lexington, MA: Ginn.

Johnson, D., & Pearson, P. D. (1984). *Teaching reading vocabulary* (2nd ed.). New York: Holt, Rinehart, & Winston.

Johnson, D., Toms-Bronowski, S., & Pittelman, S. (1982). *An investigation of the effectiveness of se-*

mantic mapping and semantic feature analysis with intermediate grade level children (Program Report No. 83–3). Madison, WI: Wisconsin Center for Education Research.

Johnson, R., Liddell, S., & Erting, C. (1989). *Unlocking the curriculum: Principles for achieving access in deaf education* (Working Paper 89–3). Washington, DC: Gallaudet University, Gallaudet Research Institute.

Jones, P. (1979). Negative interference of signed language in written English. *Sign Language Studies, 24,* 273–279.

Kamil, M. (1984). Current traditions of reading research. In P. D. Pearson, R. Barr, M. Kamil, & P. Mosenthal (Eds.), *Handbook of reading research* (pp. 39–62). White Plains, NY: Longman.

Kane, M., & Khattri, N. (1995). Assessment reform: A work in progress. *Phi Delta Kappan, 77*(1), 30–32.

Kavanaugh, J. (1986). *Otitis media and child development.* Parkton, MD: York Press.

Kelly, L. (1995). Processing of bottom-up and top-down information by skilled and average deaf readers and implications for whole language instruction. *Exceptional Children, 61,* 318–334.

King, C. (1981). *An investigation of similarities and differences in the syntactic abilities of deaf and hearing children learning English as a first or second language.* Unpublished doctoral dissertation, University of Illinois, Champaign-Urbana.

King, C., & Quigley, S. (1985). *Reading and deafness.* Austin, TX: Pro-Ed.

Kintsch, W., & van Dijk, T. (1978). Toward a model of text comprehension and production. *Psychological Review, 85,* 363–394.

Klecan-Aker, J. (1988). *Developing a reliable means of coding stories.* Unpublished manuscript, University of Houston, Houston.

Klecan-Aker, J., & Blondeau, R. (1990). An examination of the written stories of hearing-impaired school-age children. *Volta Review, 92,* 275–282.

Klecan-Aker, J., & Hedrick, D. (1985). A study of the syntactic language abilities of normal middle school children. *Language, Speech and Hearing Services in the Schools, 16,* 187–198.

Klima, E., & Bellugi, U. (1966). Syntactic regularities in the speech of children. In J. Lyons & R. Wales (Eds.), *Psycholinguistic papers: The proceedings*

of the 1966 Edinburgh conference (pp. 183–219). Edinburgh, Scotland: Edinburgh University Press.

Klima, E., & Bellugi, U. (1979). *The signs of language.* Cambridge, MA: Harvard University Press.

Kluwin, T., Getson, P., & Kluwin, B. (1980). The effects of experience on the discourse comprehension of deaf and hearing adolescents. *Directions, 1*(3), 49.

Kluwin, T., & Kelly, A. (1991). The effectiveness of dialogue journal writing in improving the writing skills of young deaf writers. *American Annals of the Deaf, 136,* 284–291.

Kragler, S. (1996). Vygotsky and at-risk readers: Assessment and instructional implications. In L. Dixon-Krauss (Ed.), *Vygotsky in the classroom: Mediated literacy instruction and assessment* (pp. 149–160). White Plains, NY: Longman.

Krashen, S. (1981). *Second language acquisition and second language learning.* Oxford, England: Pergamon.

Krashen, S. (1982). *Principles and practices of second language acquisition.* Oxford, England: Pergamon.

Krashen, S. (1985). *The input hypothesis: Issues and implications.* White Plains, NY: Longman.

Kretschmer, R., & Kretschmer, L. (1978). *Language development and intervention with the hearing impaired.* Baltimore: University Park Press.

Kroll, B. (Ed.). (1990). *Second language writing: Research insights for the classroom.* New York: Cambridge University Press

Kucera, H., & Francis, N. (1967). *Computational analysis of present-day American English.* Providence, RI: Brown University Press.

Kuhn, T. (1970). *The structure of scientific revolutions* (2nd ed.). Chicago: University of Chicago Press.

LaBerge, D., & Samuels, S. J. (1974). Toward a theory of automatic information processing in reading. *Cognitive Psychology, 6,* 293–323.

LaBerge, D., & Samuels, S. J. (1985). Toward a theory of automatic information processing in reading. In H. Singer & R. Ruddell (Eds.), *Theoretical models and processes of reading* (3rd ed.) (pp. 689–721). Newark, DE: International Reading Association.

Laine, C., & Schultz, L. (1985). Composition theory and practice: The paradigm shift. *Volta Review, 87, Learning to write and writing to learn* (pp. 9–20). [Special Issue, R. R. Kretschmer (Ed.)].

Lambert, W. (1972). A social psychology of bilingualism. In W. Lambert (Ed.), *Language, psychology, and culture* (pp. 212–235). Stanford, CA: Stanford University Press.

Lambert, W., & Tucker, G. (1972). *The bilingual education of children: The St. Lambert experiment.* Rowley, MA: Newbury House.

Lambie, R., & Daniels-Mohring, D. (1993). *Family systems within educational contexts: Understanding students with special needs.* Denver, CO: Love.

Lane, H. (1984). *When the mind hears: A history of the deaf.* New York: Random House.

Lane, H. (1988). Is there a "psychology of the deaf"? *Exceptional Children, 55,* 7–19.

Lane, H., & Baker, D. (1974). Reading achievement of the deaf: Another look. *Volta Review, 76,* 489–499.

Lane, H., Hoffmeister, R., & Bahan, B. (1996). *A journey into the DEAF-WORLD.* San Diego, CA: DawnSign Press.

Larsen-Freeman, D. (1991). *An introduction to second language acquisition research.* New York: Longman.

LaSasso, C. (1985). Visual matching test-taking strategies used by deaf readers. *Journal of Speech and Hearing Research, 28,* 2–7.

LaSasso, C., & Davey, B. (1987). The relationship between lexical knowledge and reading comprehension for prelingually, profoundly hearing-impaired students. *Volta Review, 89,* 211–220.

Lehr, F., & Osborn, J. (Eds.). (1994). *Reading, language, and literacy: Instruction for the twenty-first century.* Hillsdale, NJ: Erlbaum.

Lemley, P. (1993). *Deaf readers and engagement in the story world: A study of strategies and stances.* Unpublished doctoral dissertation, The Ohio State University, Columbus.

Letourneau, N. (1972). *The effect of multiple meanings of words on the reading comprehension of intermediate grade deaf children: A comparison of two methods of teaching multiple meanings of words and their effect on reading comprehension.* New York: Unpublished doctoral dissertation, New York University.

Levin, J., & Pressley, M. (1981). Improving children's prose comprehension: Selected strategies that seem to succeed. In C. Santa & B. Hayes (Eds.), *Children's prose comprehension* (pp. 44–71). Newark, DE: International Reading Association.

Leybaert, J. (1993). Reading in the deaf: The roles of phonological codes. In M. Marschark & M. D. Clark (Eds.), *Psychological perspectives on deafness* (pp. 269–309). Hillsdale, NJ: Erlbaum.

Liberman, I., Shankweiler, D., & Liberman, A. (1989). The alphabetic principle and learning to read. In D. Shankweiler & I. Liberman (Eds.), *Phonology and reading disability: Solving the reading puzzle* (pp. 1–33). Ann Arbor, MI: University of Michigan Press.

Lichtenstein, E. (1984). Deaf working memory processes and English language skills. In D. Martin (Ed.), *International symposium on cognition, education, and deafness: Working papers* (Vol. 2, pp. 331–360). Washington, DC: Gallaudet University Press.

Lichtenstein, E. (1985). Deaf working memory processes and English language skills. In D. Martin (Ed.), *Cognition, education, and deafness: Directions for research and instruction* (pp. 111–114). Washington, DC: Gallaudet University Press.

Liddell, S. (1980). *American Sign Language syntax.* The Hague: Mouton.

Lillo-Martin, D., Hanson, V., & Smith, S. (1991). Deaf readers' comprehension of complex syntactic structure. In D. Martin (Ed.), *Advances in cognition, education, and deafness* (pp. 146–151). Washington, DC: Gallaudet University Press.

Lillo-Martin, D., Hanson, V., & Smith, S. (1992). Deaf readers' comprehension of relative clause structure. *Applied Psycholinguistics, 13*(1), 13–30.

Lincoln, Y., & Guba, E. (1985). *Naturalistic inquiry.* Beverly Hills, CA: Sage.

Lipson, M., & Wixson, K. (1991). *Assessment and instruction of reading disability: An interactive approach.* New York: HarperCollins.

Livingston, S. (1989). Revision strategies of deaf student writers. *American Annals of the Deaf, 134,* 21–26.

Loban, W. (1976). *Language development: Kindergarten through grade twelve.* Urbana, IL: National Council of Teachers of English.

Locke, J., & Locke, V. (1971). Deaf children's phonetic, visual, and dactylic coding in a grapheme recall task. *Journal of Experimental Psychology, 89,* 142–146.

Looney, P., & Rose, S. (1979). The acquisition of inflectional suffixes by deaf youngsters using written and fingerspelled modes. *American Annals of the Deaf, 124,* 765–769.

Lott, D. (1983). Analyzing and counteracting interference errors. *English Language Teaching Journal, 37,* 256–261.

Lucas, C. (Ed.). (1990). *Sign language research.* Washington, DC: Gallaudet University Press.

Luckasson, R., Coulter, D., Polloway, E., Reiss, S., Schalock, R., Snell, M., Spitalnik, D., & Stark, J. (1992). *Mental retardation: Definition, classification and systems of supports.* Washington, DC: American Association of Mental Retardation.

Luetke-Stahlman, B. (1983). Using bilingual instructional models in teaching hearing-impaired students. *American Annals of the Deaf, 128,* 873–877.

Luetke-Stahlman, B. (1988a). The benefit of oral English-only as compared with signed input to hearing-impaired students. *Volta Review, 90,* 349–361.

Luetke-Stahlman, B. (1988b). Documenting syntactically and semantically incomplete bimodal input to hearing-impaired subjects. *American Annals of the Deaf, 133,* 230–234.

Luetke-Stahlman, B., & Luckner, J. (1991). *Effectively educating students with hearing impairments.* White Plains, NY: Longman.

Luetke-Stahlman, B., & Weiner, F. (1982). Assessing language and/or system preferences of Spanish-deaf preschoolers. *American Annals of the Deaf, 127,* 789–796.

Mace-Matluck, B., & Dominguez, D. (1981). Teaching reading to bilingual children: Effects of interaction of learner characteristics and type of reading instruction on the reading achievement of bilingual children. *NCBE Forum, 4,* 3–4.

MacGinitie, W. (1969). Flexibility in dealing with alternative meanings of words. In J. Rosenstein & W. MacGinitie (Eds.), *Verbal behavior of the deaf child: Studies of word meanings and associations* (pp. 45–55). New York: Columbia University, Teachers College Press.

Macnamara, J. (1966). *Bilingualism and primary education: A study of Irish experience.* Chicago: Aldine.

Madsen, H. (1983). *Techniques in testing.* New York: Oxford University Press.

Manzo, A. (1969). The ReQuest procedure. *Journal of Reading, 13,* 123–126, 163.

Marbury, N., & Mackinson-Smyth, J. (1986). *ASL and English: A partnership.* Paper presented at the American Sign Language Research and Teaching Conference, Newark, California, April.

Marrow, A. (1969). *The practical theorist: The life and work of Kurt Lewin.* New York: Basic Books.

Marshall, W., & Quigley, S. (1970). *Quantitative and qualitative analysis of syntactic structure in the written language of deaf students.* Urbana, IL: University of Illinois, Institute for Research on Exceptional Children.

Mason, J. (Ed.). (1989). *Reading and Writing Connections.* Needham Heights, MA: Allyn & Bacon.

Mason, J., & Allen, J. (1986). A review of emergent literacy with implications for research and practice in reading. In E. T. Rothkopf (Ed.), *Review of research in education* (pp. 3–47). Washington, DC: American Educational Research Association.

Mason, J., & Au, K. (1986). *Reading instruction for today.* Glenview, IL: Scott, Foresman.

Mason, J., Kniseley, E., & Kendall, J. (1979). Effects of polysemous words on sentence comprehension. *Reading Research Quarterly, 15,* 49–65.

Massaro, D. (1976). Review of *The Psychology of Reading* by E. Gibson and H. Levin. *American Journal of Psychology, 89,* 161–172.

Massaro, D. (1984). Building and testing models of reading processes: Examples from word recognition. In P. D. Pearson, R. Barr, M. Kamil, & P. Mosenthal (Eds.), *Handbook of reading research* (pp. 111–146). White Plains, NY: Longman.

Mather, S. (1990). Home and classroom communication. In D. Moores & K. Meadow-Orlans (Eds.), *Educational and developmental aspects of deafness* (pp. 232–254). Washington, DC: Gallaudet University Press.

Matthews, P. (1991). *Morphology* (2nd ed.). Cambridge, MA: Cambridge University Press.

Maxwell, M. (1984). A deaf child's natural development of literacy. *Sign Language Studies, 42–45,* 191–224.

Mayer, C., & Wells, G. (1996). Can the linguistic interdependence theory support a bilingual-bicultural model of literacy education for deaf students? *Journal of Deaf Studies and Deaf Education, 1*(2), 93–107.

McAnally, P., Rose, S., & Quigley, S. (1994). *Language learning practices with deaf children* (2nd ed.). Austin, TX: Pro-Ed.

McCarthey, S., & Raphael, T. (1992). Alternative research perspectives. In J. Irwin & M. Doyle (Eds.), *Reading/writing connections: Learning from research* (pp. 2–30). Newark, DE: International Reading Association.

McCormick, C., Busching, B., & Potter, E. (1992). Children's knowledge about writing: The development and use of evaluative criteria. In M. Pressley, K. Harris, & J. Guthrie (Eds.), *Promoting academic competence and literacy in school* (pp. 311–336). New York: Academic Press.

McCormick, S. (1987). *Remedial and clinical reading instruction.* Columbus, OH: Merrill.

McCormick, T. (1988). *Theories of reading in dialogue: An interdisciplinary study.* New York: University Press of America.

McGill-Franzen, A., & Gormley, K. (1980). The influence of context on deaf readers' understanding of passive sentences. *American Annals of the Deaf, 125,* 937–942.

McKee, P., Harrison, M., McCowen, A., Lehr, E., & Durr, W. (1966). *Reading for meaning* (4th ed.). Boston: Houghton Mifflin.

McLaughlin, B. (1982). Second-language learning and bilingualism in children and adults. In S. Rosenberg (Ed.), *Handbook of applied psycholinguistics* (pp. 217–256). Hillsdale, NJ: Erlbaum.

McLaughlin, B. (1984). *Second-language acquisition in childhood: Vol. 1. Preschool children* (2nd ed.). Hillsdale, NJ: Erlbaum.

McLaughlin, B. (1985). *Second-language acquisition in childhood: Vol. 2. School-age children* (2nd ed.). Hillsdale, NJ: Erlbaum.

McLaughlin, B. (1987). *Theories of second-language learning.* Baltimore: Edward Arnold.

Meadow, K. (1968). Early manual communication in relation to the deaf child's intellectual, social, and communicative functioning. *American Annals of the Deaf, 113,* 29–41.

Messerly, C., & Aram, D. (1980). Academic achievement of hearing-impaired students of hearing parents and of hearing-impaired parents: Another look. *Volta Review, 82,* 25–32.

Meyerhoff, W. (1986). *Disorders of hearing.* Austin, TX: Pro-Ed.

Mezynski, K. (1983). Issues concerning the acquisition of knowledge: Effects of vocabulary training on reading comprehension. *Review of Educational Research, 53,* 253–279.

Miller, G. (1985). The effects of general and specific self-instruction training on children's comprehension monitoring performances during reading. *Reading Research Quarterly, 20,* 616–628.

Miller, G. (1987). The influence of self-instruction on the comprehension monitoring performance of average and above-average readers. *Journal of Reading Behavior, 19,* 303–317.

Miller, G., Giovenco, A., & Rentiers, K. (1987). Fostering comprehension monitoring in below-average readers through self-instruction training. *Journal of Reading Behavior, 19,* 379–394.

Milner, E. (1963). A study of the relationship between reading readiness in grade one school children and patterns of parent-child interaction. *The 62nd Yearbook of the National Society for the Study of Education* (pp. 108–143). Chicago: University of Chicago Press.

Mitchell, D. (1982). *The process of reading: A cognitive analysis of fluent reading and learning to read.* New York: Wiley.

Montague, M. (1990). *Computers, cognition, and writing instruction.* Albany: State University of New York Press.

Moores, D. (1987). *Educating the deaf: Psychology, principles, and practices* (3rd ed.). Boston: Houghton Mifflin.

Moores, D. (1996). *Educating the deaf: Psychology, principles, and practices* (4th ed.). Boston: Houghton Mifflin.

Moores, D., Kluwin, T., Johnson, R., Cox, P., Blennerhassett, L., Kelly, L., Ewoldt, C., Sweet, C., & Fields, L. (1987). *Factors predictive of literacy in deaf adolescents.* Project No. NIH-NINCDS-83-19. Final Report. National Institute of Neurological and Communicative Disorders and Stroke.

Morrow, L. (1988). Young children's responses to one-to-one story readings in school settings. *Reading Research Quarterly, 23,* 89–107.

Mosenthal, P., Tamor, L., & Walmsley, S. (Eds.). (1983). *Research on writing: Principles and methods.* White Plains, NY: Longman.

Mukattash, L. (1980). Yes/no questions and the contrastive analysis hypothesis. *English Language Teaching Journal, 34,* 133–145.

Myklebust, H. (1960). *The psychology of deafness.* New York: Grune & Stratton.

Myklebust, H. (1964). *The psychology of deafness* (2nd ed.). New York: Grune & Stratton.

Nagy, W. (1988). *Teaching vocabulary to improve reading comprehension.* Newark, DE: International Reading Association.

Nagy, W., & Anderson, R. (1984). How many words are there in printed school English? *Reading Research Quarterly, 19,* 304–330.

Nagy, W., Herman, P., & Anderson, R. (1985). Learning words from context. *Reading Research Quarterly, 20,* 233–253.

Nagy, W., & Scott, J. (1990). Word schemas: Expectations about the form and meaning of new words. *Cognition and Instruction, 7,* 105–127.

Nagy, W., Winsor, P., Osborn, J., & O'Flahavan, J. (1994). Structural analysis: Some guidelines for instruction. In F. Lehr & J. Osborn (Eds.), *Reading, language, and literacy: Instruction for the twenty-first century* (pp. 45–58). Hillsdale, NJ: Erlbaum.

Natalicio, D., & Natalicio, L. (1971). A comparative study of English pluralization by native and non-native English speakers. *Child Development, 42,* 1302–1306.

Neuroth-Gimbrone, C., & Logiodice, C. (1992). A cooperative bilingual language program for deaf adolescents. *Sign Language Studies, 74,* 79–91.

Newport, E., & Meier, R. (1985). The acquisition of American Sign Language. In D. Slobin (Ed.), *The crosslinguistic study of language acquisition: Volume 1. The data* (pp. 881–938). Hillsdale, NJ: Erlbaum.

Nicholson, T. (1993). Reading without context. In G. B. Thompson, W. Tunmer, & T. Nicholson (Eds.), *Reading acquisition processes* (pp. 105–122). Philadelphia: Multilingual Matters LTD.

Nickerson, R. (1986). Literacy and cognitive development. In M. Wrolstad & D. Fisher (Eds.), *Toward a new understanding of literacy* (pp. 5–38). New York: Praeger.

Nolen, S., & Wilbur, R. (1985). The effects of context on deaf students' comprehension of difficult sentences. *American Annals of the Deaf, 130,* 231–235.

Nystrand, M., & Knapp, J. (1987). *Review of selected national tests of writing and reading.* University of Wisconsin, National Center on Effective Secondary Schools, School of Education, Madison. [Unpublished manuscript].

Odom, P., Blanton, R., & McIntire, C. (1970). Coding medium and word recall by deaf and hearing subjects. *Journal of Speech and Hearing Research, 13,* 54–58.

Olson, D. (1989). Literate thought. In C. K. Leong & B. Randhawa (Eds.), *Understanding literacy and cognition* (pp. 3–15). New York: Plenum Press.

O'Neill, M. (1973). *The receptive language competence of deaf children in the use of the base structure rules of transformational generative grammar.* Unpublished doctoral dissertation, University of Pittsburgh, Pennsylvania.

Orlando, A., & Shulman, B. (1989). Severe-to-profound hearing-impaired children's comprehension of figurative language. *Journal of Childhood Communication Disorders, 12*(2), 157–165.

O'Rourke, J. (1974). *Toward a science of vocabulary development.* The Hague: Mouton.

Otheguy, R., & Otto, R. (1980). The myth of static maintenance in bilingual education. *Modern Language Journal, 64,* 350–356.

Padden, C. (1980). The Deaf community and the culture of Deaf people. In C. Baker & R. Battison (Eds.), *Sign language and the Deaf community: Essays in honor of William C. Stokoe* (pp. 89–103). Silver Spring, MD: National Association of the Deaf.

Padden, C., & Ramsey, C. (1993). Deaf culture and literacy. *American Annals of the Deaf, 138,* 96–99.

Page, S. (1981). *The effect of idiomatic language in passages on the reading comprehension of deaf and hearing students.* Unpublished doctoral dissertation, Ball State University, Indiana (Abstract).

Paris, S., Cross, D., & Lipson, M. (1984). Informed strategies for learning: A program to improve children's reading awareness and comprehension. *Journal of Educational Psychology, 76,* 1239–1252.

Paris, S., & Jacobs, J. (1984). The benefits of informed instruction for children's reading awareness and comprehension skills. *Child Development, 55,* 2083–2093.

Paris, S., Wasik, B., & Turner, J. (1991). The development of strategic readers. In R. Barr, M. Kamil, P. Mosenthal, & P. D. Pearson (Eds.), *Handbook of reading research* (2nd ed.) (pp. 609–640). White Plains, NY: Longman.

Paul, P. (1984). *The comprehension of multimeaning words from selected frequency levels by deaf and hearing subjects.* Unpublished doctoral dissertation, University of Illinois, Urbana-Champaign.

Paul, P. (1987). *Deaf children's comprehension of multimeaning words: Research and implications.* Based on a paper presented at the Indiana Association for Children and Adults with Learning Disabilities (IACLD), 13th Annual Conference, Indianapolis, Indiana, October, 1987. (ERIC Document Reproduction Service ED 301 983).

Paul, P. (1989). Depth of vocabulary knowledge and reading: Implications for hearing impaired and learning disabled students. *Academic Therapy, 25,* 13–24.

Paul, P. (1990). Using ASL to teach English literacy skills (invited article). *The Deaf American, 40*(1–4), 107–113.

Paul, P. (1991). ASL to English: A bilingual minority-language immersion program for deaf students. In S. Polowe-Aldersley, P. Schragle, V. Armour, & J. Polowe (Eds.), *Conference Proceedings of the 1991 CAID/CEASD Convention* (pp. 53–56). New Orleans, LA: Convention of American Instructors of the Deaf.

Paul, P. (1993a). Deafness and text-based literacy. *American Annals of the Deaf, 138,* 72–75.

Paul, P. (1993b). Toward an understanding of deafness and reading. *Bulletin of Special Education and Rehabilitation, 3,* 117–129.

Paul, P. (1994a). Deafness paradigms in conflict. *BRIDGE: Bridging Research into Deaf and General Education, 13*(3), June, 2, 9.

Paul, P. (1994b). Toward an understanding of deafness and literacy. TELA themes: Newsletter of the Teachers of English and Language Arts Section of the Convention of American Instructors of the Deaf, *IV*(1), Fall, 3–5.

Paul, P. (1994c). *Language development of deaf students.* A paper presented at the 24th Southwest Regional Institute on Deafness Conference, Louisville, Kentucky, November.

Paul, P. (1995a). *Literacy or literate thought? Which way for deaf students?* Invited presentation at Boston University, Deaf Studies Program, Deaf Awareness Week Lecture Series, Boston, Massachusetts, April 24.

Paul, P. (1995b). *Is there a psychology of deafness?: Perspectives on language and literacy.* Invited presentation at the University of Massachusetts, Amherst, Department of Communication Disorders, Seminar Series: Early Intervention and Assessment, April 25.

Paul, P. (1996). Reading vocabulary knowledge and deafness. *Journal of Deaf Studies and Deaf Education, 1*:1, 3–15.

Paul, P., Bernhardt, E., & Gramly, C. (1992). Use of ASL in teaching reading and writing to deaf students: An interactive theoretical perspective. In *Conference Proceedings: Bilingual Considerations in the Education of Deaf Students: ASL and English* (pp. 75–105). Washington, DC: Gallaudet University, Extension and Summer Programs.

Paul, P., & Gustafson, G. (1991). Hearing-impaired students' comprehension of high-frequency multimeaning words. *Remedial and Special Education* (RASE), *12*(4), 52–62.

Paul, P., & Jackson, D. (1993). *Toward a psychology of deafness: Theoretical and empirical perspectives.* Boston: Allyn & Bacon.

Paul, P., & O'Rourke, J. (1988). Multimeaning words and reading comprehension: Implications for special education students. *Remedial and Special Education* (RASE), *9*(3), 42–52.

Paul, P., & Quigley, S. (1990). *Education and deafness.* White Plains, NY: Longman.

Paul, P., & Quigley, S. (1994a). *Language and deafness* (2nd ed.). San Diego, CA: Singular Publishing Group.

Paul, P., & Quigley, S. (1994b). American Sign Language/English bilingual education. In P. McAnally, S. Rose, & S. Quigley, *Language learning practices with deaf children* (2nd ed.) (pp. 219–253). Austin, TX: Pro-Ed.

Paul, P., & Ward, M. (1996). Inclusion paradigms in conflict. *Theory into Practice, Inclusive Schools: The Continuing Debate, 35*(1), 4–11.

Payne, J-A. (1982). *A study of the comprehension of verb-particle combinations among deaf and hearing subjects.* Unpublished doctoral dissertation, University of Illinois, Urbana-Champaign.

Payne, J-A., & Quigley, S. (1987). Hearing-impaired children's comprehension of verb-particle combinations. *Volta Review, 89,* 133–143.

Pearson, P. D. (1986). Twenty years of research in reading comprehension. In T. Raphael (Ed.), *The con-*

texts of school-based literacy (pp. 43–62). New York: Random House.

Pearson, P. D., Barr, R., Kamil, M., & Mosenthal, P. (Eds.). (1984). *Handbook of reading research.* White Plains, NY: Longman.

Pearson, P. D., & Dole, J. (1987). Explicit comprehension instruction: A review of research and a new conceptualization of instruction. *Elementary School Journal, 88* (2), 151–165.

Pearson, P. D., & Fielding, L. (1991). Comprehension instruction. In R. Barr, M. Kamil, P. Mosenthal, & P. D. Pearson (Eds.), *Handbook of reading research* (2nd ed.) (pp. 815–860). New York: Longman.

Pearson, P. D., & Gallagher, M. (1983). The instruction of reading comprehension. *Contemporary Educational Psychology, 8,* 317–344.

Pearson, P. D., & Johnson, D. (1978). *Teaching reading comprehension.* New York: Holt, Rinehart, & Winston.

Pearson, P. D., & Stallman, A. (1994). Resistance, complacency, and reform in reading assessment. In F. Lehr & J. Osborn (Eds.), *Reading, language, and literacy: Instruction for the twenty-first century* (pp. 239–251). Hillsdale, NJ: Erlbaum.

Pearson, P. D., & Valencia, S. (1986). *Assessment, accountability, and professional prerogative.* Paper presented at the 1986 National Reading Conference in Austin, Texas, December.

Perfetti, C. (1985). *Reading ability.* New York: Oxford University Press.

Petitto, L., & Marentette, P. (1991). Babbling in the manual mode: Evidence for the ontogeny of language. *Science, 251,* 1493–1496.

Phelps-Gunn, T., & Phelps-Terasaki, D. (1982). *Written language instruction: Theory and remediation.* Rockville, MD: Aspen.

Piaget, J. (1971). *Psychology and epistemology.* New York: Vintage Books.

Piaget, J. (1977). *The development of thought: Equilibration of cognitive structures.* New York: Viking.

Piaget, J. (1980). *Six psychological studies.* Brighton, Sussex, England: Harvester Press.

Piatelli-Palmarini, M. (Ed.). (1980). *Language and learning.* Cambridge, MA: Harvard University Press.

Pinker, S. (1994). *The language instinct: How the mind creates language.* New York: William Morrow & Company.

Pintner, R. (1918). The measurement of language ability and language progress of deaf children. *Volta Review, 20,* 755–764.

Pintner, R. (1927). The survey of schools for the deaf— V. *American Annals of the Deaf, 72,* 377–414.

Pintner, R., & Paterson, D. (1916). A measurement of the language ability of deaf children. *Psychological Review, 23,* 413–436.

Pintner, R., & Paterson, D. (1917). The ability of deaf and hearing children to follow printed directions. *American Annals of the Deaf, 62,* 448–472.

Poizner, H., Klima, E., & Bellugi, U. (1987). *What the hands reveal about the brain.* Cambridge, MA: MIT Press.

Politzer, R. (1971). Toward individualization in foreign language teaching. *Modern Language Journal, 55,* 207–212.

Popper, K. (1959). *The logic of scientific discovery.* New York: Basic Books.

Popper, K. (1972). *Objective knowledge: An evolutionary approach.* Oxford, England: Oxford University Press.

Porter, R. (1977). A cross-sectional study of morpheme acquisition in first language learners. *Language Learning, 27,* 47–62.

Power, D., & Quigley, S. (1973). Deaf children's acquisition of the passive voice. *Journal of Speech and Hearing Research, 16,* 5–11.

Prabhu, N. (1990). There is no best method—why? *TESOL Quarterly, 24,* 161–176.

Pressley, M., Goodchild, F., Fleet, J., Zajchowski, R., & Evans, E. (1989). The challenges of classroom strategy instruction. *Elementary School Journal, 89* (3), 301–342.

Priest, J. (1991). *Theories of the mind.* Boston: Houghton Mifflin.

Pugh, C. (1946). Summaries from appraisal of the silent reading abilities of acoustically handicapped children. *American Annals of the Deaf, 91,* 331–349.

Quigley, S. (1969). *The influence of fingerspelling on the development of language, communication, and educational achievement in deaf children.* Urbana, IL: University of Illinois, Institute for Research on Exceptional Children.

Quigley, S., & Frisina, R. (1961). *Institutionalization and psychoeducational development of deaf children* (CEC Research Monograph). Washington, DC: Council of Exceptional Children.

Quigley, S., & King, C. (1981). *Reading milestones.* Beaverton, OR: Dormac.

Quigley, S., & King, C. (1982). *Reading milestones.* Beaverton, OR: Dormac.

Quigley, S., & King, C. (1983). *Reading milestones.* Beaverton, OR: Dormac.

Quigley, S., & King, C. (1984). *Reading milestones.* Beaverton, OR: Dormac.

Quigley, S., & Kretschmer, R. (1982). *The education of deaf children: Issues, theory, and practice.* Austin, TX: Pro-Ed.

Quigley, S., & Paul, P. (1986). A perspective on academic achievement. In D. Luterman (Ed.), *Deafness in perspective* (pp. 55–86). San Diego, CA: College-Hill Press.

Quigley, S., & Paul, P. (1989). English language development. In M. Wang, M. Reynolds, & H. Walberg (Eds.), *The handbook of special education: Research and practice* (Vol. 3, pp. 3–21). Oxford, England: Pergamon.

Quigley, S., & Paul, P. (1990). *Language and deafness.* San Diego, CA: Singular Publishing Group.

Quigley, S., & Paul, P. (1994). Reflections. In P. McAnally, S. Rose, & S. Quigley, *Language learning practices with deaf children* (2nd ed.) (pp. 255–272). Austin, TX: Pro-Ed.

Quigley, S., Paul, P., McAnally, P., Rose, S., & Payne, J-A. (1990). *The reading bridge: Teacher's guide: Mosaic.* San Diego, CA: Dormac.

Quigley, S., Paul, P., McAnally, P., Rose, S., & Payne, J-A. (1991). *The reading bridge: Teacher's guide: Patterns.* San Diego, CA: Dormac.

Quigley, S., Power, D., & Steinkamp, M. (1977). The language structure of deaf children. *Volta Review, 79,* 73–83.

Quigley, S., Power, D., Steinkamp, M., & Jones, B. (1978). *Test of syntactic abilities.* Beaverton, OR: Dormac.

Quigley, S., Smith, N., & Wilbur, R. (1974). Comprehension of relativized sentences by deaf students. *Journal of Speech and Hearing Research, 17,* 325–341.

Quigley, S., Steinkamp, M., Power, D., & Jones, B. (1978). *Test of syntactic abilities.* Beaverton, OR: Dormac.

Quigley, S., Wilbur, R., & Montanelli, D. (1974). Question formation in the language of deaf students. *Journal of Speech and Hearing Research, 17,* 699–713.

Quigley, S., Wilbur, R., & Montanelli, D. (1976). Complement structures in the language of deaf students. *Journal of Speech and Hearing Research, 19,* 448–457.

Quigley, S., Wilbur, R., Power, D., Montanelli, D., & Steinkamp, M. (1976). *Syntactic structures in the language of deaf children* (Final Report). Urbana, IL: University of Illinois, Institute for Child Behavior and Development. (ERIC Document Reproduction Service No. ED 119 447).

Raffin, M. (1976). *The acquisition of inflectional morphemes by deaf children using seeing essential English.* Unpublished doctoral dissertation, University of Iowa, Iowa City.

Raffin, M., Davis, J., & Gilman, L. (1978). Comprehension of inflectional morphemes by deaf children exposed to a visual English sign system. *Journal of Speech and Hearing Research, 21,* 387–400.

Raimes, A. (1983). *Techniques in teaching writing.* New York: Oxford University Press.

Raphael, T. (1984). Teaching learners about sources of information for answering comprehension questions. *Journal of Reading, 27,* 303–311.

Raphael, T., & McKinney, J. (1983). An examination of fifth-and eighth-grade children's question-answering behavior: An instructional study in metacognition. *Journal of Reading Behavior, 15* (1), 67–86.

Raphael, T., & Pearson, P. D. (1985). Increasing students' awareness of sources of information for answering questions. *American Educational Research Journal, 22,* 217–236.

Raphael, T., & Wonnacut, C. (1985). Heightening fourth-grade students' sensitivity to sources of information for answering comprehension questions. *Reading Research Journal, 20,* 282–296.

Ray, W. (1984). *Literary meaning: From phenomenology to deconstruction.* Oxford, England: Basil Blackwell.

Reagan, T. (1985). The deaf as a linguistic minority: Educational considerations. *Harvard Educational Review, 55,* 265–277.

Reagan, T. (1990). Cultural considerations in the education of deaf children. In D. Moores & K. Meadow-Orlans (Eds.), *Educational and development aspects of deafness* (pp. 73–84). Washington, DC: Gallaudet University Press.

Regis, E. (1987). *Who got Einstein's office? Eccentricity and genius at the institute for advanced study.* Reading, MA: Addison-Wesley.

Reich, P. (1986). *Language development*. Englewood Cliffs, NJ: Prentice-Hall.

Richards, J. (1974a). Error analysis and second language strategies. In J. Schumann & N. Stenson (Eds.), *New frontiers in second language learning* (pp. 32–53). Rowley, MA: Newbury House.

Richards, J. (1974b). *Error analysis: Perspectives on second language acquisition*. London: Longman.

Richards, J. (1974c). A non-constrastive approach to error analysis. In J. Richards (Ed), *Error analysis: Perspectives on second language acquisition* (pp. 172–188). London: Longman.

Richards, J. (1976). The role of vocabulary teaching. *TESOL Quarterly, 10,* 77–90.

Ritzer, G. (1991). *Metatheorizing in sociology*. Lexington, MA: Lexington Books.

Ritzer, G. (Ed.). (1992). *Metatheorizing*. Newbury Park: Sage.

Robbins, N., & Hatcher, C. (1981). The effects of syntax on the reading comprehension of hearing-impaired children. *Volta Review, 83,* 105–115.

Robinson, J. (1990). *Conversations on the written word: Essays on language and literacy*. Portsmouth, NH: Boynton/Cook.

Rosansky, E. (1976). Methods and morphemes in second language acquisition. *Language Learning, 26,* 409–425.

Rosenblatt, L. (1989). Writing and reading: The transactional theory. In J. Mason (Ed.), *Reading and writing connections* (pp. 153–176). Boston: Allyn & Bacon.

Rosier, P., & Farella, M. (1976). Bilingual education at Rock Point—Some early results. *TESOL Quarterly, 10,* 379–388.

Rubin, A., & Hansen, J. (1986). Reading and writing: How are the first two R's related? In J. Orasanu (Ed.), *Reading comprehension: From research to practice* (pp. 163–170). Hillsdale, NJ: Erlbaum.

Ruddell, R., & Haggard, M. (1985). Oral and written language acquisition and the reading process. In H. Singer & R. Ruddell (Eds.), *Theoretical models and processes of reading* (3rd ed.) (pp. 63–80). Newark, DE: International Reading Association.

Rumelhart, D. (1977). Toward an interactive model of reading. In S. Dornic (Ed.), *Attention and performance VI* (pp. 573–603). New York: Academic Press.

Rumelhart, D. (1980). Schemata: The building blocks of cognition. In R. Spiro, B. Bruce, & W. Brewer (Eds.), *Theoretical issues in reading comprehension* (pp. 33–58). Hillsdale, NJ: Erlbaum.

Rumelhart, D., McClelland, J., and the PDP Research Group. (1986). *Parallel-distributed processing: Explorations in the microstructure of cognition: Vol. 1. Foundations*. Cambridge, MA: The MIT Press.

Russell, W., Quigley, S., & Power, D. (1976). *Linguistics and deaf children*. Washington, DC: Alexander Graham Bell Association for the Deaf.

Salvia, J., & Ysseldyke, J. (1991). *Assessment* (5th ed.). Boston: Houghton Mifflin.

Samuels, S. J., & Kamil, M. (1984). Models of the reading process. In P. D. Pearson, R. Barr, M. Kamil, & P. Mosenthal, (Eds.), *Handbook of reading research* (pp. 185–224). White Plains, NY: Longman.

Sarachan-Deily, A. (1982). Hearing-impaired and hearing readers' sentence processing errors. *Volta Review, 84,* 81–95.

Sarachan-Deily, A. (1985). Written narratives of deaf and hearing students: Story recall and inference. *Journal of Speech and Hearing Research, 28,* 151–159.

Scardamalia, M., Bereiter, C., & Goelman, H. (1982). The role of production factors in writing ability. In M. Nystrand (Ed.), *What writers know: The language, process, and structure of written discourse* (pp. 173–210). New York: Academic Press.

Schachter, J., & Celce-Murcia, M. (1977). Some reservations concerning error analysis. *TESOL Quarterly, 11,* 441–451.

Schatz, E., & Baldwin, R. (1986). Context clues are unreliable predictors of word meanings. *Reading Research Quarterly, 21,* 439–453.

Schirmer, B. (1994). *Language and literacy development in children who are deaf*. New York: Maxwell Macmillan International.

Schleper, D. (1995). Reading to deaf children: Learning from deaf adults. *Perspectives in Education and Deafness, 13*(4), 4–8.

Schmitt, P. (1969). *Deaf children's comprehension and production of sentence transformation and verb tenses*. Unpublished doctoral dissertation, University of Illinois, Urbana-Champaign.

Schulze, B. (1965). An evaluation of vocabulary development by thirty-two deaf children over a three-year period. *American Annals of the Deaf, 110,* 424–435.

Scott, J., Hiebert, E., & Anderson, R. (1994). Research as we approach the millennium: Beyond becoming a nation of readers. In F. Lehr & J. Osborn (Eds.), *Reading, language, and literacy: Instruction for the twenty-first century* (pp. 253–280). Hillsdale, NJ: Erlbaum.

Scovel, T. (1982). Questions concerning the application of neurolinguistic research to second language learning/teaching. *TESOL Quarterly, 16,* 323–331.

Scovel, T. (1988). Multiple perspectives make singular teaching. In L. Beebe (Ed.), *Issues in second language acquisition: Multiple perspectives* (pp. 169–190). New York: Newbury House.

Searle, J. (1976). A classification of illocutionary acts. *Language in Society, 5,* 1–23.

Searle, J. (1992). *The rediscovery of the mind.* Cambridge, MA: The MIT Press.

Searls, E., & Klesius, K. (1984). 99 multiple meaning words for primary students and ways to teach them. *Reading Psychology: An International Quarterly, 5,* 55–63.

Seidenberg, M. (1990). Lexical access: Another theoretical soupstone? In D. Balota, G. B. Flores d' Arcais, & K. Rayner (Eds.), *Comprehension processes in reading* (pp. 33–71). Hillsdale, NJ: Erlbaum.

Seldes, G. (1985). *The great thoughts.* New York: Ballantine Books.

Selinker, L. (1972). Interlanguage. *IRAL, 10,* 209–231.

Shankweiler, D., & Liberman, I. (Eds.). (1989). *Phonology and reading disability: Solving the reading puzzle.* Ann Arbor, MI: The University of Michigan Press.

Shuy, R. (1981). A holistic view of language. *Research in the Teaching of English, 15,* 101–112.

Silva, T. (1990). Second language composition instruction: Developments, issues, and directions in ESL. In B. Kroll (Ed.), *Second language writing: Research insights for the classroom* (pp. 11–23). New York: Cambridge University Press.

Silvaroli, N. (1990). *Classroom reading inventory* (6th ed.). Dubuque, IA: William. C. Brown.

Silverman-Dresner, T., & Guilfoyle, G. (1972). *Vocabulary norms for deaf children: The Lexington School for the Deaf education series, book VII.* Washington, DC: Alexander Graham Bell Association for the Deaf.

Simmons, A. (1963). *Comparison of written and spoken language from deaf and hearing children at five age levels.* Unpublished doctoral dissertation, Washington University, St. Louis, MO.

Singer, H., & Ruddell, R. (Eds.). (1985). *Theoretical models and processes of reading.* Newark, DE: International Reading Association.

Smith, F. (1971). *Understanding reading.* New York: Holt, Rinehart, & Winston.

Smith, F. (1975). *Comprehension and learning: A conceptual framework for teachers.* New York: Holt, Rinehart, & Winston.

Smith, F. (1978). *Understanding reading* (Rev. ed.). New York: Holt, Rinehart, & Winston.

Smith, T., Polloway, E., Patton, J., & Dowdy, C. (1995). *Teaching students with special needs in inclusive settings.* Boston: Allyn & Bacon.

Snyder, L. (1984). Cognition and language development. In R. Naremore (Ed.), *Language science* (pp. 107–145). San Diego, CA: College-Hill Press.

Sommers, N. (1980). Revision strategies of student writers and experienced adult writers. *College Composition and Communication, 31,* 378–388.

Spencer, P., & Gutfreund, M. (1990). Directiveness in mother-infant interactions. In D. Moores & K. Meadow-Orlans (Eds.), *Educational and developmental aspects of deafness* (pp. 350–365). Washington, DC: Gallaudet University Press.

Sridhar, S. (1980). Contrastive analysis, error analysis, and interlanguage. In K. Croft (Ed.), *Readings on English as a second language: For teachers and teacher trainees* (2nd ed.) (pp. 91–119). Boston: Little, Brown.

Stahl, S. (1986). Three principles of effective vocabulary instruction. *Journal of Reading, 29,* 662–668.

Stahl, S., & Fairbanks, M. (1986). The effects of vocabulary instruction: A model-based meta-analysis. *Review of Educational Research, 56,* 72–110.

Stainback, W., & Stainback, S. (Eds.) (1992). *Support networks for inclusive schooling: Interdependent integrated education.* Baltimore: Brookes.

Stanley, N. (1996). Vygotsky and multicultural assessment and instruction. In L. Dixon-Krauss (Ed.), *Vygotsky in the classroom: Mediated literacy instruction and assessment* (pp. 133–148). White Plains, NY: Longman.

Stanovich, K. (1980). Toward an interactive-compensatory model of individual differences in the development of reading fluency. *Reading Research Quarterly, 16,* 32–71.

Stanovich, K. (1986). Matthew effects in reading: Some consequences of individual differences in the acquisition of literacy. *Reading Research Quarterly, 21*, 360–407.

Stanovich, K. (1991). Word recognition: Changing perspectives. In R. Barr, M. Kamil, P. Mosenthal, & P. D. Pearson (Eds.), *Handbook of reading research* (2nd ed.) (pp. 418–452). White Plains, NY: Longman.

Stanovich, K. (1992). Speculations on the causes and consequences of individual differences in early reading acquisition. In P. Gough, L. Ehri, & R. Treiman (Eds.), *Reading acquisition* (pp. 307–342). Hillsdale, NJ: Erlbaum.

Stein, N., & Glenn, C. (1979). An analysis of story comprehension in elementary school children. In R. O. Freedle (Ed.), *New directions in discourse processing* (Vol. 2, pp. 53–120). Norwood, NJ: Ablex.

Steinberg, D. (1982). *Psycholinguistics: Language, mind, and the world.* White Plains, NY: Longman.

Sternberg, R., & Powell, J. (1983). Comprehending verbal comprehension. *American Psychologist, 38*, 878–893.

Stewart, D. (1985). Language dominance in deaf students. *Sign Language Studies, 49*, 375–385.

Stoodt, B. (1989). *Reading instruction* (2nd ed.). New York: Harper & Row.

Strassman, B. (1992). Deaf adolescents' metacognitive knowledge about school-related reading. *American Annals of the Deaf, 137*, 326–330.

Strickland, D., & Cullinan, B. (1990). Afterword. In M. Adams, *Beginning to read: Thinking and learning about print* (pp. 425–433). Cambridge, MA: The MIT Press.

Strong, M. (1988a). A bilingual approach to the education of young deaf children: ASL and English. In M. Strong (Ed.), *Language learning and deafness* (pp. 113–129). New York: Cambridge University Press.

Strong, M. (Ed.). (1988b). *Language learning and deafness.* New York: Cambridge University Press.

Stuckless, E. R. (1991). Reflections on bilingual, bicultural education for deaf children: Some concerns about current advocacy and trends. *American Annals of the Deaf, 136*, 270–272.

Stuckless, E. R., & Birch, J. (1966). The influence of early manual communication on the linguistic development of deaf children. *American Annals of the Deaf, 111*, 452–460, 499–504.

Stuckless, E. R., & Marks, C. (1966). *Assessment of the written language of deaf students.* Pittsburgh, PA: University of Pittsburgh, School of Education.

Swain, M., & Lapkin, S. (1982). *Evaluating bilingual education: A Canadian example.* Clevedon, England: Multilingual Matters, Ltd.

Taylor, L. (1969). *A language analysis of the writing of deaf children.* Unpublished doctoral dissertation, Florida State University, Tallahassee.

Taylor, L. (1990). *Teaching and learning vocabulary.* Englewood Cliffs, NJ: Prentice Hall.

Templeton, S., & Bear, D. (Eds.). (1992). *Development of orthographic knowledge and the foundations of literacy: A memorial Festschrift for Edmund H. Henderson.* Hillsdale, NJ: Erlbaum.

Templin, M. (1950). *The development of reasoning in children with normal and defective hearing.* Minneapolis, MN: University of Minnesota.

Tierney, R., Carter, M., & Desai, L. (1991). *Portfolio assessment in the reading-writing classroom.* Norwell, MA: Christopher-Gordon.

Tierney, R., & Cunningham, J. (1984). Research on teaching reading comprehension. In P. D. Pearson, R. Barr, M. Kamil, & P. Mosenthal (Eds.), *Handbook of reading research* (pp. 609–655). White Plains, NY: Longman.

Tierney, R., & Pearson, P. D. (1983). Toward a composing model of reading. *Language Arts, 60*, 568–580.

Tompkins, G. (1990). *Teaching writing: Balancing process and product.* Columbus, OH: Merrill.

Travers, R. (1978). *An introduction to educational research* (4th ed.). New York: Macmillan.

Trybus, R., & Karchmer, M. (1977). School achievement scores of hearing-impaired children: National data on achievement status and growth patterns. *American Annals of the Deaf, 122*, 62–69.

Tucker, J. A. (1985). Curriculum-based assessment: An introduction. *Exceptional Children, 52*, 199–204.

Turnbull, A., & Turnbull, H.R. (1990). *Families, professionals, and exceptionality: A special partnership* (2nd ed.). New York: Maxwell Macmillian.

Tyler, A., & Nagy, W. (1989). The acquisition of English derivational morphology. *Journal of Memory and Language, 28*, 649–667.

Tzeng, S-J. (1993). *Speech recoding, short-term memory, and reading ability in immature readers with severe to profound hearing impairment.* Unpublished doctoral dissertation, The Ohio State University, Columbus.

Van Cleve, J., & Crouch, B. (1989). *A place of their own.* Washington, DC: Gallaudet University Press.

Venezky, R. (1984). The history of reading research. In P. D. Pearson, R. Barr, M. Kamil, & P. Mosenthal (Eds.), *Handbook of reading research* (pp. 3–38). White Plains, NY: Longman.

Verghese, C. P. (1989). *Teaching English as a second language.* Green Park Extension, New Delhi, India: Sterling Publishers Private Limited.

Verhoeven, L. (1992). Assessment of bilingual proficiency. In L. Verhoeven & J. de Jong (Eds.), *The construct of language proficiency: Applications of psychological models to language assessment* (pp. 125–136). Philadelphia: Benjamins.

Vygotsky, L. (1962). *Thought and language.* Cambridge, MA: MIT Press.

Vygotsky, L. (1978). *Mind in society: The development of higher psychological processes.* Cambridge, MA: Harvard University Press.

Wagner, D. (1986). When literacy isn't reading (and vice versa). In M. Wrolstad & D. Fisher (Eds.), *Toward a new understanding of literacy* (pp. 319–331). New York: Praeger.

Walter, G. (1976). *Considerations in developing a vocabulary test for deaf students.* Rochester, NY: Unpublished manuscript, National Technical Institute for the Deaf.

Walter, G. (1978). Lexical abilities of hearing and hearing-impaired children. *American Annals of the Deaf, 123,* 976–982.

Washburn, A. (1983). Seeing essential English: The development and use of a sign system over two decades. *Teaching English to Deaf and Second-Language Students, 2*(1), 26–30.

Weiner, B. (1974). *Achievement motivation and attribution theory.* Morristown, NJ: General Learning Press.

Whitman, W. (1980). *Leaves of grass.* New York: Signet.

Wiggins, G. (1991). Standards, not standardization: Evoking quality student work. *Educational Leadership, 48,* 18–25.

Wilbur, R. (1977). An explanation of deaf children's difficulty with certain syntactic structures in English. *Volta Review, 79,* 85–92.

Wilbur, R. (1987). *American Sign Language: Linguistics and applied dimensions* (2nd ed.). Boston: Little, Brown.

Wilbur, R., Fraser, J., & Fruchter, A. (1981). *Comprehension of idioms by hearing-impaired students.* Paper presented at the American Speech-Language-Hearing Association Convention, Los Angeles, CA.

Wilbur, R., Goodhart, W., & Fuller, D. (1989). Comprehension of English modals by hearing-impaired children. *Volta Review, 91,* 5–18.

Wilcox, S., & Wilcox, P. (1991). *Learning to see: American Sign Language as a second language.* Englewood Cliffs, NJ: Prentice Hall Regents.

Williams, C. (1994). The language and literacy worlds of three profoundly deaf preschool children. *Reading Research Quarterly, 29*(2), 124–155.

Williams, C. (1996). *Response to literature as a pedagogical approach: An investigation of young deaf children's response to picturebook reading.* Abstract of a paper presented at the 1996 American Educational Research Association, New York, New York, April. [Paper presented by C. Williams and passage taken from abstract; see also Williams & McLean, 1996].

Williams, C., & McLean, M. (1996). *Response to literature as a pedagogical approach: An investigation of young deaf children's response to picturebook reading.* Paper presented at the annual meeting of the American Educational Research Association in New York, April.

Wixson, K., Bosky, A., Yochum, M., & Alvermann, D. (1984). An interview for assessing students' perceptions of classroom reading tasks. *Reading Teacher, 37,* 346–352.

Wolk, S., & Schildroth, A. (1984). Consistency of an associational strategy used on reading comprehension tests by hearing-impaired students. *Journal of Research in Reading, 7,* 135–142.

Wong-Fillmore, L. (1989). Teachability and second language acquisition. In M. Rice & R. Schiefelbusch (Eds.), *The teachability of language* (pp. 311–332). Baltimore: Paul H. Brookes.

Wray, D., & Medwell, J. (1991). *Literacy and language in the primary years.* New York: Routledge.

Wrightstone, J., Aronow, M., & Moskowitz, S. (1963). Developing reading test norms for deaf children. *American Annals of the Deaf, 108,* 311–316.

Yaden, D., Smolkin, L., & MacGillivray, L. (1993). A psychogenetic perspective on children's understanding about letter associations during alphabet book readings. *Journal of Reading Behavior, 25*(1), 43–68.

Yamashita, C. (1992). *The relationships among prior knowledge, metacognition, and reading comprehension for hearing-impaired students.* Unpublished master's thesis, The Ohio State University, Columbus.

Yoshinaga-Itano, C., & Snyder, L. (1985). Form and meaning in the written language of hearing-impaired children. *Volta Review, 87,* 75–90.

Index

Adams, M., 24, 27, 31, 33–34, 38–42, 47–50, 88, 93, 101, 129, 132–133, 140, 182, 186, 189, 197, 199–200, 204, 245, 264, 291–292, 305

Assessment
controlled-response items in, 107, 109–110, 286
criterion-referenced issues and, 283
curriculum-based types of, 293–294
ecological models of, 294–295
effects on instruction, 277–278
formal types of, 285–286
free-response items in, 107, 109–110, 286
general issues of, 277–279
improvement of, 291
informal types of, 285–289
issues related to deafness, 280–282
mediated learning and, 295–296
need for reform of, 277
norm-referenced issues and, 283, 290
on writing, 289–291
practicality issues in, 284–285
purpose and use of, 279–280
reliability issues in, 284
unobtrusive (alternative) measures of, 285–286, 292–296
validity issues in, 284–285

Best method
affected by, 16
and critical theory, 140
and qualitative research, 183
validity of, 241–242

Bilingualism
academic proficiency in, 148, 153
analyses of errors and, 160–162
ASL/English, 15, 147, 149
ASL and English-based signed systems and, 148–149
basic tenets of some prominent ASL/English models for, 146
communication mode and parental acceptance as variables in, 164–165

communicative proficiency in, 148, 153
contrastive approaches to error analysis and, 160, 172
deaf children of deaf parents/deaf children of hearing parents and, 163
Deaf English and, 167–168
description of, 148–149
effects of ASL on subsequent development of English and, 162–166
English/Spanish and deaf children and, 169–170
establishment of ASL/English programs for, 171–174
focus on metalinguistic ability in programs for, 173–174
interference in, 160
interlanguage approaches to error analysis and, 160
L1 bilingual immersion and, 175–176
L2 bilingual immersion and, 175–176
L2 monolingual immersion and, 175–176
L2 submersion and, 175–176
noncontrastive approaches to error analysis in, 160
notion of English is L2 for most deaf students in, 166–171
notion of transfer in, 176–177
perception on errors in ASL/English situations of, 160
reasons for controversial findings in error analyses in, 160–161
synthesis of research on type of program for, 175–176
the all or nothing phenomenon of, 148
type of student and language goal for, 174–175

Bradley-Johnson, S., 276, 289, 296

Chomsky, N., 13, 17, 31, 35, 77, 93, 99, 109, 112, 151, 159–160, 283

Clinical view
and reading-comprehensive perspective, 136–137
and text-based literacy, 140–141
and writing, 117
of deafness, 20–21
of reading and deafness, 63

Comprehension
as top-down processing, 8